Progress in Epileptic Disorders
Volume 3

**From First Unprovoked Seizure
to Newly Diagnosed Epilepsy**

Progress in Epileptic Disorders
International Advisory Board

Aicardi Jean, *France*
Arzimanoglou Alexis, *France*
Baumgartner Christoph, *Austria*
Brodie Martin, *UK*
Cross Helen, *UK*
Duchowny Michael, *USA*
Elger Christian, *Germany*
French Jacqueline, *USA*
Glauser Tracy, *USA*
Gobbi Giuseppe, *Italy*
Guerrini Renzo, *Italy*
Hirsch Edouard, *France*
Kahane Philippe, *France*
Luders Hans, *USA*
Meador Kimford, *USA*
Moshé Solomon L., *USA*
Noachtar Soheyl, *Germany*
Noebels Jeffrey, *USA*
Palmini André, *Brazil*
Perucca Emilio, *Italy*
Pitkanen Asla, *Finland*
Ryvlin Philippe, *France*
Scheffer Ingrid, *Australia*
Schmitz Bettina, *Germany*
Schmidt Dieter, *Germany*
Serratosa José, *Spain*
Shorvon Simon, *UK*
Tinuper Paolo, *Italy*
Thomas Pierre, *France*
Tuxhorn Ingrid, *Germany*
Wolf Peter, *Denmark*

Progress in Epileptic Disorders
Volume 3

From First Unprovoked Seizure to Newly Diagnosed Epilepsy

Philippe Ryvlin
Ettore Beghi
Peter Camfield
Dale Hesdorffer

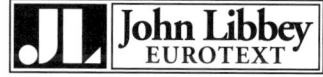

ISBN: 978-2-74-200656-4
ISSN: 1777-4284
Vol. 3.

Published by
Éditions John Libbey Eurotext
127, avenue de la République, 92120 Montrouge, France
Tél. : 01 46 73 06 60
Site internet : http://www.jle.com

John Libbey Eurotext
42-46 High Street
Esher, Surrey
KT10 9KY
United Kingdom

© 2007, John Libbey Eurotext. All rights reserved.

Unauthorized duplication contravenes applicable laws.
Il est interdit de reproduire intégralement ou partiellement le présent ouvrage sans autorisation de l'éditeur ou du Centre Français d'Exploitation du Droit de Copie, 20, rue des Grands-Augustins, 75006 Paris.

Contents

Foreword VII

Workshop participants IX

Section I:
Setting the scene

From first unprovoked seizure to newly diagnosed epilepsy: definitions and diagnostic issues at epilepsy onset
  Alexis Arzimanoglou 3

Commentary by *Dorotée Kasteleijn Nolst Trenité*: Provoked and unprovoked? ... 11

How restricted is the spectrum of epilepsies observed in prospective cohorts of first unprovoked seizure?
  Willem Arts, Hans Stroink, Cees van Donselaar 13

Section II:
Back to the future

Natural evolution of first unprovoked epileptic seizure
  Pierre Jallon, S. Perrig, Anne T. Berg 27

Risk factors for developing epilepsy after a first unprovoked seizure
  Sheril R. Haut, Christine O'Dell, Shlomo Shinnar 37

Section III:
Epileptogenesis and disease progression: the example of febrile seizures

"Complex" febrile seizures and the epilepsy: information from an experimental model
  Céline Dubé, Tallie Z. Baram 49

Febrile seizures as a risk factor for the development of epilepsy: human data
  Peter Camfield, Carol Camfield 59

Section IV:
Novel approaches of medical risk factors for unprovoked seizures and cryptogenic epilepsy

Comorbidity of epilepsy and neuropsychiatric disorders: epidemiological considerations
  Dale C. Hesdorffer 71

Commentary by *Andres M. Kanner* 95

Epileptic seizures in the context of the dysimmune syndromes
  Sean T. Hwang, Frank G. Gilliam 107

Section V:
From randomized controlled trials to patient-oriented decision making

From randomized controlled trials to patient-oriented therapy: methodology and clinical issues
  Philippe Ryvlin 147

Treatment of first unprovoked seizure
  Ettore Beghi 157

Treatment of newly diagnosed epilepsy
  Antony G. Marson 169

Bridging the gap between clinical guidelines and individualized patient treatment
  John M. Pellock 187

Section VI:
Future Challenges

What types of trials and studies do we need for early treatment of epilepsy?
  Elinor Ben Menachem, Fredrick Azstely 203

From prediction of medical intractability to early surgical treatment
  Jerome Engel Jr, Anne T. Berg 209

Foreword

Important progress has recently been made in the field of new onset seizures and epilepsy, prompting a timely closed meeting held in March 2007 in Roma and this new volume of the book series dedicated to *"Progress in Epileptic Disorders"*.

Thanks to the participation of the international experts that contributed to discussions of these advances, the present book addresses a number of important issues and hot topics, covering fields that extend *"From first unprovoked seizure to newly diagnosed epilepsy"*.

The first section of the book includes an up to date review of epidemiological data, encompassing the natural evolution of single unprovoked seizures, risk factors for recurrent seizures, and the potential for comorbid conditions such as depression, migraine, ADHD, and dysimmune metabolic disorders to promote the development of epilepsy. The impact of febrile convulsions on long-term brain hyperexcitability is also discussed.

The second section concentrates on therapeutic issues, concerning the management of single unprovoked seizures and newly diagnosed epilepsy. These include the impact of immediate versus deferred treatment and the choice of the most appropriate antiepileptic drug therapy.

Several methodological issues are addressed in parallel with the chapters, providing new insights into domains, such as the representativeness of the patient population in the studies under consideration, as well as the limitations and pitfalls of most randomised controlled trials. The value of these trials in the development of treatment guidelines is also discussed.

On behalf of the scientific committee we sincerely thank all the participants for their valuable contributions to the debate and UCB for the unrestricted educational grant that supported this project proposed by the journal *Epileptic Disorders*. We are confident that this book will offer perspectives for addressing future challenges in the field.

Philippe Ryvlin, Ettore Beghi, Peter Camfield, Dale Hesdorffer

Workshop on
"From First Unprovoked Seizure to Newly Diagnosed Epilepsy"
Rome, March 2007

Scientific Committee:
Alexis Arzimanoglou (France), Ettore Beghi (Italy), Peter Camfield (Canada), Dale Hesdorffer (USA), Edouard Hirsch (France), Philippe Kahane (France), Philippe Ryvlin (France)

List of Participants

Andermann Frederick, MD,OC, FRCP, Professor of Neurology and Pediatrics, McGill University; Director, Epilepsy Service, Montreal Neurological Hospital, 3801 University St., Room 127, Montreal, Quebec H3A 2B4, Canada
andermannf@qc.aibn.com

Andermann Eva, MD, Ph.D.,FCCMG,Director, Neurogenetics Unit, Montreal Neurological Hospital & Institute; Professor, Departments of Neurology & Neurosurgery and Human Genetics, McGill University, 3801 University,Rm.127, Montreal, Quebec, H3A 2B4 Canada
andermannf@qc.aibn.com

Arts Willem, Prof., Department of Paediatric Neurology, Erasmus Medical Centre – Sophia Children's Hospital, P.O. Box 260,3000 CB Rotterdam,The Netherlands
w.f.m.arts@erasmusmc.nl

Arzimanoglou Alexis, MD, Epileptic Disorders Editor-in-Chief, Head of the Epilepsy Program, Child Neurology & Metabolic Diseases Department, University Hospital Robert Debré, 48 Boulevard Sérurier, 75935 Paris Cedex 19, and Institute for Children and Adolescents with Epilepsy IDEE, Lyon, France
alexis.arzimanoglou@rdb.aphp.fr

Azstely Fredrik, M.D. Ph.D., Assoc. Prof., Epilepsy Research Group, Section of Clinical Neuroscience and Rehabilitation, Institute of Neuroscience and Physiology, Sahlgrenska Academy, 413 45 Göteborg, Sweden
fredrik.azstely@neuro.gu.se

Baram Tallie Z, Prof. Pediatrics,Anatomy & Neurobiology and Neurology, Danette Shepard Professor of Neurological Sciences, Med. Sci. I; ZOT 4475, University of California at Irvine, Irvine,CA 92697-4475, USA
tallie@uci.edu

Beghi Ettore, Laboratorio Malattie Neurologiche, Istituto "Mario Negri", Via Eritrea 62, 20157 Milano, Italy
beghi@marionegri.it

Benbadis Selim, Department of Neurology and Neurosurgery, Comprehensive Epilepsy Program and Clinical Neurophysiology Laboratory, University of South Florida and University of South Florida and Tampa General Hospital, 4202 E. Fowler Avenue,Tampa, FL 33620, USA
sbenbadi@hsc.usf.edu

Ben-Menachem Elinor, MD, PhD, Institute for Clinical Neuroscience and Physiology, Göteborgs University, Sahögrenska University Hospital, 413 45 Göteborg, Sweden
ebm@neuro.gu.se

Berquin Patrick, Pediatric Neurology, Departments of Pediatrics, University Hospital, 80054 Amiens, France
berquin.patrick@chu-amiens.fr

Besag Frank, Consultant Neuropsychiatrist, FRCP FRCPsych FRCPCH, Bedfordshire and Luton Community NHS Trust,Twinwoods Health Resource Centre, Milton Road, Bedford, Beds MK41 6AT,UK
Fbesag@aol.com

Bova Stefania Maria, MD, Child Neurology Unit, ICP – Children Hospital V Buzzi,Via Castelvetro 22-32, 20154 Milano, Italy
stefania.bova@icp.mi.it

Camfield Carole, IWK Health Centre, PO Box 9700, 5850 University Ave, Halifax, Nova Scotia, B3K 6R8 Canada
Camfield@dal.ca

Camfield Peter, IWK Health Centre, PO Box 9700, 5850 University Ave, Halifax, Nova Scotia, B3K 6R8 Canada
Camfield@dal.ca

Cramer Joyce, Associate Research Scientist, Department of Psychiatry,Yale University School of Medicine, 950 Campbell Ave. (151D),West Haven,CT 06516-2770, US
joyce.cramer@yale.edu

Cross Helen Dr,MB ChB PhD FRCP FRCPCH, Child Neurologist, Institute of Child Health, University College London, London WC1N 2AP, United Kingdom
hcross@ich.ucl.ac.uk

Dubeau François, Montreal Neurological Hospital, 3801, Université, room 138, Montreal, Qc, H3A 2B4, Canada
francois.dubeau@muhc.mcgill.ca

Engel Pete, Jonathan Sinay Distinguished Professor of Neurology, Neurobiology, and Psychiatry and Biobehavioral Sciences; Director, UCLA Seizure Disorder Center, David Geffen School of Medicine at UCLA, 710 Westwood Plaza, Los Angeles, CA 90095-1769, USA
engel@ucla.edu

Fogarasi Andras, MD, PhD, Bethesda Children's Hospital, Epilepsy Center, Bethesda Street 3, 1146 Budapest, Hungary
fogarasi@bethesda.hu

Francione Stefano, Centro per la Chirurgia dell'Epilessia "Claudio Munari", Dipartimento di Scienze Neurologiche,Ospedale Niguarda Ca' Granda, Piazza Ospedale Maggiore 3, 20162 Milano, Italy
stefano.francione@ospedaleniguarda.it

Gilliam Franck,The Neurological Institute, 7th Floor, Columbia University, 710 West 168th Street, New York, NY 10032, USA
fgilliam@neuro.columbia.edu

List of participants

Gobbi Giuseppe, Neuropsichiatria Infantile, Dipartimento Materno-Infantile, Ospedale Maggiore "Pizzardi", Largo Nigrisoli 2, 40133 Bologna, Italy
Giuseppe.Gobbi@ausl.bologna.it

Guekht Alla, Department of Neurology and Neurosurgery, Russian State Medical University 117049, Leninsky prospect 8 bl., 8 Moscow Russia
a.shpak@g23.relcom.ru

Haut Sheryl, M.D.,Associate Professor of Clinical Neurology; Director, Adult Epilepsy,Montefiore Medical Center,Albert Einstein College of Medicine, 111 East 210th St., Bronx, NY 10467, USA
haut@aecom.yu.edu

Hesdorffer Dale, Ph.D.,Assistant Professor of Epidemiology, Columbia University, GH Sergievsky Center, 630 W 168th, P & S Unit 16, New York,NY 10032,USA
dch5@columbia.edu

Hirsch Edouard, Professor, Neurologist-Neurophysiologist, Epileptology Service, Neurology Department, University Hospitals, 1 Place de l'Hôpital, 67091 Strasbourg Cedex, and Institute for Children and Adolescents with Epilepsy IDEE, Lyon, France
Edouard.Hirsch@chru-strasbourg.fr

Jallon Pierre, Unité d'Epileptologie clinique et d'EEG, Hôpital Cantonal de Genève, 1211. Genève 14, Switzerland
pierre.jallon@hcuge.ch

Kahane Philippe, MD, PhD, Epilepsy Unit, Neurology Department and INSERM U704, University Hospital, BP 217X, 38043 Grenoble Cedex, and Institute for Children and Adolescents with Epilepsy IDEE, Lyon, France
philippe.kahane@ujf-grenoble.fr

Kanner Andres, M.D., Professor of Neurological Sciences, Rush Medical College Director, Laboratory of Electroencephalography and Video-EEGTelemetry and Associate Director, Section of Epilepsy and Clinical Neurophysiology and Rush Epilepsy Center, Rush University Medical Center, Department of Neurological Sciences, 1653 West Congress Parkway, Chicago, Illinois 60612, USA
akanner@rush.edu

Kasteleijn-Nolst Trenité Dorothée, Neurologist, Department of Medical Genetics,University Medical Centre Utrecht (UMCU),Locatie Wilhelmina Kinderziekenhuis, Lundlaan 6, de Uithof, 3584 EA Utrecht, The Netherlands
Dorothee.Kasteleijn@uniroma1.it

Kotagal Prakashl, M.D.,Head, Pediatric Epilepsy Section, Desk S-51, Cleveland Clinic Foundation, 9500 Euclid Avenue,Cleveland, Ohio, 44195, USA
kotagap@ccf.org

Lagae Lieven, MD PhD, Epilepsy Clinical Neurophysiology, University Hospitals of Gasthuisberg, Herestraat 49, 3000 Leuven, Belgium
lieven.lagae@uz.kuleuven.ac.be

Luders Hans, M.D., Ph.D., Professor and Director, Epilepsy Center,The Neurological Institute, Case Medical Center, 11100 Euclid Avenue, Lakeside, Suite 3200, Cleveland, OH 44106-6058
hans.luders@UHhospitals.org

Marson Tony,The Walton Centre, Lower Lane, Fazakerley, Liverpool, L9 7LJ, United Kingdom
a.g.marson@liv.ac.uk

Mikati Mohamad, MD, Director,Adult and Pediatric Epilepsy Program, Professor and Chairman Department of Pediatrics,American University of Beirut, POBox 11-0236/B53, Riad El Solh Beirut 1107 2020, Lebanon
mamikati@aub.edu.lb

Nashef Lina, Consultant Neurologist, Neurology Department, King's College Hospital, Denmark Hill, London SE5 9RS, United Kingdom
lina.nashef@kingsch.nhs.uk

Noachtar Soheyl, Associate Professor of Neurology, University of Munich; Head, Epilepsy Center and Neurological Sleep Center, Dept of Neurology, Klinikum Grosshadern, University of Munich, Marchioninistr. 15, 81377 Munich, Germany
noa@med.uni-muenchen.de

Nordli Douglas, Jr., MD, Children's Memorial Hospital and Feinberg School of Medicine, Northwestern University, Children's Memorial Hospital, 2300 Children's Plaza, no. 29, Chicago, IL 60614, USA
DNordli@childrensmemorial.org

Pellock Jack, Professor and Chairman, Division of Child Neurology, Medical College of Virginia, VCU Health Systems, 1001 East Marshall Street, Box 980211, Richmond, VA 23298-0211, USA
jpellock@gems.vcu.edu

Picot Marie-Christine, Unit of Clinical Research and Epidemiology, Department of Medical Information, University Hospital of Montpellier, 34295 Montpellier Cedex 5, France
mc-picot@chu-montpellier.fr

Rosenow Felix, MZ Nervenheilkunde, Neurologische Klinik mit Poliklinik, Interdisziplinäres Epilepsie-Zentrum am Klinikum der Philipps-Universität Marburg, Rudolf-Bultmann Str.8, 35033 Marburg, Germany
Rosenow@mailer.uni-marburg.de

Ryvlin Philippe, Department of Functional Neurology and Epileptology, Neurology University Hospital, 59 Boulevard Pinel, 69677 Bron, and Institute for Children and Adolescents with Epilepsy IDEE, Lyon, France
ryvlin@cermep.fr

Sainte-Rose Christian, Professor and Head of the Pediatric Neurosurgery Dpt., University Hospital Necker-Enfants Malades, 149 rue de Sèvres, 75015 Paris, France
christian.sainte-rose@nck.aphp.fr

Sallaz Monique, Neurobiologist, Project Leader Institute for Children and Adolescents with Epilepsy IDEE, Lyon, France
monique.sallaz@fondation-idee.fr

Semah Franck, Head of the Nuclear Medicine and Clinical Resaerch Unit (UMNRC), CEA, Service Hospitalier Frédéric Joliot, 4 place du Général Leclerc, 91401 Orsay Cedex, France
semah@shfj.cea.fr

Serratosa José, Unidad de Epilepsia, Servicio de Neurologia, Fundacion Jimenez Diaz, Universidad Autonoma de Madrid, Avda Reyes Catolicos, 2, 28040 Madrid, Spain
serratosa@telefonica.net

Shields Donald, Division of Pediatric Neurology, David Geffen School of Medicine at UCLA, 10833 LeConte Avenue, Los Angeles, CA 90095-1752
wshields@mednet.ucla.edu

Sillanpää Matti, MD PhD, Professor, Senior Research Scientist, Depts. Public Health and Child Neurology, University of Turku, Turku, Finland
matti.sillanpaa@utu.fi

Thomas Pierre, MD, PhD, Professor of Neurology, UF-EEG-Epileptology Unit, Department of Neurology, Pasteur Hospital, Avenue de la Voie romaine, BP 69, 06002 Nice Cedex, France
piertho@wanadoo.fr

Trinka Eugen, Head of Epilepsy Service and EEG Laboratory, University Hospital Innsbruck, Anichstrasse 35, 6020 Innsbruck, Austria
eugen.trinka@uklibk.ac.at

Tuxhorn Ingrid, Dr, MD, Neurologist, Epilepsy Center Bethel, Clinic Mara, Maraweg 21, 33617 Bielefeld, Germany
Ingrid.Tuxhorn@evkb.de

Valenti Maria-Paola, Neurology Department, University Hospitals, 1 Place de l'Hôpital, 67091 Strasbourg Cedex, France
mapival@wanadoo.fr

Veggiotti Pierangielo, Dipartimento di Clinica Neurologica e Psichiatrica dell'Età Evolutiva, Laboratorio EEG dell'età evolutiva, Fondazione "Istituto Neurologico Casimiro Mondino", Via Ferrata 6, 27100 Pavia, Italy
pveggiot@unipv.it

Vigevano Federico, Divisione de Neurologia, Ospedale Pediatrico Bambino Gesu, Piazza S. Onofrio 4, 00165 Roma, Italy
vigevano@opbg.net

Wheless James, M.D., Professor and Chief of Pediatric Neurology, Neuroscience Institute & LeBonheur Comprehensive Epilepsy Program, LeBonheur Children's Medical Center, Clinical Chief & Director of Pediatric Neurology, St Jude Children's Research Hospital, 777 Washington Avenue, P250 Memphis, TN 38105, USA
jwheless@utmem.edu

Workshop supported by an unrestricted educational grant from UCB

Section I:
Setting the scene

From first unprovoked seizure to newly diagnosed epilepsy: definitions and diagnostic issues at epilepsy onset

Alexis Arzimanoglou

University Hospital Robert Debré (APHP), Paris and CTRS-IDEE, Lyon, France

---

To develop optimal approaches for the investigation, diagnosis and treatment of epilepsy, to evaluate the effectiveness of treatment strategies, and, more importantly, to identify interventions that may prevent the development of epilepsy, valid information regarding the frequency, cause, and natural history of the condition is still necessary.

A "first unprovoked seizure" almost automatically generates the need for a number of diagnostic investigations, raises numerous questions on evolution and prognosis and necessitates treatment (or no treatment) decisions. As a result a large body of literature on "First seizure", and even more on "Newly diagnosed epilepsy", is nowadays available.

The single term "first seizure" normally applies to a very large spectrum of clinical presentations. Similarly, the term "newly diagnosed epilepsy" can make reference to the innumerable possible patterns of seizure recurrences and epilepsy syndromes. Consequently, such single terms that are used for so many clinical pictures are bound to be unsatisfactory.

To better highlight the meaning, and underscore the limits, of the terms to be used in the chapters that follow, some definitions are necessary. Issues related to "diagnosis" of a first paroxysmal event, preferably an epileptic seizure, will be discussed in this introductory chapter.

■ First epileptic seizure: definition and diagnostic difficulties

Epileptic seizures or attacks are defined as **transient clinical events** that result from the abnormal, excessive activity of a more or less extensive population of cerebral neurons. The clinical events that constitute epileptic seizures can be extremely diverse, and no single manifestation is essential (Engel, 2006). Seizures may appear as attacks of involuntary muscle contractions, that can be sustained (tonic), interrupted (clonic) or both (tonic-clonic).

The term "convulsion" is also used to design some of these episodes. It does not imply a specific mechanism and in fact "convulsions" may be either epileptic or non-epileptic. Epileptic seizures may also manifest as disturbances of consciousness only; they may consist of sensory or visceral sensations, motor signs; or they may present as perversions of ideation, emotion, or mood. The symptoms may be so slight or so trivial that a seizure may escape recognition unless it is authenticated by simultaneous EEG recording. Finally, epileptic seizures are often difficult to distinguish from other paroxysmal events such as syncope, movement disorders, and behavioral non-epileptic manifestations.

In theory, the distinction implies the presence or absence of an epileptic discharge. When trying to differentiate the epileptic nature of a first paroxysmal event from a non-epileptic transient clinical phenomenon, the presence of such a discharge can only be assumed[1].

In fact, a first episode will be characterized as epileptic exclusively on the basis of available information on the circumstances, the temporal sequence of the events as described by eyewitnesses and/or the patient, family history, personal history, data from somatic and neurologic examination.

From a diagnostic point view, a comprehensive diagnostic work-up is unavoidable following a first paroxysmal, transient episode. Current available data suggests that somatic and neurologic examination and a good quality EEG (with the exception of febrile convulsions) are the minimum. On the basis of available (or not available) description of the clinical symptom (seizure) and the degree of confidence of the treating physician, work-up will be completed or not by neuroimaging investigations (CTscan, MRI or both). If further investigations are required (lumbar puncture, metabolic screening, indication for a biopsy, more sophisticated neuroimaging techniques, evoked potentials, neuro-ophthalmologic examination, 24H EEG, video-EEG, etc.) will depend, as always in medical practice, on *careful and knowledgeable analysis and synthesis of associated signs and symptoms* (family and personal history, fever, mental status, focal neurological signs, etc.).

A special problem is that of cases in which paroxysmal EEG activity (often intense) is not associated with clinical seizures in the conventional meaning of the term but with non-paroxysmal, lasting clinical changes. Such changes involve mainly cognitive functions or behaviour, and the individual presents with intellectual dysfunction

---

1. To push the complexity of the issue further, even from a theoretical standpoint, the differentiation of an epileptic discharge from other paroxysmal activities may be difficult. For example, tonic seizures occurring with acute anoxia usually are interpreted as a release phenomenon that results from the interruption of the inhibitory influences from the cortex, which is more sensitive than the brainstem reticular formation to the lack of oxygen (Stephenson, 1990; Gastaut, 1974; Lombroso and Lerman, 1967). In such a situation, one must ask what the nature of the excessive activity of the brainstem neurons responsible for tonic contraction is. Could this activity be considered an excessive discharge in the gray matter? Other such examples could be given (e.g., the paroxysmal dyskinesias), but debate on this problem is beyond the scope of the present chapter.

or deterioration, as well as learning difficulties, sometimes associated with psychiatric overtones. The deterioration may be global, or it may affect only specific functions, especially language; however, it may also manifest as disturbances in perception (gnosias) or executive functions. The issue of "paroxysmal EEG activity" that precedes a "first clinical episode" is usually left out from all studies concerning the "first seizure". Strangely enough, although for obvious reasons, this applies even to studies related to the process of epileptogenesis.

All the above mentioned difficulties probably explain why available studies on "First unprovoked seizure" almost exclusively concern a first episode of a tonic-clonic seizure (secondarily or primarily generalized) or, occasionally, a first episode of a focal motor seizure or of status. Distinguishing a first generalized tonic-clonic episode from a first secondarily generalized seizure may also prove to be impossible, or may only be based upon indirect indications (an EEG focus or the presence of a lesion on neuroimaging studies).

All other types of seizures (typical or atypical absences, myoclonias, epileptic spasms, tonic or atonic-astatic seizures) virtually never occur as a single attack and they have a high frequency of repetition. They are almost never investigated by a physician following a "first episode". Consequently, **available results of studies on "first seizure" or "newly diagnosed epilepsy" are not applicable** to neonatal seizures, to the majority of generalized symptomatic epilepsies of childhood, to syndromes such as the myoclonic epilepsies of early childhood or childhood absence epilepsy.

■ Occasional seizure, unprovoked seizures, epilepsy: a continuum?

To consider a first epileptic seizure as the first manifestation of "epilepsy", two relatively related conditions are required:
- an *isolated seizure*[2], considered as a response to a provoking factor such as an acute cerebral pathology or other extracerebral disturbances, **must be excluded**;
- the paroxysmal epileptic event has to be considered as *unprovoked*, in other words not induced by given circumstances, but **occurring "spontaneously"**.

Diagnosing a "first epileptic seizure" as an "isolated" (provoked) event is not always easy. In fact isolated (occasional) seizures can have a recognizable cause, or they can apparently be unprovoked. On the other hand, commonsense thinking indicates that, for all seizures, factors that precipitate the attack and factors that contribute to arresting it must exist. Some of the precipitating factors, such as intermittent photic stimulation, certain sounds, or lack of sleep, are known. Many more precipitating factors are as yet unknown, or they are only imperfectly described, while still others are only suspected. Stress, psychologic factors, and fatigue are probably responsible for precipitating a sizeable proportion of epileptic seizures, but the exact nature of these stimuli and their mechanisms of action in producing epilepsy remain unexplored. A certain degree of confusion is also due to the fact that the terms "provoked" and "triggered" are sometimes used as if they were interchangeable. As discussed by

---

2. The ambiguous term "occasional seizure" is also used in some cases implying that although this is an isolated event (and cannot be considered as epilepsy) it can recur from time to time.

Pohlmann-Eden et al. (2006) provoking factors include fever, head injury, excessive alcohol intake, withdrawal from alcohol or drugs, hypoglycemia, electrolyte disturbance, brain infection, ischemic stroke, intracranial hemorrhage and proconvulsive drugs. Seizures that follow severe psychological stress or considerable sleep deprivation are not considered as "acute symptomatic" but instead "triggered" by these factors in susceptible individuals with an underlying epilepsy disorder. Reflex seizures are also considered as triggered by a given stimuli (stroboscopic lights, reading, etc.)

In fact, most seizures likely have a multifactorial origin. Patients with a focal brain lesion may convulse only when excessive or abnormal sensory stimulation is applied to the part of the body corresponding to the lesion (e.g., a stump after the amputation of one limb [Symonds, 1959]). In general, the production of a seizure probably requires a brain injury, a genetic predisposition, or both, with its resulting hyperexcitability on the one hand and afferent stimuli of either cerebral or extracerebral origin on the other. The severity, location and spatial dimension of the injury are other modifying factors. The state of the brain and its excitability is therefore influenced by both intrinsic factors, such as circadian rhythms, stress, or the state of vigilance, and extrinsic factors that may be neural or of another nature. The source of some of those extrinsic influxes may well be extracerebral. Therefore, a fever, a disturbance in an individual's water balance; or hormonal factors, for example those seen with the ovulatory cycle in women (Mattson et al., 1981; Schmidt, 1981) can provoke or inhibit the occurrence of seizures in certain patients with epilepsy.

When observed from this perspective, the dividing line between isolated (or occasional provoked) and unprovoked epileptic seizures becomes immaterial. However, under different circumstances – for example a seizure due to meningitis that will be complicated by epilepsy in only 3% of the cases – the distinction provoked/unprovoked is of great importance.

In practice, the proper classification of a number of seizures is often arbitrary. An adolescent with a first attack occurring in response to flickering lights or television and bilateral synchronous SW discharges on his EEG receives a diagnosis of photogenic epilepsy, whereas, in a 7 months old baby a prolonged unilateral clonic seizure triggered by fever would probably raise the suspicion of Dravet syndrome, would also lead to the elimination by high quality MRI of a structural brain lesion but at that stage would be classified as "isolated or occasional". Arguments supporting either the "occasional" or the "unprovoked" nature of such events can certainly be found. The major difficulty derives from the fact that a definite answer cannot be given immediately after the first provoked/unprovoked episode. In fact, recurrence risks must also be taken into account (see chapter by Haut et al.).

Such difficulties indicate that **"unprovoked seizures" are not necessarily an all-or-none phenomenon**. Rather, a continuous variation in the threshold for seizures exists, with the severe repeated type representing one end (considered to be "epilepsy") and the occasional seizure, the other.

■ Diagnosing "new" epilepsy

The definition of *epilepsy* is fraught with many difficulties. First, the number of seizures and the duration necessary to satisfy the definition of a *recurrent and enduring condition* is an arbitrary determination. Most physicians would not make a diagnosis of epilepsy in an individual who has a cluster of seizures within a single episode over one day, even if no obvious precipitant was found. Such episodes, however, may well be the first manifestation of a chronic seizure disorder. This also applies to the occurrence of an isolated seizure.

On the other hand, most epileptologists do not hesitate to diagnose epilepsy in an individual after a single seizure as long as the attack has the typical features of those observed in well-defined epilepsy syndromes and it is associated with the corresponding typical EEG manifestations. For example, a single seizure occurring on awakening in a child who is five to 10 years of age that is marked by gurgling noises, drooling, and aphemia and that is associated with a spike focus in one centro-temporal area would be diagnosed as Rolandic epilepsy (Arzimanoglou et al., 2004).

In other circumstances diagnosis of epilepsy after a first seizure may prove more difficult or arbitrary. For example, following a first convulsive episode with a notion of some focal signs would lead to the realization of neuroimaging investigations. A normal MRI would then lead to classify this first episode as a *possible epilepsy onset*. The presence of a lesion even vaguely suggesting a relationship to the focal signs described would be, at least for some physicians, a sufficiently strong element in favor of the diagnosis of *definite epilepsy*. This would then lead to initiation of AED treatment if not surgery[3].

The duration of the seizure-free period that is necessary to consider the probability of a single seizure is also difficult to determine. The incidence of single seizures can be determined only by studying the relapse rate after a first seizure, which is the inverse expression of the likelihood of its remaining isolated. In most cases, the issue of whether a first seizure will remain isolated or whether it marks the onset of epilepsy is resolved within one or 2 years (Haut and Shinnar, 2007). This statement is probably applicable to epilepsy with relatively frequent attacks. Clearly, late recurrences are possible after several years. Usually, long seizure-free intervals indicate that the seizures, even if recurrent, will remain infrequent and that they thus may be considered "occasional." The common epidemiologic definition of epilepsy as two or more unprovoked seizures is arbitrary, and, for practical purposes, rare seizures have different consequences for the patient.

A related issue is the so-called *"silent period"*. As pointed out by Engel and Pedley (1998), Gowers (1881) recognized more than 100 years ago, that there is almost always a seizure-free interval between a causative cerebral injury and onset of symptomatic epilepsy. The latency of occurrence of posttraumatic seizures is one of the best examples. Another example, most probably implicating different pathophysiological mechanisms is the Hemiconvulsions-Hemiplegia-Epilepsy syndrome (Arzimanoglou and Dravet, 2001). In approximately three-fourths of patients, hemiconvulsion-hemiplegia syndrome evolve to the secondary appearance of partial seizures that

---

3. The issue of "surgery", although not in the scope of the present chapter, needs some explanation. Strictly speaking a child with a first focal seizure clearly due to a dysembryoplastic neuroepithelial tumour, for example, do not yet has "epilepsy". However, because the lesion is known to be highly epileptogenic, some teams would directly suggest surgery despite of the fact that the lesion is not considered as progressive. Patients with this profile are often included in surgery publications discussing epilepsy outcome following surgery.

are clearly different from the initial hemiclonic attack (Gastaut et al., 1974). In a proportion of the patients, partial seizures may appear even after the hemiplegia has completely cleared. The average interval from initial convulsions to chronic epilepsy was one to 2 years, with 85% of the epilepsies having started within three years of the initial hemiconvulsion in one study (Aicardi et al., 1969). However, this series was biased in favor of the early onset of complex partial seizures, and these often occur five to 10 years after the initial episode.

The presence of "*a silent period*" also raises important questions about the process of epileptogenesis, which in turn are important when evaluating how much "meaningful" can current approaches of the "role of the first seizure" be.

The clinical data suggest that epileptogenensis is a dynamic and evolving process that progressively alters neuronal excitability, establishes critical interconnections, and perhaps requires critical structural changes before the first clinical seizure appears. What may be an essential sequence is that first, a small neuronal aggregate is injured, in one of probably a multitude of ways, so that it becomes abnormally excitable and potentially epileptogenic. Second, the necessary anatomic and physiologic relations develop in this region to establish an epileptogenic network of sufficient size that seizures are expressed clinically. Although demonstrated in experimental animal models, what is lacking in humans, of course, is evidence of a subclinical epileptogenic abnormality preceding the appearance of clinical seizures. Thus, if it were possible to have depth electrodes placed in the hippocampus from the time of the epileptogenic injury, it is likely that epileptiform changes would be detected long before any clinical hint of epilepsy. That this sequence in fact occurs is suggested by the occasional observation of focal EEG spikes in patients with a brain tumor or vascular malformation, even in the absence of clinical seizures (Engel and Pedley, 1998). Similar questions can be raised with reference to highly epileptogenic congenital lesions, such as DNETs or gangliogliomas.

Because of the great variability in latent periods seen among patients, there must be both intrinsic and acquired modifying factors unique to each individual. One of these is undoubtedly genetic background, which is an inherent determinant of a person's susceptibility to seizures ("seizure threshold"). Another factor is location and spatial dimension of the injury and a third is the severity of the injury, which may be expressed in terms of the effect a specific lesion has on adjacent or displaced brain tissue.

As discussed in another chapter (Beghi, 2007) the aforementioned difficulties have an obvious impact on the decision to treat. The problem posed by a first seizure is one of secondary prevention rather than one of therapy.

Discrepancies among the figures of *recurrence rate* after a first seizure likely result from sampling and methodologic differences. The rate is generally lower in series from the general population than it is in hospital-based series (Hopkins et al., 1988). Some patients with an isolated seizure may never be seen in a specialized center or even by a doctor (Costeff and Avni, 1982), which may result in an apparent increase in recurrence rate. On the other hand, some series may include patients with nonepileptic seizures, thus lowering the recurrence rates because these are not likely to be followed by continuing epilepsy. The issue of recurrence rate is complex because time factors (*i.e.* how early after the event the patient is seen), the circumstances of occurrence (*i.e.* how certain is the absence of precipitating factors), antecedents (personal and familial), and the type of seizure and syndrome are involved.

In several epidemiologic studies (Sander and Sillanpää, 1998; Hauser *et al.*, 1991; Hauser and Kurland, 1975), the occurrence of two seizures, provided they did not occur during the same morbid episode, was accepted as the operational definition of epilepsy. This definition, though convenient, is obviously arbitrary. In other studies (Todt, 1984), the threshold for a diagnosis of epilepsy was set at three attacks. Camfield *et al.* (1985) clearly showed that most children who experience a second seizure experience further seizures, suggesting that two seizures are a sufficient epidemiological criterion for the definition of epilepsy. This was also confirmed by Shinnar *et al.* (2000).

Most studies on *remission rates* are confronted with similar difficulties. Methodologic differences, especially in the criteria of inclusion (exclude or not those with febrile convulsions or seizures associated with acute systemic disorders; normal *versus* abnormal global neurologic status; etiology, etc.) and duration of follow-up, are important.

■ A concluding remark

For patients and clinicians the crucial questions to be answered by studies on "first unprovoked seizure" are related to prognosis (in terms of risk of recurrence) and to therapeutic strategies, including prevention of neuronal damage. Epidemiologists are mainly interested by the predictors of seizure recurrence and by the underlying etiologies. Health authorities, but also clinicians, hope to define through these studies the optimal diagnostic strategies, those with a minimal cost that would avoid diagnostic errors.

A number of questions on treatment issues follow: does immediate AED therapy prevents the development of "chronic epilepsy"? What is the impact of immediate *versus* deferred AED treatment? Can we apply the results of available studies to all forms of epilepsies and epilepsy syndromes?

As discussed above current available studies on "First seizure" are limited to tonic-clonic seizures (primarily or secondarily generalized) and status epilepticus as the first manifestation. Data is not available for all other types of seizures, although they usually represent the clinical expression of those epilepsies that will lead to an encephalopathy.

The division between "provoked" and "unprovoked" seizure is often artificial. However, the notion of "occasional or isolated provoked" seizure is important and should be maintained. Designs used up to now to study both the prognostic and therapeutic issues related to a "first seizure" probably yielded the maximum they could provide. Novel approaches, integrating underlying pathologies, are needed particularly if our wish is to identify as early as possible those patients that run a high risk of a first unprovoked seizure. Preventing such an event will then be our next challenge.

References

Aicardi J, Amsli J, Chevrie JJ. Acute hemiplegia in infancy and childhood. *Dev Med Child Neurol* 1969; 11: 162-73.

Arzimanoglou A, Dravet C. Hemiconvulsion-Hemiplegia-epilepsy syndrome. In: Gilman S, editor. MedLink Neurology. San Diego: MedLink Corporation. Available at www.medlink.com.

Arzimanoglou A, Guerrini R, Aicardi J. *Aicardi's Epilepsy in Children*, (3rd edition) 2004. Philadelphia: Lippincott Williams & Wilkins.

Beghi E. Treatment of first unprovoked seizure. In: P. Ryvlin, E. Beghi, P. Camfield, D. Hesdorffer, eds. *From first unprovoked seizure to newly diagnosed epilepsy*. Progress in Epileptic Disorders 3; 2007; Paris: John Libbey Eurotext, pp. xx-yy.

Camfield PR, Camfield CS, Dooley JM, Tibbles JA, Fung T, Garner B. Epilepsy after a first unprovoked seizure in childhood. *Neurology* 1985; 35 (11): 1657-60.

Costeff H, Avni A. Reported seizures in early childhood: a 14-year follow-up. *Dev Med Child Neurol*. 1982; 24 (4): 472-8.

Engel J Jr, Pedley TA, eds. *Epilepsy: a comprehensive textbook*, 1998; Philadelphia: Lippincott-Williams and Wilkins.

Engel J Jr. Report of the ILAE classification core group. *Epilepsia* 2006; 47 (9): 1558-68.

Gastaut H. 1974. Syncopes: generalized anoxic seizures. In: Vinken PJ, Bruyn GW, eds. Handbook of clinical neurology, Vol. 15. Amsterdam: North Holland, 815-35.

Gastaut H, Broughton R, Tassinari CA *et al*. Unilateral epileptic seizures. In: Vinken PJ, Gruyn GW. Eds. *The epilepsies*. Handbook of clinical Neurology, 1974; Vol. 15. Amsterdam Elsevier, 235-45.

Gowers WR. Epilepsy and Other Chronic Convulsive Diseases: Their Causes, Symptoms and Treatment. London: J & A Churchill; 1881.

Hauser WA, Kurland LT. The epidemiology of epilepsy in Rochester, Minnesota, 1935 through 1967. *Epilepsia* 1975; 16 (1): 1-66.

Hauser WA, Annegers JF, Kurland LT. Prevalence of epilepsy in Rochester, Minnesota: 1940-1980. *Epilepsia* 1991; 32 (4): 429-45.

Haut S, Shinnar S. Risk factors for developing epilepsy after a first unprovoked seizure. In: P. Ryvlin, E. Beghi, P. Camfield, D. Hesdorffer, eds. *From first unprovoked seizure to newly diagnosed epilepsy. Progress in Epileptic Disorders* 3; 2007; Paris: John Libbey Eurotext, pp. xx-yy.

Hopkins A, Garman A, Clarke C. The first seizure in adult life. Value of clinical features, electroencephalography, and computerised tomographic scanning in prediction of seizure recurrence. *Lancet* 1988; 1 (8588): 721-6.

Lombroso CT, Lerman P. Breathholding spells (cyanotic and pallid infantile syncope). *Pediatrics* 1967; 39 (4): 563-81.

Mattson RH, Cramer JA, Caldwell BV *et al*. Seizure frequency and the menstrual cycle: a clinical study. *Epilepsia* 1981; 22: 242-7.

Pohlmann-Eden B, Beghi E, Camfield C, Camfield P. The first seizure and its management in adults and children. *BMJ* 2006; 332 (7537): 339-42.

Sander JW, Sillanpää M. Natural history and prognosis. In: Engel J Jr, Pedley TA, eds. *Epilepsy: a comprehensive textbook*, 1998; Vol. 1. Philadelphia: Lippincott-Williams and Wilkins, 69-86.

Schmidt D. Effect of antiepileptic drugs on estrogen and progesterone metabolism and on oral contraception. In: Dam M, Gram L, Penry JK, eds. *Advances in epileptology, XIIth Epilepsy International Symposium*. 1981; New York: Raven Press, 423-31.

Shinnar S, Berg AT, O'Dell C, Newstein D, Moshe SL, Hauser WA. Predictors of multiple seizures in a cohort of children prospectively followed from the time of their first unprovoked seizure. *Ann Neurol*. 2000; 48 (2): 140-7.

Stephenson JB. 1990. *Fits and faints*. MacKeith, London.

Symonds C. Excitation and inhibition in epilepsy. *Proc R Soc Med* 1959; 52 (6): 395-402.

Todt H. The late prognosis of epilepsy in childhood: results of a prospective follow-up study. *Epilepsia* 1984; 25 (2): 137-44.

■ Commentary by Dorothée Kasteleijn Nolst Trenité: Provoked and unprovoked?

There are many provocative factors that either induce seizures or make the seizures become worse in terms of duration and frequency. Seizures can be provoked by both physical and mental stress. Physical stress includes fever, sleep deprivation, hyperventilation, drug or alcohol withdrawal, menstruation and physical exercise. Mental stress is more difficult to specify, although many patients will mention this as a factor that influences the epilepsy.

In a recent prospective questionnaire survey among 1,677 patients in Denmark, Norway and the USA with a mixed epilepsy background, 53% reported at least one seizure-precipitating factor, while 30% claimed to have experienced two or more such factors. Emotional stress, sleep deprivation, and tiredness were the three most frequently reported precipitants. Flickering lights were also often mentioned. When seizures seem to be provoked by visual stimuli like flickering lights, TV, videogames, patterns, etc., or by other specific factors, they are however considered to be reflex seizures. Reflex seizures are often classified according to the nature of the seizure-trigger, partly because the seizures themselves do not differ from those encountered in other forms of epilepsy. Thus reflex seizures include generalised convulsive and non-convulsive seizures, focal or myoclonic seizures.

According to the 2001 Task Force classification proposal, typical precipitants include visual stimuli, thinking, music, eating, praxis, somatosensory and proprioceptive factors, reading, hot water and startle. More exotic factors are also described – tooth brushing, telephone, etc.

Detection of precipitants depends on a variety of factors:
– awareness of the patients and relatives (knowledge about the possibility of provocation in general and of specific factors);
– type of seizure(retrograde amnesia, retaining consciousness);
– frequency of seizures (likelihood of recognition of a pattern);
– duration of epilepsy (likelihood of recognition of a pattern);
– exposure to one or more potentially provocative factors at a time (disco, sleep deprivation, specific videogames or TV programmes);
– age (fever);
– available time for history taking;
– open mind of the physician.

For all above reasons, a "diagnosis" of provoked seizures can be made, while that of unprovoked may not. It might even be that "unprovoked" in sensu stricto does not exist at all and that all seizures are triggered by factors including many so far unknown ones.

Maybe it would be better to avoid the term "unprovoked".

Reference

Nakken KO, Solaas MH, Kjeldsen MJ, Friis ML, Pellock JM, Corey LA. Which seizure-precipitating factors do patients with epilepsy most frequently report? *Epilepsy Behav* 2005; 6: 185-9.

Editorial note: This comments refers to patients with established epilepsy and raises the issue of provoking factors on some occasions. The issue of "triggering versus provoking factor" is addressed in the paper by Pohlmann-Eden *et al.* (see Arzimanoglou paper reference list).

How restricted is the spectrum of epilepsies observed in prospective cohorts of first unprovoked seizure?

Willem Arts[1], Hans Stroink[2], Cees van Donselaar[3]

[1] Department of Paediatric Neurology, Erasmus Medical Centre – Sophia Children's Hospital, Rotterdam
[2] Department of Neurology, St. Elisabeth Hospital, Tilburg
[3] Department of Neurology, Medical Centre Rijnmond-Zuid, Rotterdam
The Netherlands

Whether provoked or unprovoked, a solitary (single) seizure (SS) is usually generalized tonic-clonic or tonic, with or without (simple or complex) partial onset (Practice Parameter, 2000). The ILAE definition of epilepsy (1989) holds that one single seizure does not constitute epilepsy. Only after the occurrence of two or more unprovoked seizures, the diagnosis of epilepsy may be made (Commission on Classification, ILAE, 1989). Strictly speaking, this means that one can only define the type of seizure in patients with a SS, and, by definition, prospective follow-up studies after a SS can only determine the type of epilepsy after a second seizure has occurred (the classification 4.2 "isolated seizures or isolated status epilepticus" does not constitute a specific syndrome). Considering the discussions following its publication, the recent proposal to redefine epilepsy as a condition of the brain characterized by a continuous disposition to generate epileptic seizures after a single seizure has occurred (Fisher 2005), seems as yet to be too premature and controversial to replace the old, widely used and still well-established definition.

Indeed, studies and meta-analyses that tried to identify variables predictive of seizure recurrence after a SS, usually examined aetiology, positive findings at neurological and/or imaging studies, and EEG abnormalities, but not epilepsy type or syndrome. One could conclude, therefore, that the question asked in the title of this chapter can only be answered for those patients with a solitary seizure who also had a second seizure. But then the question remains which proportions of patients with various epilepsy syndromes and types actually do have only one seizure, as compared to the proportions having one or more recurrences. It seems to be perfectly possible, for instance, to make the diagnosis of benign partial epilepsy of childhood with rolandic spikes on the basis of just one typical single seizure and the appropriate EEG pattern.

Although most children with benign rolandic epilepsy will not be treated, it would be worthwhile for prognostic purposes to know how many of these children have at least one recurrence and so, by definition, develop the full syndrome. The same holds true even more for other syndromes, since the prognosis resulting from a syndrome diagnosis could influence the decision to start treatment even after the first seizure. In this paper, we want to discuss whether an electroclinical syndrome diagnosis can be made after just one seizure, and how extended (or restricted) is the spectrum of epilepsies and syndromes that become obvious at that moment. To that end, we examine how various authors dealt with the problem of classification and syndrome diagnosis after a SS, present their results and try to formulate recommendations for future research in this area.

■ Which syndromes?

The exploratory method implicit in the title of this chapter suggests that we analyze which syndromes prevail in the prospective follow-up studies of unprovoked single seizures. However, it may be helpful to first look at the problem the other way round: look at the 1989 ILAE classification of epilepsy types and syndromes, and identify the syndromes that would be expected to present with a single, solitary seizure (Table I). At present, this "old" classification is still in use for clinical-epidemiological purposes, but one may of course include syndromes that have been defined since then (e.g. nocturnal frontal lobe epilepsy). All epilepsy types with partial seizures may present with a SS, whether they be idiopathic (1.1), remote symptomatic (1.2) or cryptogenic (1.3). If they remain partial, most patients will have had several seizures before coming to medical attention. Commonly, presentation with a single seizure is marked by partial onset and secondary generalization. An exception might be a complex partial status epilepticus. The generalized epilepsies are more heterogeneous. In the idiopathic group (2.1), presentation with a single generalized tonic-clonic seizure is limited mainly to the categories "idiopathic generalized epilepsy, not otherwise defined", "epilepsy with generalized tonic-clonic seizures on awakening" and "epilepsies with seizures elicited by specific modes of precipitation". In the former, one finds among others the GEFS-plus syndrome (and we may here include Dravet syndrome as well) in which the first seizure is not necessarily always provoked by fever; and the group with only sporadic tonic-clonic seizures, which probably is a separate syndrome. In the latter (the "reflex epilepsies"), it may be difficult to prove that no other epileptic incidents, like absences, myoclonic jerks or subjective photosensitive phenomena have occurred. Apart from generalized tonic-clonic seizures, the first manifestation may be an absence status in rare cases of childhood or juvenile absence epilepsy. However, it is never certain whether short absences did not precede this. Most "symptomatic or cryptogenic generalized epilepsies" (2.2 and 2.3), of which the best-known types are West or Lennox-Gastaut syndrome, will not present with solitary seizures. In the, admittedly rare, Landau-Kleffner syndrome (classified as "epilepsy with both generalized and focal features", 3.1), the first seizure (if it occurs: some children with this syndrome never have epileptic seizures at all) may be solitary partial or generalized, although other, always recurring seizures like atypical absences or myoclonic seizures are probably more frequent. As we will see, various studies

Table I. ILAE classification (bold: syndromes that may present with an unprovoked solitary seizure)

1. Localization-related epilepsies
   1.1. **Idiopathic** (*e.g.* benign childhood epilepsy with rolandic spikes, early onset benign epilepsy with occipital spikes [Panaiyotopoulos], late onset benign epilepsy with occipital spikes [Gastaut], autosomal dominant nocturnal frontal lobe epilepsy, familial temporal lobe epilepsy)
   1.2. **Symptomatic**
   1.3. **Cryptogenic**
2. Generalized epilepsies
   2.1. Idiopathic
      Benign familial neonatal seizures
      Benign familial and non-familial infantile seizures
      Benign myoclonic epilepsy in infancy
      Childhood absence epilepsy
      Juvenile absence epilepsy
      Juvenile myoclonic epilepsy
      Epilepsy with grand mal seizures on awakening
      Other generalized idiopathic epilepsies (a.o. GEFS+, Dravet syndrome, Epilepsy with generalized tonic-clonic seizures only)
      Epilepsies with seizures precipitated by specific modes of activation
   2.2. Cryptogenic and/or symptomatic
      West syndrome
      Lennox-Gastaut syndrome
      Epilepsy with myoclonic absences
      Epilepsy with myoclonic-astatic seizures
   2.3. Symptomatic
      Early myoclonic encephalopathy
      Ohtahara syndrome
      Other symptomatic generalized epilepsies
      Specific syndromes (a.o. progressive myoclonus epilepsies)
3. Undetermined whether focal or generalized
   3.1. Epilepsy with both generalized and focal features (**Acquired epileptic aphasia**, CSWS syndrome)
   3.2. **Epilepsy without unequivocal generalized or focal features**
4. Special syndromes
   4.1. Situation-related
   4.2. **Isolated seizures and isolated status epilepticus**

conclude that many solitary unprovoked seizures cannot be classified, and they use the category "epilepsy without unequivocal generalized or focal features" (3.2) for these cases. Finally, authors who do not wish at all to classify the epilepsy types of their patients with a solitary seizure usually use category 4.2 ("isolated unprovoked seizures or status epilepticus"). However, the way authors use these classifications, may differ. When analysing the results of our first seizure in childhood study (Stroink *et al.*, 1998), we found that in cases of generalized tonic-clonic seizures in the absence of focal EEG abnormalities, we had usually used the classification 2.1 (idiopathic generalized not otherwise defined) rather than the probably better 3.2 (unclear whether focal or generalized) as used by Shinnar (1999).

■ Methodological issues

Having limited the battlefield to the epilepsy types and syndromes enumerated above, we have to address methodological issues that could confuse comparison of the results of the various prospective studies done in the past, and some still continuing. Particularly, they concern the accuracy and reliability of the diagnosis of a SS or epilepsy. The accuracy concerns the patient selection, history (earlier non-convulsive seizures?), interval between seizure and intake, definitions used, work-up, need for reclassification after follow-up and the like. The reliability deals with inter-observer agreement. Our group assessed the accuracy and reliability of the diagnosis of a solitary seizure both in adults (whatever its cause; Van Donselaar, 1989; Van Donselaar, 1990) and in children (Stroink, 2003; Stroink, 2004). It is evident that both prognosis and syndrome classification may be influenced by a false-positive or false-negative diagnosis of epilepsy or a single seizure. In these cohorts, the proportion of a false-positive diagnosis amounted to about 5%, and of a false-negative diagnosis to between 5 and 10%. Since the methodology of ascertaining the diagnosis in these cohorts was very strict, involving panels of independent experts, and following on the patients with an unclear diagnosis, we may assume that in other SS cohorts the proportion of incorrect positive or negative diagnoses has been even larger. Others agree with this concept (Camfield, 2003), bringing forward findings in adults (Smith, 1999) and children (Berg, 1999). Attempts to classify the epilepsy syndrome in a cohort of patients after only a few seizures are also bound to contain about 10% (Berg, *Epilepsia*, 2000; Middendorp, 2003) to almost 20% (Shinnar, 1999) misclassifications. Even using videotapes of seizures does not yield complete agreement between independent observers (Parra, 2001). Moreover, not many prospective cohort studies of epilepsy or single seizures actually reclassified their patients after follow-up. However, independent classification after *e.g.* two years of follow-up is bound to contain a number of reclassifications (Stroink, 1998). It is evident that incorrect diagnoses, whether false-positive or false-negative, will be made in every series in a substantial proportion, and this will undoubtedly influence the results of studies on prognosis as well as on aetiology and classification.

We also have to consider the influence of different inclusion criteria on studies of prognosis and syndrome diagnosis. A status epilepticus as a first unprovoked seizure was accepted by some (Shinnar, 1990, 1996, 2000; Jallon, 2001), but not by others (FIRST group 1993, Stroink, 1998 – the latter for purely practical reasons: children with SE were in those days uniformly treated with AED, and the investigators wanted to look at a cohort that was not treated). Multiple seizures on one and the same day were accepted as a first seizure by Shinnar (1990), Jallon (2001) and by the ILAE Commission on Epidemiology (1993), but not by Hopkins (1988), the National General Practice Study of Epilepsy (NGPSE, 1990), the FIRST group (1993), Stroink (1998), and Camfield (2000). The latter authors found that multiple seizures on one day have exactly the same prognosis as seizures occurring with one or more day(s) interval, and they conclude that multiple seizures on one day are sufficient to make the diagnosis of epilepsy. In children, a problem could also be the inclusion in SS cohorts of children with a history of febrile seizures. Most authors studying SS cohorts in children also included children with previous febrile seizures, suggesting that this entry criterion has never been considered a controversial issue. A history of other, mainly non-convulsive, epileptic events has stirred more discussion. Such events include absences, myoclonic jerks, atonic or astatic falls, auras (Van Donselaar, 1990) and other partial seizures mistaken for non-epileptic events (*e.g.* the bizarre seizures sometimes occurring in nocturnal frontal lobe epilepsy, resembling night terrors in the eyes of the unschooled bystander). In the epilepsy syndromes in which sporadic tonic-clonic seizures co-exist with other seizure types, the tonic-clonic seizures are often not the first to occur (*e.g.* in myoclonic-astatic epilepsy) or they usually occur with fever like in Dravet syndrome. In most prospective cohort studies of solitary seizures the relevant syndromes have been excluded after taking a thorough history; however, not all authors have followed this policy (King, 1998; see below), and this of course bears on their results.

■ Clinical presentation and supplementary examinations

Let us return now to the patient presenting with a single seizure. When a person presents with a solitary convulsion and diagnostic doubts as to the nature of the event have been overcome, it is imperative to establish whether the seizure really was unprovoked. We will not discuss this question here, except for noting that especially a status epilepticus has a very high risk of being acute symptomatic, as others have also remarked (Chin, 2006; Riviello, 2006). Appropriate diagnostic methods are available to demonstrate or refute an acute symptomatic aetiology and their use should be guided by the clinical circumstances. Most current guidelines on seizures and epilepsy discuss the way they should be applied. In daily practice, the diagnosis of a first unprovoked seizure is usually made by exclusion.

The next step will be to classify the seizure into one of the different seizure types, take a thorough history to find out whether earlier epileptic events might have occurred, and perform a physical examination to establish a possible causal diagnosis. An important issue arising immediately after taking the history and performing the physical examination is whether to perform an EEG and at which moment, early after the seizure or later. For many years, epileptiform EEG abnormalities have been known to act as a significant determinant for the recurrence risk both in adults (Van Donselaar, 1992) and children (Stroink, 1998). In addition, the EEG helps to classify the epilepsy type. Based upon clinical description alone, Stroink (1998) classified 91% of the first seizures in their cohort as generalized and 9% as partial. After the EEG, the distribution was 54% generalized tonic-clonic, 40% partial and 6% unclear, well in accordance with the findings of Shinnar (1990). The EEG also helps to differentiate a seizure from a non-epileptic event (both by an abnormal background pattern and by epileptiform abnormalities relevant to the seizure that has occurred) and guides decisions on the performance of imaging studies and future management of the seizure disorder. Sometimes, a clear diagnosis of an epilepsy syndrome becomes apparent. The AAN practice parameter (2000) therefore unambiguously recommends performing an EEG as part of the evaluation of children with a solitary seizure. The objections of Gilbert (2000) regarding the low sensitivity and specificity of the EEG and therefore its uselessness in decisions regarding treatment are certainly relevant but are neutralized if the physician ordering the EEG is aware of this, and uses the EEG in the context of the historical and clinical data (Berg, *Neurology* 2000). The same holds true for adults (Van Donselaar, 1992). In epilepsy as it is still usually defined, but not after a solitary seizure, the sensitivity and positive predictive value can be enhanced considerably when a normal standard EEG is followed by an EEG after (partial) sleep deprivation (Carpay, 1997; Schreiner, 2003). It is another question at which point in time after the seizure the EEG should be performed. Most studies maintain that an early EEG (within 24 hours) is more likely to contain epileptiform abnormalities than an EEG performed later (King, 1998). Used in this way, the combination of history, physical examination and EEG usually allows the differentiation between localization-related (possibly secondarily generalized) and primary generalized seizures, and may allow a syndrome diagnosis even after a single seizure.

After the EEG, the question of neuroimaging comes up. We will not discuss acute computed tomography of the brain when a patient with a solitary seizure without a known cause presents in the emergency department. The actual reason to perform a CT in that setting is the rapid detection of an acute symptomatic cause of the seizure. It is evident from recent series that MRI is the study of choice in patients with solitary unprovoked seizure or status epilepticus, in children (Berg, 1999), but especially in adults (Pohlmann-Eden, 2006; Sharma, 2003). However, for children most practice parameters indicate that MRI after a SS is only necessary if any alarm symptoms or signs are present, like seizure description with focal features certain skin abnormalities, focal neurological signs, mental retardation, macro- or microcephaly or other dysmorphic features. Both sensitivity and specificity of MRI are superior to those of CT. Tumours, vascular lesions, scars and congenital abnormalities are among the most frequently detected abnormalities in patients with a remote symptomatic aetiology.

■ Clinical classification

For patients with any type of solitary unprovoked seizure, these are the examinations that need to be performed. After these studies, a simple classification should be possible. Ideally, one can at this point make a distinction between seizure type (partial, secondary generalized, primary generalized), localization (generalized or partial, frontal, temporal, parietal, occipital), aetiology (idiopathic, cryptogenic or remote symptomatic), and in many cases also syndrome (according to the ILAE syndrome classification). It is fair to state that at that time the recurrence risk of the individual patient will also be known. *Tables II* (studies on patients of all ages, population-based except for the study by King [1998]) and *III* (studies on children, hospital-based) present the details of those cohort studies that tried to establish the categories of epilepsy types after just one or multiple seizures. Often, these are data collected by the same group of investigators, but not always from the same cohorts (*e.g.* the first seizure cohort assembled by Shinnar in the Bronx and the epilepsy cohort recruited by Berg in Connecticut).

Despite the different methods of classification used by the various groups, the results, especially concerning those categories containing clearly established syndromes with prognostic and therapeutic consequences, seem to agree to a large extent. Many syndromes from the category "idiopathic generalized" do not present with a single seizure. The proportion of patients in whom no definite syndrome diagnosis can be made, whether classified as 3.2 or 4.2, is, as could be expected, larger in studies on SS than in studies on patients with newly diagnosed epilepsy, with the exception of the series by King (1998). However, their first-seizure study was in many ways different from the study design used by most other investigators. They recruited patients

Table II. Epilepsy syndrome categories according to the ILAE classification (see *Table I*) in prospective (almost) population-based series of first seizure or epilepsy patients of all ages (data given as percentage of the entire cohort or of the total number of the cohorts combined)

First seizure	N	1.1	1.2	1.3	2.1	2.2	2.3	3.1	3.2	4.2
Olafsson 2005[1]	207	6	25	16	6	0	0	0.5	45	
Jallon 2001[2]	926	9	16	10	16	0	1	0.2	0	48
King 1998[3]	300	4	54[4]	[4]	23[5]	0	0.3	0	0	19
Total	1433	7	18[6]	11[6]	16	0	1			
Epilepsy										
Olafsson 2005	290	6	26	27	10	2	0	3	27	
Jallon 2001	1016	5	14	29	27	4	3	0	17	1
Total	1306	5	16	29	24	3	2	0.1	19	

[1] Classified into the category they would have been assigned to if the seizures had been recurrent
[2] A single seizure without any EEG or neuroimaging abnormality was classified as isolated seizure (4.2)
[3] Only children over 5 years were included; obvious remote symptomatic cases were excluded; 23% had previously had similar events and 24% minor epileptic events
[4] 1.2 and 1.3 taken together
[5] Of whom 13 were classified by the authors as idiopathic generalized, but with the comment that they "could not be diagnosed more precisely on completion of the clinical and EEG studies"
[6] Calculated with exclusion of the series by King et al., 1998

from emergency rooms, outpatient clinics, local general practitioners and specialists. Probably, therefore, this was not a completely representative and consecutive series. This might be illustrated by the fact that of the total study group, only 20% were children below 16. Perhaps most importantly, they also included patients who by history had experienced more seizures, very much facilitating their classification, especially the rather crude one the authors used. These methodological differences explain to a large extent the different results they present.

In the childhood cohorts *(Table III)*, idiopathic syndromes occur more often than in the cohorts with patients of all ages. Cryptogenic and symptomatic generalized epilepsy occur almost exclusively in the epilepsy and not in the first seizure group. This is the most important explanation of the concept that a child presenting with a single seizure will seldom develop catastrophic childhood epilepsy. In the cohort described by Shinnar (1999), at last follow-up five out of 407 children (all presenting with a solitary partial seizure) had Lennox-Gastaut syndrome. In the Dutch cohort, six out of 156 children were in the end classified as secondary generalized epilepsy. In the Shinnar cohort only children with a recurrence received a syndrome diagnosis, and the children without a recurrence were classified as 4.2. The Dutch study tried to classify all children in one of the syndrome categories regardless of recurrence or not. This may be one reason for the discrepant frequencies of idiopathic generalized epilepsy (more frequent when children with and without a recurrence are combined) and cryptogenic and symptomatic localized epilepsy (more frequent if only those with a recurrence are counted). An additional explanation could be that our group used category 3.2 too infrequently, as can also be seen in *Table III*.

Table III. Epilepsy syndrome categories according to the ILAE classification (see Table I) in prospective series of first seizure and epilepsy patients in childhood (data given as percentage of the entire cohort or of the total number of the cohorts combined)

First seizure	N	1.1	1.2	1.3	2.1	2.2	2.3	3.1	3.2	4.2
Shinnar 1999	407	6	13	8	5	1	0	0	12	55
Stroink 1998[1]	156	12	28[3]	3	51	3[3]	3	0	7	
Stroink 1998[2]	156	8	9	10	14	1	2	0	3	54
Total[4]	563	7	12	9	7	1	1	0	9	55
Epilepsy										
Berg 1999	613	10	32	17	21	7	2	1	12	
Arts 2004	453	6	15	19	43	7	7	0	4	
Sillanpää 2006	144	10	45	5	22	10[3]	3	3	6	
Total	1210	8	27	16	29	11[3]	3	1	8	

[7] Classification at the moment of recruitment of the patients
[8] Classification at two years of follow-up
[9] Non-idiopathic cases combined
[10] Rows 1 and 3 combined

The various epilepsy syndromes that occur in the first seizure series correspond quite well with the syndromes delineated in table I. However, recruitment variations account for the different numbers and proportions in each category, and a meta-analysis may for this reason be an illusion.

Follow-up

The Dutch Study was able to follow 156 children presenting with a solitary seizure for two years. None of them was treated after the first seizure. At two years, we counted 85 recurrences. Of the 85, we could follow 66 children for five years and 58 children for a median of 15 years. Looking at terminal remission at 5 and 15 years, the outcome was almost identical for children presenting with a solitary seizure and having one or more recurrences as compared with the children presenting with multiple seizures. After a median follow-up of 15 years, terminal remission more than 5 years was found in 71 and 72%, respectively, and terminal remission less than one year in 21 and 18%. This finding bears directly on the indication for AED treatment after a first solitary seizure. Such treatment would not change the prognosis of those with recurrence in a significant way, and children without a recurrence (almost 50%) would have been treated unnecessarily (Geerts, to be published).

Conclusions

In children presenting with a first-ever unprovoked epileptic seizure, the spectrum of epilepsy types and syndromes is restricted as compared to cohorts of patients presenting with multiple seizures. After a thorough history, physical examination, EEG and – if necessary – imaging study (preferably MRI), many patients can already after their first seizure be classified according to seizure type as well as to epilepsy syndrome.

The EEG plays a crucial role in this: if the seizure was generalized tonic-clonic without evident focal onset, and the EEG is normal, a syndrome diagnosis is very difficult and the preliminary classification "unclear whether focal or generalized" seems to be adequate. It is unusual for the seizure disorder in patients presenting with a SS to develop into any type of intractable epilepsy syndrome. A correct classification of seizure type and epilepsy syndrome after a SS will certainly influence the management of the patient, the guidance for parents, family members or carers, and eventually the decision to start pharmacological treatment, and if yes, how. These very practical consequences of a careful diagnostic process are in our view more important than a semantic discussion on the definition of epilepsy, but they do seem to affect the way the definition will be formulated. The views that epilepsy only exists after two or more seizures on the one hand, and that some epilepsy syndromes can be diagnosed after just one seizure on the other, need to be reconciliated. It is evident that an epilepsy syndrome can be present after a solitary seizure, regardless of which definition of epilepsy one uses [the "old" one of the ILAE, or the one proposed by Fisher (2005)]. Future studies will, moreover, (re)define a number of currently not well-understood syndromes on the basis of genetic disposition and pathophysiology. The results will rephrase the classification of epilepsy syndromes, and diversify the hitherto rather crude epidemiological studies based upon epilepsy as a syndromic entity. Combining epidemiological results such as those described in this chapter with recent clinical and genetic data promises to be the most fruitful approach to enhance the knowledge about childhood epilepsy.

References

Arts WFM, Brouwer OF, Peters ACB, Stroink H, Peeters EAJ, Schmitz PIM, *et al*. Course and prognosis of childhood epilepsy: 5-year follow-up of the Dutch study of epilepsy in childhood. *Brain* 2004; 127: 1774-84.

Berg AT, Shinnar S, Levy SR, Testa FM. Newly diagnosed epilepsy in children: presentation at diagnosis. *Epilepsia* 1999; 40: 445-52.

Berg AT, Shinnar S, Levy SR, Testa FM, Smith-Rapaport S, Beckerman B. How well can epilepsy syndromes be identified at diagnosis? A reassessment 2 years after initial diagnosis. *Epilepsia* 2000; 41: 1269-75.

Berg AT, Arts W, Boulloche J, Camfield CS, Camfield P, Jallon P, Loiseau J, Loiseau P, Shinnar S. An EEG should not be obtained routinely after first unprovoked seizure in childhood (letter). *Neurology* 2000; 55: 898.

Camfield P, Camfield C. Epilepsy can be diagnosed when the first two seizures occur on the same day. *Epilepsia* 2000; 41: 1230-3.

Camfield P, Camfield C. Childhood epilepsy: what is the evidence for what we think and what we do? *J Child Neurol* 2003; 8: 272-87.

Carpay JA, De Weerd AW, Schimsheimer RJ, Stroink H, Brouwer OF, Peters AC, Van Donselaar CA, Geerts AT, Arts WF. The diagnostic yield of a second EEG after partial sleep deprivation: a prospective study in children with newly diagnosed seizures. *Epilepsia* 1997; 38: 595-9.

Chin RFM, Neville BGR, Peckham C, Bedford H, Wade A, Scott RC for the NLSTEPSS Collaborative Group. Incidence, cause, and short-term outcome of convulsive status epilepticus in childhood: prospective population-based study. *Lancet* 2006; 368: 222-9.

Commission on classification and terminology of the International League Against Epilepsy. Proposal for revised classification of epilepsies and epileptic syndromes. *Epilepsia* 1989; 30: 89-99.

Commission on Epidemiology and Prognosis of the International League Against Epilepsy. Guidelines for epidemiologic studies on epilepsy. *Epilepsia* 1993; 34: 592-6.

Fisher RS, Van Emde Boas W, Blume W, Elger C, Genton P, Lee P, Engel J. Epileptic seizures and epilepsy: definitions proposed by the International League Against Epilepsy (ILAE) and the International Bureau for Epilepsy (IBE). *Epilepsia* 2005; 46: 470-2.

First Seizure Trial Group (FIRST group). Randomized clinical trial on the efficacy of antiepileptic drugs in reducing the risk of relapse after a first unprovoked tonic-clonic seizure. *Neurology* 1993; 43: 478-83.

Gilbert DL, Buncher CR. An EEG should not be obtained routinely after first unprovoked seizure in childhood. *Neurology* 2000; 54: 635-41.

Hopkins A, Garman A, Clarke C. The first seizure in adult life. *Lancet* 1988; I: 721-6.

Jallon P, Loiseau P, Loiseau J on behalf of Groupe CAROLE. Newly diagnosed unprovoked epileptic seizures: presentation at diagnosis in CAROLE study. *Epilepsia* 2001; 42: 464-75.

King MA, Newton MR, Jackson GD, Fitt GJ, Mitchell LA, Silvapulle MJ, Berkovic SF. Epileptology of the first seizure presentation: a clinical, electroencephalographic, and magnetic resonance imaging study of 300 consecutive patients. *Lancet* 1998; 352: 1007-11.

Middeldorp C, Geerts AT, Brouwer OF, Peters AC, Stroink H, Van Donselaar CA, Arts WF. Non-symptomatic generalized epilepsy in children younger than six years: excellent prognosis, but classification should be reconsidered after follow-up: the Dutch Study of Epilepsy in Childhood. *Epilepsia.* 2002; 43: 734-9.

Hart YM, Sander JWAS, Johnson AL, Shorvon SD, for the NGPSE. National General Practice Study of Epilepsy: recurrence after a first seizure. *Lancet* 1990; 336: 1271-4.

Olafsson E, Ludvigsson P, Gudmundsson G, Hesdorffer D, Kjartansson O, Hauser WA. Incidence of unprovoked seizures and epilepsy in Iceland and assessment of the epilepsy syndrome classification: a prospective study. *Lancet Neurology* 2005; 4: 627-34.

Parra J, Augustijn PB, Geerts Y, Van Emde Boas W. Classification of epileptic seizures: a comparison of two systems. *Epilepsia* 2001; 42: 476-82.

Pohlmann-Eden B, Beghi E, Camfield C, Camfield P. The first seizure and its management in adults and children. *Brit Med J* 2006; 332: 339-42.

Hirtz D, Ashwal S, Berg AT, Bettis D, Camfield C, Camfield P, Crumrine P, Elterman R, Schneider S, Shinnar S. Practice Parameter: evaluating a first nonfebrile seizure in children. *Neurology* 2000; 55: 616-23.

Riviello JJ, Ashwal S, Hirtz D, Glauser T, Ballaban-Gil K, Kelley K, Morton LD, Phillips S, Sloan E, Shinnar S. Practice parameter: diagnostic assessment of the child with status epilepticus (an evidence-based review). *Neurology* 2006; 67: 1542-50.

Schreiner A, Pohlmann-Eden B. Value of the early electroencephalogram after a first unprovoked seizure. *Clin Electroencephalogr* 2003; 34: 140-4.

Sharma S, Riviello JJ, Harper MB, Baskin MN. The role of emergent neuroimaging in children with new-onset afebrile seizures. *Pediatrics* 2003; 111: 1-5.

Shinnar S, Berg AT, Moshé SL, Petix M, Maytal J, Kang H, Goldensohn ES, Hauser WA. Risk of seizure recurrence following a first unprovoked seizure in childhood: a prospective study. *Pediatrics* 1990; 85: 1076-85.

Shinnar S, Berg AT, Moshe SL, O'Dell C, Alemany M, Newstein D, Kang H, Goldensohn ES, Hauser WA. The risk of seizure recurrence after a first unprovoked afebrile seizure in childhood: an extended follow-up. *Pediatrics* 1996; 98: 216-25.

Shinnar S, O'Dell C, Berg AT. Distribution of epilepsy syndromes in a cohort of children prospectively monitored from the time of their first unprovoked seizure. *Epilepsia* 1999; 40: 1378-83.

Shinnar S, Berg AT, O'Dell C, Newstein D, Moshe SL, Hauser WA. Predictors of multiple seizures in a cohort of children prospectively followed from the time of their first unprovoked seizure. *Ann Neurol* 2000; 48: 140-7.

Sillanpää M, Schmidt D. Natural history of treated childhood-onset epilepsy: prospective long-term population-based study. *Brain* 2006; 129: 617-24.

Smith D, Defalla BA, Chadwick DW. The misdiagnosis of epilepsy and the management of refractory epilepsy in a specialist clinic. *Quart J Med* 1999; 92: 15-23.

Stroink H, Brouwer OF, Arts WFM, Geerts AT, Peters ACB, Van Donselaar CA. The first unprovoked, untreated seizure in childhood: a hospital-based study of the accuracy of the diagnosis, rate of recurrence, and long-term outcome after recurrence. Dutch study of epilepsy in childhood. *J Neurol Neurosurg Psychiatry* 1998; 64: 595-600.

Stroink H, Van Donselaar CA, Geerts AT, Peters ACB, Brouwer OF, Arts WFM. The accuracy of the diagnosis of paroxysmal events in children. *Neurology* 2003; 60: 979-82.

Stroink H, Van Donselaar CA, Geerts AT, Peters ACB, Brouwer OF, Van Nieuwenhuizen O, De Coo RFM, Geesink H, Arts WFM. Interrater agreement of the diagnosis and classification of a first seizure in childhood. The Dutch Study of Epilepsy in Childhood. *J Neurol Neurosurg Psychiatry* 2004; 75: 241-5.

Van Donselaar CA, Geerts AT, Meulstee J, Habbema JDF, Staal A. Reliability of the diagnosis of a first seizure. *Neurology* 1989; 39: 267-71.

Van Donselaar CA, Geerts AT, Schimsheimer RJ. Usefulness of an aura for classification of a first generalized seizure. *Epilepsia* 1990; 31: 529-35.

Van Donselaar CA, Schimsheimer RJ, Geerts AT, Declerck AC. Value of the electroencephalogram in adult patients with untreated idiopathic first seizures. *Arch Neurol* 1992; 49: 231-7.

Section II:
Back to the future

Natural evolution of first unprovoked epileptic seizure

Pierre Jallon [1], S. Perrig [1], Anne T. Berg [2]

[1] Unité d'épileptologie clinique, Hopitaux Universitaires de Genève, Genève, Switzerland
[2] Dept Biology, Northern Illinois University, DeKalb, USA

A better understanding of the natural evolution of epilepsy is indispensable for developing rational and appropriate treatment strategies and planning for needed healthcare resources.

Gowers wrote that " the spontaneous cessation of seizure is an event too rare to be anticipated in any given case" and has described three modes of onset of epilepsy:
– Minor seizures which occur alone for months and years before there are severe attacks.
– Severe fits recurring without any preceding Petit Mal.
– A single severe fit and no other fit or sign of epilepsy for months and even years, when another attack occurs, after which they usually become frequent.

Between the last two forms there is gradation of varying interval between the first and the second fit. Since this description we know that epilepsy is usually a short-lived condition as the ratio of prevalence/incidence would lead us to believe it.

The risk of recurrence after a first unprovoked seizure (FUS) has been repeatedly investigated. However, the management of patients with such a seizure is still controversial in part because of a wide range of estimated recurrence rates (Beghi, 2002). The reported recurrence rates following a first unprovoked seizure have been estimated from 23 to 71% (Berg, 1991). Forty to 50% of untreated patients can expect a recurrence within two years (Berg, 1991).

We are interested in the individual who presents at the time of a first unprovoked seizure. The questions of interest are:
a) What is the underlying nature of his disorder?
b) Will he go on to have further seizures and hence meet operational definitions of epilepsy?
c) What are the factors that determine the likely course after a first unprovoked seizure?

This poses some problems because, as demonstrated in the CAROLE study (Jallon et al., 1999; CAROLE, 2000; Jallon et al., 2001), the types of epilepsy that present at the time of a first seizure are very different from those that come to medical attention once the patient clearly has epilepsy. Consequently, disorders such as childhood absence and West syndrome virtually never present at the time of a first seizure. This is both a function of the type of seizures and the type of epilepsy. By contrast, generalized tonic-clonic seizures are those most likely to be recognized and diagnosed at the time of a first seizure. Thus our ability to address these questions is limited to those types of seizures and epilepsy that can be recognized from the very first seizure.

Definitions

Epilepsy: Not all seizures are a symptom of epilepsy. Some seizures occur as an acute reaction to an abnormal event or severe disruption of homeostasis. Epilepsy is a disorder whose most dramatic manifestation is the occurrence of apparently spontaneous, unprovoked seizures. The ILAE has accepted at least a few different definitions of epilepsy. Most recently, epilepsy was defined as "a disorder characterized by *an enduring predisposition* to generate epileptic seizures and by neurobiologic, cognitive, psychological and social consequences of this condition. The definition requires the occurrence of *at least one epileptic seizure*." (Fisher et al., 2005) While conceptually appealing, this does not easily translate into a set of criterion that can be used for research or, for the most part, clinical, purposes. Consequently, epidemiologists and most clinical researchers prefer the operational definition recommended by the ILAE Commission of epidemiology and prognosis of epilepsies: "epilepsy is defined by *two or more unprovoked seizures* occurring at least 24 hours apart" (Commission, 1993). For the most part, we will use that definition.

First unprovoked seizure (FUS): Consequently, for research and clinical purposes, someone who presents at the time of the very first unprovoked seizures is not considered to have "epilepsy" proper. FUS may be categorized into two subgroups, symptomatic and idiopathic or cryptogenic.

Index seizure: This refers to the seizure that brings a patient to medical attention for the first time. It may be the first seizure or the patient may already have had two or even many seizures before seeking medical attention (Carole, 2000).

Natural evolution of First Unprovoked Seizure does exist

Some reflexions from our clinical experience.

− A first seizure can be an isolated seizure.

− A first epileptic seizure can be determined to be a symptom of epilepsy when EEG symptomatology allows identification of a well characterized epileptic syndrome, such as one of the idiopathic generalized syndromes.

− In localization-related idiopathic syndromes, such as in Benign epilepsy with centro-temporal spikes (BECTS), the course is almost always benign without treatment. Morever, certain forms of treatment are known to aggravate seizures in this syndrome.

- A first unprovoked seizure might be considered as a possible manifestation of epilepsy if there is some structural brain abnormalities which might predict an especially high risk of recurrence (Fisher et al., 2005).
- Despite the use of best available treatment, certain epileptic syndromes invariably follow a severe course, becoming chronic and pharmaco-resistant.
- Over the course of the last 20 years and despite the recent introduction of over ten new AEDs, there has been no detectable change in the proportion of patients with pharacoresistant epilepsy or in epilepsy-associated mortality.

An unusual story of epilepsy in childhood

Delphine was born, without any problem in late 1982. Just after her third birthday, Delphine had a prolonged right hemi-convulsion lasting approximately one hour. She had a right motor deficit that disappeared 48 hours after the convulsion. No treatment was given. During three years, Delphine had repeated EEGs which showed occipital paroxysms. In early 1987, she had a seizure described as follow by her mother: "She said she was in pain and complained of nausea. She looked pale, disoriented and was crying. Then she turned her head and shoulder to the right and started to convulse." At that time, A. Beaumanoir, who has perfectly described what was called Gastaut type occipital epilepsy, wrote in her conclusion: "this EEG record and the symptomatology are consistent with a benign occipital epilepsy, but the child is a little too young." In retrospect, it was probably Panayiotopoulos syndrome not yet described at the time. Delphine went on to have a series of seizures during the next two years despite treatment with sodium valproate. In October 1988, during an EEG, Delphine had two absence seizures with palpebral myoclonias. The mother thought that Delphine was simply "on the moon". In April 1989, she had a seizure early in the morning with right facial myoclonias and she was unable to speak. The EEG at that time showed left centro-temporal spikes associated with some bilateral paroxysmal discharges. Delphine did not have any more seizure, and we were beginning to discontinue her treatment when her mother mentioned that Delphine was having a lot of difficulties in her school work. Perhaps not surprisingly, her sleep EEG showed a typical ESES, that was treated with clobazam for three years. When Delphine was 18 year old, her EEG was normal. About that time, she had her first MRI, which showed a left mesio-temporal sclerosis associated with a discrete T2 dysplasia. Delphine has never had any more seizures. She left regular school and is now an attractive young woman, who is model in a fashion agency and was married last year.

So, Delphine has presented with no less than six true epileptic syndromes each of which has had its own presentation and evolution. Prescribed treatments did not seem to have modified the evolution of these epilepsies during 15 years (Figure 1)!

Lessons from epidemiological studies

As Sander has underlined in many papers (Sander, 1993; Sander and Sillanpää, 1997; Sander, 2003; Kwan and Sander, 2004), the natural history of untreated epileptic seizures is difficult to assess from many of the observational studies because patients

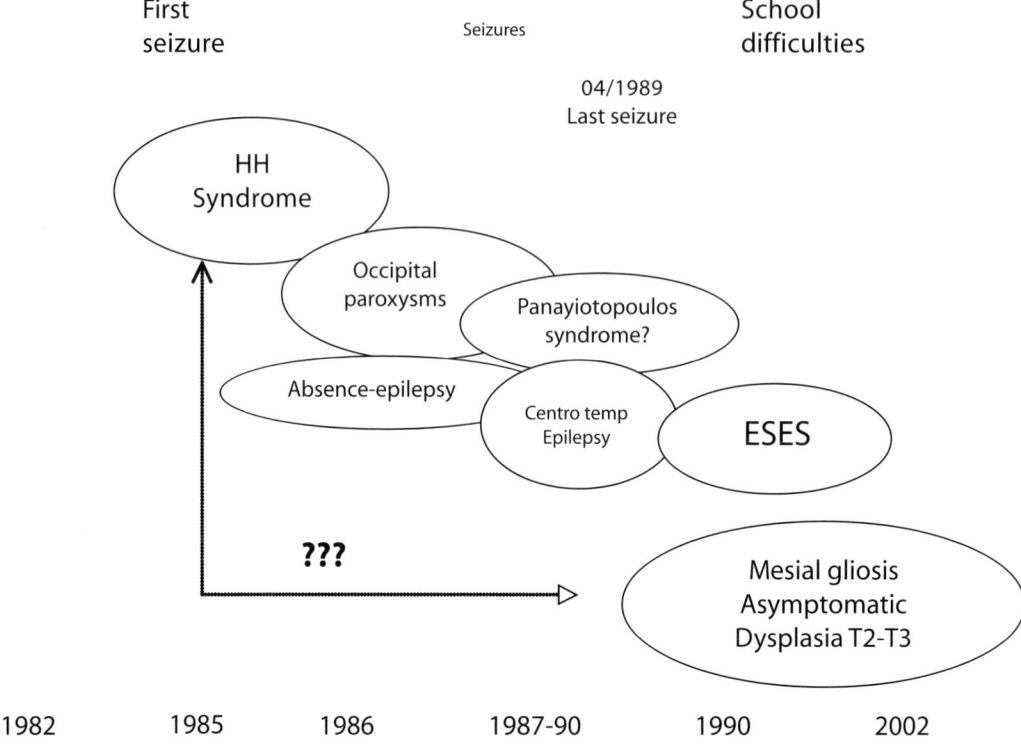

Figure 1. An unusual story of epilepsy: six syndromes observed in one patient.

are typically treated (Sillanpää, 2000). Circumstantial evidence about the possibility of spontaneous remission has emerged from studies in developing countries where the treatment gap could be around 80%. (Meinardi et al., 1998)

In any truly chronic condition cumulative incidence rate should be similar to the prevalence rate, the difference being explained by death rates and/or AED-induced remission (Juul-Jensen and Foldspang, 1983). Assuming that incidence rates for epilepsy are similar in developed and developing countries, and that failure to give an adequate treatment may facilitate the evolution of epilepsy into an intractable condition, prevalence rates in developing countries would be much higher than those reported in developed world. This is not usually the case (Placencia et al., 1992; Wang et al., 2003) although some studies have reported high prevalence rates in some selected or isolated populations (Goudsmit, 1983; Gracia et al., 1990). The hypothetic high mortality rate of epilepsy and shorter life expectancy in developing countries cannot explain alone by these epidemiological features. Case ascertainment for active epilepsy could not have been optimal, patients in remission being missing. A spontaneous remission of epilepsy in some patients seems a plausible explanation.

Lessons from observational studies

On average, the observational studies, taken as a whole, provide an estimate of the two year recurrence risk in range of 40%, depending aspects of the study design (Berg and Shinnar, 1991). All the long term observational studies of first seizures demonstrate the risk of recurrence is highest during the period immediately after the initial seizure: 80 to 90% of the patients who recur do so within two years of the initial seizure.

Some studies with untreated patients

Lindsten et al. (2001) evaluated the recurrence rate of a total of 107 patients aged > 17 years followed with a median follow up of 10.3 years. The cumulative recurrence rate over 3 years was 24% in patients not treated and 67% in treated patients. However multivariate analysis confirmed that the treatment variable was not an independent predictor of seizure recurrence.

Stroink (1998): overall recurrence rate is 54% at 2 years after a 1st UPS in 156 Dutch children aged 1 month to 16 years. A terminal remission of at least 12 months was present in 121 out of the 156 children. The indication for starting long term anticonvulsivant treatment after a single seizure in childhood is weak because the risk of developing intractable epilepsy is already low. It seems advisable to delay long term anticonvulsivant therapy until recurrent seizures are adversely affecting children life without signs of spontaneous remission.

Two recent studies in developing countries show the same results as Mani in 1993 (37%) and Placencia, 1992 (31%):
– In Hong Kong, Hui (2001) in a retrospective study concerning 132 non treated patients 13 to 86 years with a FUS showed that the cumulative probability of a second seizure at 1, 2 3 and 4 years was 30, 27, 42, 37% respectively.
– In Brazil, Scotoni (2004) 213 Brazilian patients aged from 1 month to 17 years were enrolled after a FUS non treated cryptogenic seizure. Mean follow up was 25.7 months. Recurrence occurred in 34% of patients.

Lessons from Randomized Control Trials (RCTs) studies

To study the natural course of epilepsy requires that patients not be treated. The two large-scale RCTs that have been done, do just that. They provide the best estimates of the outcomes after a first untreated unprovoked seizure and the impact of treatment on the longer-term outcome.

The first study is a multi-center study from Italy (First Seizure Trial Group, 1993). The trial involved 397 patients ranging in age from 2 to 70 years. Subjects seen within 7 days after a first TC seizure with or without partial onset were randomized to immediate treatment (CBZ, PHT, VPA, Pb) or to treatment with the same drug only after recurrence. One hundred and ninety three patients were randomized to deferred treatment only in the event of a second seizure (i.e. initially untreated). The reported recurrence risk was 18%, 28% 41% and 51% at 3, 5, 12 and 24 months after the initial seizure vs 7%, 8%, 17% and 25% in the treated group. The risk of relapse was 2.8 times higher for untreated subjects.

The European-wide Multicenter Epilepsy and Single Seizure study or MESS (Marson et al., 2005) included both first seizures and newly recognized epilepsy. In this study, 408 patients with a first unprovoked seizure were randomized to the deferred treatment group. The risk of recurrence at 6 months, 2, 5 and 8 years after randomization was 26%, 39%, 51% and 52%. Vs 18%, 32%, 42% and 46%. The overall hazards ratio was provided for the entire trial and was 1.4 for untreated vs treated arms. This translates into a treatment effect about 30%.

Together, these studies provide a very consistent estimate of the risk of a seizure recurrence following a first unprovoked seizure, about 50% after two years of follw-up. They also provide estimates of the impact of treatment in reducing this risk, although the estimates differ somewhat between the two studies. With extended follow-up, however, both of these studies demonstrated that there was no difference in remission rates between immediate and deferred treatment groups, suggesting that the early suppression of seizures with treatment did not alter the longer-term course of the disorder.

In fact, this same basic finding is seen repeatedly in other settings in which patients at high risk of seizures are randomized to treatment and non-treatment arms. Treatment suppresses immediate recurrence risk but does not seem to alter long-term outcomes.

■ Pragmatic considerations

The concept of single isolated seizure

All epilepsies begin with a first seizure. This 1st seizure may turn out to be an isolated event-usually symptomatic of a pathologic condition or indicative of an inherent increased risk for development of epilepsy-and the need to prevent such a development (Beghi, 1997).

P. Wolf (1997) defined single seizure: "as solitary seizure events that may occur once in the lifetime or very rarely, at lengthy intervals. Isolated seizures apart from the febrile seizures of early childhood may not be a separate syndrome but rather represent across syndromes the group of patients having the most benign course and the lowest risk for seizures".

Pierre Loiseau first reported in 1978 a study of 83 patients aged 10-20 years a description of what presents not as an epilepsy syndrome but as a seizure susceptibility syndrome: Isolated partial seizures of adolescence (IPSA) (Loiseau et al., 2005). The frequency of IPSA however is difficult to determine, a long follow-up for to eliminate a recurrence is mandatory. IPSA would represent one-quarter of first unprovoked seizure partial seizure occurring between 12 and 18 years of age. However, no population-based study documents this figures. In the French observational study of newly diagnosed seizures (Jallon et al., 2001) 85 patients aged 12-19 years seen after a first unprovoked seizure were included. Two years later, no recurrence was noted in 66 of them. By definition, the seizures are partial but nearly 60% are secondary generalized. Combined symptoms are noted in 57% of seizures: They are mainly motor signs (versive) or sensory symptoms (visual). Psychic symptoms are very rare. They are never post-ictal symptomatology such as motor or psychic deficits. EEG is normal or with theta changes over the centro-parietal regions (Capovilla *et al.*, 2001).

Does medical treatment influence the outcome of epilepsy?

"AEDs have greatly improved the lives of patients with epilepsy. The resulting impact on psycho-social, educational and other quality of life measures is substantial and is a strong justification for their rational use". (Shinnar and Berg, 1996).

However, the treatment of a single seizure is no longer automatic. Many factors have to be weighted including the effect of treatment on recurrence and the effect of treatment on the long term prognosis of epilepsy Such factors include a documented etiology or an abnormal EEG. In some circumstances, postponement of treatment may be the best course of action, for example for a pregnant women.

The Italian multicentre randomized trial comparing the treatment of the FUS with the treatment of recurrence demonstrates that the long term effects of the two strategies are similar. The chance of achieving 1-year remission was 82% in patient treated at the first seizure and 84% in patients at the time of seizure relapse. Similarly, the chance of achieving 2-years remission was 60% and 59% (Musicco, 1994).

These findings seems confirmed by studies in developing countries where most patients with epilepsy are left untreated because drugs are nor available or too expensive or receive drugs (and often only Phenobarbital) after a prolonged disease course and repeated seizures. In these studies, untreated patients tend to achieve seizure remission in similar proportions to those of patient with treatment (Feksi, 1991).

The concept that early administration of AEDs can influence the prognosis of epilepsy is not unanimously accepted. The start of the treatment leads to a proportion of successes and failures similar to that of early treated patients. Three studies in developing countries involving more than 1 000 patients with chronic epilepsy and who had never received AED treatment found that neither the duration of the condition nor the number of seizures before treatment were predictors of outcome (Watts, 1992; Feksi, 1991; Placencia, 1993).

After more than a decade of clinical use of "new" AEDs for the treatment of epilepsy, one third of the patients with chronic epilepsy are still resistant to pharmacotherapy. (Blume, 2006; Schmidt, 2002)

The treatment does not seem to influence the secular trend of epilepsy mortality.

The natural evolution of epilepsy may be probably one of the major risk factor of pharmaco-resistance.

References

Beghi E. Prognosis of first seizure. In *Prognosis of epilepsies*. Jallon *et al.* Paris: John Libbey, 2002, 21-8.

Beghi E, Berg AT, Hauser WA. The treatment of single seizures. In *Epilepsy: a comprehensive textbook*. Engel Jr, Pedley TA ed. Philadephia: Lippincott-Raven Publishers, 1997: 1287-94.

Berg AT, Shinnar S. The risk of seizure recurrence following a first unprovoked seizure: a quantitative review. *Neurology* 1991; 41: 965-72.

Blume W. The progression of epilepsy. *Epilepsia* 2006; 47: 71-8.

Camfield P, Camfield C, Cooley J, Smith E, Garner B. A randomized study of carbamazepine *versus* no medication after a first unprovoked seizure in childhood. *Neurology* 1989; 39: 851-2.

Capovilla G, Gambardella A, Romeo A *et al*. Benign partial epilepsies of adolescence: a report of 27 new cases. *Epilepsia* 2001; 42: 15: 49-52.

Carole G. Délais évolutifs des syndromes épileptiques avant leur diagnostic: résultats descriptifs de l'enquête CAROLE. *Rev Neurol* 2000; 156: 481-90.

Cockerell O, Johnson A, Sander J, Shorvon S. Prognosis of epilepsy: A review and further analysis of the first nine years of the British National General Practice Study of Epilepsy, a prospective population-based study. *Epilepsia* 1997; 38: 31-46.

Commission on Epidemiology and Prognosis, International League Against Epilepsy. Guidelines for epidemiologic studies on epilepsy. *Epilepsia* 1993; 34: 592-6.

Feksi AT, Kaamugishi J, Sander JWAS, Gatiti S. Comprehensive primary health care antiepileptic drug treatment programme in rural and semi-urban Kenya. *Lancet* 1991; 337: 406-9.

First SeizureTrial Group. Randomized clinical trial of the efficacy of antiepileptic drugs in reducing the risk of relapse after a first unprovoked tonic-clonic seizure. *Neurology* 1993; 43: 478-83.

Fisher RS, van Emde Boas W, Blume W, Elger C, Genton P, Lee P *et al*. Epileptic seizures and epilepsy: Definitions proposed by the International League Against Epilepsy (ILAE) and the International Bureau for Epilepsy (IBE). *Epilepsia* 2005; 46: 470-2.

Foy PM, Chadwick DW, Rajgopalan N, Johnson AL, Shaw MDM. Do Prophylactic anticonvulsant drugs alter the pattern of seizures after craniotomy. *J Neurol Neurosurg Psychiatry* 1992; 55: 753-7.

Goudsmit J, van der Waals F, Gajdusek D. Epilepsy in the Gbawein and Wroghbarh Clan of Grand Bassa County, Liberia: The endemic occurrence of "See-ee" in the native population. *Neuroepidemiology* 1983; 2: 24-34.

Gracia F, Loo de Lao S, Castillo L, Larreategui M, Archbold C, Majela Brenes M, Reeves W.C. Epidemiology of Epilepsy in Guaymi Indians from Bocas del Toro Province, Republic of Panama. *Epilepsia* 1990;31: 718-23.

Hauser WA, Lee JR. Do seizures beget seizures. *Prog Brain Res* 2002; 135: 215-9.

Hauser WA, Rich SS, Annegers JF, Anderson VE. Seizure recurrence after a 1st unprovoked seizure: an extended follow up. *Neurology* 1990; 40: 1163-70.

Hui ACF, Tang A, Wong KS, Mok V, Kay R. Recurrence after a first untreated seizure in the Hong Kong Chinese population. *Epilepsia* 2001; 42: 94-7.

Jallon P, Loiseau J, Loiseau P, de Zélicourt M, Motte J, Vallée L and the CAROLE *group. The risk of recurrence after a first unprovoked epileptic seizure in teenagers. Epilepsia* 1999; 40 (suppl 9): 87-8.

Jallon P, Loiseau P, Loiseau J. on behalf of groupe CAROLE (Coordination Active du Reseau Observatoire de l'Epilepsie). Newly diagnosed unprovoked epileptic seizures: presentation at diagnosis in CAROLE study. *Epilepsia* 2001; 42: 464-75.

Juul-Jensen P, Foldspang A. Natural history of epileptic seizures. *Epilepsia* 1983; 24: 297-312.

Keranen T, Riekkinen PJ. Remission of seizures in untreated epilepsy. *British Medical Journal* 1993; 307: 483.

Kwan P, Sander JWAS. The natural history of epilepsy: an epidemiological view. *J Neurol Neurosurg Psychiatry* 2004; 75: 1376-81.

Lindsten H, Stenlund H, L F. Remission of seizures in a population-based adult cohort with a newly diagnosed unprovoked epileptic seizure. *Epilepsia* 2001; 42: 1025-30.

Loiseau P, Orgogozo JM. An unrecognized syndrome of benign focal epileptic seizures in teenagers? *Lancet* 1978; 2: 1070-1.

Loiseau P, Jallon P, Wolf P. Isolated partial seizures in adolescence. In *Epileptic syndromes in children and adolescence*. Roger J, Bureau M, Dravet Ch, Genton P, Tassinari CA, Wolf P. ed. Paris: John Libbey Eurotext, 2005: 359-63.

Marson A, Jacoby A, Johnson A, Gamble C, Chadwick D. Immediate *versus* deferred antiepileptic drug treatment for early epilepsy and single seizures: a randomised controlled trial. *Lancet* 2005;365: 2007-13.

Musicco M, Beghi E, Solari A, for the First Seizure Trial Group. Treatment of a first tonic-clonic seizure does not improve the prognosis of epilepsy. *Neurology* 1997; 49: 991-8.

Placencia M, Paredes V, Cascante S *et al*. Epileptic seizures in Andean region of Ecuador: prevalence and incidence and regional variation. *Brain* 1992; 115: 771-82.

Placencia M, Sander JWAS, Roman M, Madera A, Crespo F, Cascante S, Shorvon SD. The characteristics of epilepsy in a largely untreated population in rural Ecuador. *Neurol, Neurosurg, and Psychiatry* 1994; 57; 320-5.

Sander JW. The epidemiology of epilepsy revisited. *Curr Opin Neurol* 2003; 16: 165-70.

Sander JWAS. Some aspects of prognosis in the epilepsies: a review. *Epilepsia* 1993; 34 (6): 1007-16.

Sander JWAS, Sillapää M. Natural history and prognosis. In *Epilepsy: a comprehensive textbook*. Engel Jr, Pedley TA ed. Philadephia: Lippincott-Raven Publishers, 1997: 69-89.

Sander JWAS. The natural history of epilepsy in the era of new antiepileptic drugs and surgical treatment. *Epilepsia* 2003; 44: 17-20.

Schachter SC. Current evidence indicates that antiepileptic drugs are anti ictal, not anti-epileptic. *Epilepsy Res* 2002; 50: 67-70.

Schmidt D. The clinical impact of new antiepileptic drugs after a decade of use in epilepsy. *Epilepsy Research* 2002; 15: 1-132.

Scotoni AE, Manreza MLG, Guerreiro M. Recurrence after a first Unprovoked cryptogenic/idiopathic seizure in children: a prospective study from Sao Paulo, Brazil. *Epilepsia* 2004; 45: 166-70.

Semah F, Picot MC, Adam C, Broglin D, Arzimanoglou A, Bazin B, Cavalcanti D, Baulac M. Is the underlying cause of epilepsy a major prognosis factor for recurrence? *Neurology* 1998, 51: 1256-62.

Shinnar S, Berg AT, Moshe SL, O'Dell C, Alemany M, Newstein D *et al*. The risk of seizure recurrence after a first unprovoked afebrile seizure in childhood: an extended follow-up. *Pediatrics* 1996; 98: 216-25.

Shinnar S, Berg AT. Does antiepileptic drug therapy prevent the development of "chronic" epilepsy? *Epilepsia* 1996; 37: 701-8.

Sillanpää M. Long-term outcome of epilepsy. *Epileptic Disorders* 2000; 2: 79-88.

Stroink H, Brouwer OF, Arts WF, Geerts AT, Peters AC, van Donselaar CA. The first unprovoked, untreated seizure in childhood: a hospital based study of the accuracy of the diagnosis, rate of recurrence, and long term outcome after recurrence. Dutch study of epilepsy in childhood. *J Neurol Neurosurg Psychiatry* 1998; 64 (5): 595-600.

Temkin NR. Antiepileptogenesis and Seizure Prevention Trials with Antiepileptic Drugs: Meta-Analysis of Controlled Trials. *Epilepsia* 2001; 42: 515-24.

Wang WZ, Wu JZ, Wang DS, Dai XY, Yang B, Wang TP *et al*. The prevalence and treatment gap in epilepsy in China: An ILAE/IBE/WHO study. *Neurology* 2003; 60: 1544-5.

Watts AE. The natural history of untreated epilepsy in a rural community in Africa. *Epilepsia* 1992; 33: 464-8.

Wolf P. Isolated seizures. In Epilepsy: a comprehensive textbook. Engel Jr, Pedley TA ed. Philadephia: Lippincott-Raven Publishers, 1997: 2475-81.

Risk factors for developing epilepsy after a first unprovoked seizure

Sheryl R. Haut, Christine O'Dell[1], Shlomo Shinnar[2]

Departments of Neurology, Pediatrics and The Comprehensive Epilepsy Management Center[1,2], Montefiore Medical Center, Albert Einstein College of Medicine, Bronx, New York, USA.

One of the challenges in the treatment of seizures and epilepsy is the approach to a first unprovoked seizure. While many children and adults with seizures present to medical attention with a history of prior events, approximately one third to one half will present following a single seizure (Sander *et al.*, 1990; Group CAROLE, 2001). The therapeutic decisions to follow have important implications for health and quality of life. In an era of increasing awareness and concern about medication side effects, the impact of initiating potential long-term therapy may be substantial. Alternately, the possibility that each seizure may increase the risk of subsequent seizures and development of epilepsy suggests a mandate of initial aggressive therapy. Thus any exploration of the approach to a first unprovoked seizure requires an understanding of the natural history and prognosis of the disorder, including to a large degree risk factors for recurrence and the development of epilepsy.

■ A first unprovoked seizure: Definition

A first unprovoked seizure is defined as a seizure occurring in a person over one month of age with no prior history of unprovoked seizures (Commission, 1993). The definition excludes neonatal seizures, febrile seizures, or seizures in the setting of acute precipitating causes such as head trauma, infection, or metabolic derangements. Conversely, provoked implies an insult such as those listed, sufficient to alter brain function in any individual. Factors such as sleep deprivation or strobe lights that can trigger seizures in susceptible individuals are considered triggers but for purposes of first seizures these events would still be considered unprovoked (Commission, 1993). Most studies define a first unprovoked seizure in accordance with International League Against Epilepsy (ILAE) guidelines, to include either a single seizure or a flurry of seizures within 24 hours with return to baseline between seizures (Commission, 1993). The choice of accepting two seizures within 24 hours as equivalent to one seizure has been debated (Shinnar *et al.*, 1990, 1996; Camfield and Camfield, 2000; Kho *et al.*, 2006). As discussed in more detail below, the majority of studies have found no difference in recurrence risks in children or adults who present with a flurry of seizures in one day compared to those who present with a single seizure justifying the ILAE epidemiological definitions. Furthermore, studies of adults with refractory partial epilepsy being evaluated for epilepsy surgery in monitoring units demonstrate that seizure flurries or clusters do not represent independent seizures (Haut et al., 1997) and also support this definition. In approximately 10-12% of cases, the first unprovoked seizure will be status epilepticus (seizure with duration ≥ 30 minutes or a series of seizures lasting ≥ 30 minutes without regaining of consciousness in between) and this is not considered an exclusion criterion (Commission, Shinnar et al., 1990, 2001; Hauser et al., 1982).

■ Recurrence risk after a first unprovoked seizure

Over the past few decades, many studies have attempted to address the recurrence risk following a first unprovoked seizure using a variety of recruitment and identification techniques (Annegers et al., 1986; Berg et al., 1991; Camfield et al., 1985, 1989; Hauser et al., 1982, 1990, 1998; Hopkins et al., 1988; Shinnar et al., 1990, 1996, 2002; Stroink et al., 1998; van Donselaar et al., 1990, 1992, 1997; Elwes et al., 1985; FIRST, 1993; Hirtz et al., 1984, 2000; Lindsten et al., 2001, more). It is almost impossible to do prospective population based studies of first seizures as many first seizures are unrecognized and/or unwitnessed, and the majority of patients do not present for medical attention unless the first seizure is convulsive. Therefore many population-based studies rely on retrospective identification, a fact that limits the results.

The reported overall recurrence risk following a first unprovoked seizure in children and adults varies from 27% to 71%, although studies that carefully exclude those with prior seizures generally report a range of 27-52%. These rates appear constant across gender, age and geographic location (Hui et al., 2001; Daoud et al., 2004; Das et al., 2000). In two meta-analyses, recurrence rates in prospective studies (40% at two years) were reported to be lower than retrospective studies (51-52% at two years) (Berg and Shinnar, 1991; Wiebe, 2002). There are now a number of large prospective class 2 studies (not population based but otherwise well designed prospective studies) in both children and adults (Hauser et al., 1982; Shinnar et al., 1990; FIRST, 1993, Stroink et al., 1998; van Donselaar et al., 1990, 1992, 1997; Hopkins et al., 1988; Marson et al., 2005). While study populations are often heterogeneous, with different distributions of demographic and prognostic factors, which may contribute to the variability noted the main variability has been the methodologies and definitions. Studies that are prospective have shown remarkably similar recurrence risks. This is especially true of the more recent prospective studies where many patients were not treated following the first seizure (Marson et al., 2005).

Time to recurrence

While the absolute recurrence risk reported in different studies varies considerably, the time course of recurrence is remarkably similar among all studies (Berg and Shinnar, 1991). The majority of recurrences occur early, with approximately 50% of recurrences occurring within 6 months of the initial seizure (Berg and Shinnar, 1991, Shinnar 1996). Eighty percent of the five-year recurrence risk appears to be realized by 2 years after the initial seizure (Berg and Shinnar, 1991; Wiebe, 2002). Late recurrences are unusual, but they have occurred up to 10 years after the initial seizure (Shinnar, 1996, 2000). In one prospective study with long term follow-up, the cumulative risk of a second seizure was 29%, 37%, 43% and 46% at 1, 2, 5 and 10 years respectively (Shinnar, 2000). This time course is true both in studies that report low and high recurrence risks (Annegers et al., 1986; Berg and Shinnar, 1991; Camfield et al., 1985, 1989; Hauser et al., 1982, 1990, 1998; Shinnar et al., 1990, 1996, 2002; Elwes et al., 1985; FIRST, 1993; Hirtz et al., 1984).

Risk factors for recurrence

In contrast to the variability in recurrence risk, risk factors for recurrence are highly preserved across studies. A relatively small number of factors appear to be associated with a differential recurrence risk. The most important of these are the etiology of the seizure, the electroencephalogram (EEG), and whether the first seizure occurred in wakefulness or sleep. These factors are consistent across most studies regardless of the absolute risk of recurrence reported in the individual study (Annegers et al., 1986; Berg and Shinnar, 1991; Camfield et al., 1985; Hauser et al., 1982, 1990, 1998; Hopkins et al., 1988; Shinnar et al., 1990, 1996, 2000; Stroink et al., 1998; Pohlmann-Eden et al., 2006; Kim et al., 2006). Factors not associated with a significant change in the recurrence risk include age of onset, the duration of the initial seizure in children, and multiple seizures at first seizure presentation. Selected risk factors are discussed below.

Etiology

In the ILAE classification, etiology of seizures is classified as remote symptomatic, cryptogenic or idiopathic (Commission, 1993). Remote symptomatic seizures are those without an immediate cause but with an identifiable prior brain injury or the presence of a static encephalopathy such as mental retardation or cerebral palsy, which are known to be associated with an increased risk of seizures. Cryptogenic seizures are those occurring in otherwise normal individuals with no clear etiology. Idiopathic is reserved for seizures occurring in the context of the presumed genetic epilepsies such as benign Rolandic and childhood absence (Commission, 1989; Roger et al., 2002). However, much of the literature on the recurrence risk following a first unprovoked seizure considers idiopathic and cryptogenic together as idiopathic, using a prior classification (Hauser et al., 1982).

A remote symptomatic first seizure confers a higher recurrence risk than a cryptogenic first seizure, for both children and adults. A meta-analysis of the studies published up to 1990, found that the relative risk of recurrence following a remote symptomatic first seizure was 1.8 (95% confidence interval 1.5, 2.1) compared to those with a cryptogenic first seizure (Berg and Shinnar, 1991). Comparable findings are reported in more recent studies (Shinnar et al., 1996; Stroink et al., 1998; Hirtz et al., 2000; Lindsten et al., 2001). It should be noted that a remote symptomatic seizure is associated with both a higher risk of recurrence, a higher risk of multiple recurrences and a lower probability of long-term remission (Shinnar et al., 2002). This is similar to the predictive value of etiology in newly diagnosed epilepsy (Berg et al., 2001a, b). Many of these studies were performed in the previous decade; with continued improvement in MRI resolution, cases previously classified as cryptogenic may well represent remote symptomatic. However, even recent studies of newly diagnosed epilepsy find a low rate of imaging abnormalities in children who are neurologically normal. (Berg AT, et al., 2000).

The occurrence of a first idiopathic unprovoked seizure, defined as a first seizure associated with a consistently abnormal EEG (Commission, 1989; Roger et al., 2002), may be consistent with a diagnosis of an epilepsy syndrome, as discussed below. First idiopathic seizures occur almost exclusively in children or adolescents, and the recurrence risk is actually comparable to those with a remote symptomatic first seizure (Shinnar et al., 1996). This is because, by definition an idiopathic first seizure is associated with an EEG signature of focal spikes or generalized spike and wave and as described below, an epileptiform EEG is a key risk factor for recurrence, especially in children. It should be noted that while the risk of a second seizure is also high in idiopathic syndromes, the risks of multiple seizures as well as long term prognosis is low in the idiopathic cases (Shinnar et al., 2002).

Electroencephalogram

EEG performed within 48 hours of a first unprovoked seizure shows abnormalities in up to 70% of cases (Schreiner and Pohlmann-Eden 2003). The EEG is an important predictor of recurrence, particularly in cases that are not remote symptomatic and in children (Berg and Shinnar, 1991; Camfield et al., 1985; Hauser et al., 1982; Hauser et al., 1990; Hopkins et al., 1988; Shinnar et al., 1990, 1994, 1996; Stroink et al., 1998; van Donselaar et al., 1990, 1992, 1997; Hirtz et al., 2000; Kim et al., 2006). All studies of recurrence risk following a first seizure in childhood report that the presence of an abnormal EEG confers a higher recurrence risk than a normal EEG (Berg and Shinnar, 1991; Camfield et al., 1985; Shinnar et al., 1990, 1994, 1996, 2002; Stroink et al., 1998; Hirtz et al., 2000). EEG is therefore considered a standard in the diagnostic evaluation of a first unprovoked seizure in children (Hirtz et al., 2000). While some studies have reported that only epileptiform abnormalities increase the recurrence risk in children (Camfield et al., 1985), in our data, any clearly abnormal EEG patterns including generalized spike and wave, focal spikes, and focal or generalized slowing increased the risk of recurrence in cases that were not remote symptomatic (Shinnar et al., 1994, 1996). The risk of seizure recurrence by 24 months for children with an idiopathic/cryptogenic first seizure in our study was 25% for those with a normal EEG, 34% for those with nonepileptiform abnormalities and 54% for those with epileptiform abnormalities (Shinnar et al., 1994, 1996).

In adults, the majority of studies also find an increased recurrence risk associated with an abnormal EEG (Berg and Shinnar, 1991; Hauser et al., 1990, 1998; van Donselaar et al., 1992; Kim et al., 2006) though one study failed to find a significant effect (Hopkins et al., 1988), and one study found that only generalized spike and wave patterns, not focal spikes, were predictive of recurrence (Hauser et al., 1982). A meta-analysis of these studies concluded that the overall data do support an association between abnormal EEG and an increased recurrence risk in adults (Berg and Shinnar,

1991), though which EEG patterns besides generalized spike and wave are important remains unclear (Berg and Shinnar, 1991; Hauser et al., 1990, 1998; van Donselaar et al., 1992). Recent results from the MESS trial also support the association between any EEG abnormality and an increased recurrence risk (Kim et al., 2006).

Sleep state at time of first seizure

The association between sleep and seizure involves both sleep state and time of sleep. In children, whose sleep patterns may include daytime naps, the association is between sleep state (rather than time of day) and seizure recurrence risk (Shinnar et al., 1993, 1996), while in adults, seizures that occur at night are associated with a higher recurrence risk than those that occur in the daytime (Hopkins et al., 1988). These represent complimentary findings. In children, especially young children, one cannot presume that afternoon is an awake period so one has to ask about awake or asleep. Furthermore, if the first seizure occurs in sleep, there is a high likelihood that the second one, should it occur, will also occur during sleep (Shinnar et al., 1993). In our series, the 2-year recurrence risk was 53% for children whose initial seizure occurred during sleep compared with 30% for those whose initial seizure occurred while awake (Shinnar et al., 1996). From a therapeutic point of view, the implication of a seizure in sleep is unclear. While the recurrence risk is higher, recurrences will tend to occur in sleep, which is associated with a lower morbidity than a daytime seizure.

Seizure Classification

Most first unprovoked seizures are convulsive; other seizure types such as absence, complex partial seizure and myoclonic seizures typically occur more than once before the patient is brought to medical attention (Hirtz et al., 2000; Pohlmann-Eden et al., 2006). The risk of recurrence following a first unprovoked seizure is reported to be higher in subjects with a partial seizure than in those with a generalized first seizure (Berg and Shinnar, 1991). However, this association is mostly found on univariate analysis and disappears once the effect of etiology and the EEG are accounted for (Berg and Shinnar, 1991; Hauser et al., 1982; Shinnar et al., 1990, 1996). Partial seizures are more common in those with a remote symptomatic first seizure and in children with an abnormal EEG (Shinnar et al., 1990). Generalized seizures that present to medical attention at the time of the first seizure are usually tonic-clonic (Shinnar et al., 1996).

Duration of Initial Seizure

In children, the duration of the first seizure, including status epilepticus, appears not to be associated with a differential recurrence risk. In our study, 48 (12%) of 407 children (38 cryptogenic/idiopathic, 10 remote symptomatic) presented with status epilepticus (duration $\geq$ 30 minutes) as their first unprovoked seizure (Shinnar et al., 1996). The recurrence risk in these children was not different than in children whose first seizure was briefer. However, if a recurrence did occur it was likely to be prolonged (Shinnar et al., 1996, 2001). Of the 24 children with an initial episode of status who experienced a seizure recurrence, 5 (21%) recurred with status. Of the 147 children who presented with an initial brief seizure and experienced a seizure recurrence, only 2 (1%) recurred with status epilepticus (p < 0.001). In general there are data that indicate that there is a subgroup of children with a predisposition to prolonged seizures (Shinnar et al., 2001). Similar data have been reported in febrile seizures where an initial prolonged febrile seizure does not alter the risk of another febrile seizure but should another one occur it is likely to be prolonged (Berg and Shinnar, 1996). In adults there is a suggestion that a prolonged first seizure, particularly in remote symptomatic cases is associated with a higher risk of recurrence (Hauser et al., 1990).

Number of seizures at "first seizure" presentation

As discussed above, the definition of a first unprovoked seizure allows for a cluster of seizures within 24 hours to be considered as a single first seizure. In most studies, recurrence risk is not increased for more than one seizure at initial presentation), even for the occurrence of multiple seizures at first seizure onset (Hauser et al., 1982; Shinnar et al., 1990, 1996; Kho et al., 2006). In the MESS study, number of seizures at presentation was associated with an increased recurrence risk (Kim et al., 2006), but this included any prior seizures and not necessarily multiple seizures at "first seizure" presentation. Similarly, the study by the Camfields compared children whose first two seizures occurred on the same day to children whose first two seizures occurred on different days, and was not strictly speaking a comparison of the impact of the number of seizures in one day on recurrence risk. The impact of the number of seizures in one day on recurrence risk is important, as a significant number of cases present in this fashion. Shinnar et al., reported 23% of first unprovoked seizures in children were multiple on one day whereas Kho et al. (2006) reported 14% of adults presented in this fashion. In fact, the very high rate of recurrence reported by Elwes et al. (1985) is largely explained by their considering two seizures in one day as a recurrence which accounted for almost 20% of their cases. The preponderance of evidence at this time is that there is no clear difference in recurrence risk between those who present with a single event or a flurry of seizures as their first unprovoked seizure. This supports the ILAE view and also has therapeutic implications. Interestingly, one can think of both a prolonged seizure and a flurry of seizures in one day as a failure of the inhibitory mechanisms that ordinarily terminate a seizure (Shinnar et al., 2001). Thus is makes sense that either both or neither will be risk factors for recurrence and that is indeed the case.

■ What happens after two seizures?

Recent studies in adults (Hauser et al., 1998) and children (Shinnar et al., 2000) have examined what happens after a second seizure. In both adults and children the recurrence risk after a second seizure is approximately 70% (Hauser et al., 1998; Shinnar et al., 2000). Those with a remote symptomatic etiology and those whose second seizure occurs within six months of the first have a higher recurrence risk (Shinnar et al., 2000). However, unlike the case with a first unprovoked seizure, there are no identifiable subgroups with a low recurrence risk. Interestingly, in most studies, factors that predict an initial recurrence such as an abnormal EEG and sleep state at the time of the seizure are no longer associated with a differential risk of further seizures once a second seizure has occurred. The likely explanation is that those factors such as an abnormal EEG indicate a tendency to seizures, but that once a second one occurred, thus confirming this tendency, these factors are no longer predictive. Etiology on the other hand predicts not just a second seizure but an increased risk of many seizures (Shinnar et al., 2000). Interestingly in our study, the treatment effects were similar to those in the randomized clinical trials after a first seizure. Following a second seizure, on univariate analysis, treatment did not alter the risk of a third seizure. But on multivariable analysis, the risk was reduced in half (Shinnar et al., 2000). Not surprisingly, children whose second seizure occurred soon after the initial one and children with remote symptomatic etiology were more likely to be treated. This confounder may also explain why in observational studies following a first seizure, treatment does not seem to affect recurrence risk whereas randomized trials show a 50% reduction in recurrence risk.

Risk Allocation Models

A number of studies have combined risk factor analysis to present risk allocation models for seizure recurrence. Camfield et al. (1985) examined the risk of seizure recurrence in various combinations of the variables significant in that study: EEG, abnormal neurological examination, and seizure classification. More recently, the MESS trial (Kim et al., 2006) presented a risk allocation model for seizure recurrence using a regression model that includes etiology, total number of seizures at time of randomization, and the presence of an abnormal EEG. Utilizing this model, risk levels can be calculated based on these variables potentially guiding treatment decisions. A history of two seizures was consistent with moderate risk, while a history of three seizures was consistent with high risk for recurrence (Kim et al., 2006).

▪ Diagnosis of "epilepsy" after a first seizure

The accepted definition of epilepsy requires two unprovoked seizures 24 hours apart (Commission 93). An epilepsy syndrome, however, may be diagnosed even after a single seizure (Shinnar et al., 1999), for example the diagnosis of benign rolandic epilepsy in the setting of a first nocturnal seizure and rolandic spikes on EEG. More recently, a definition of epilepsy has been proposed by the ILAE/IBE (Fisher et al., 2005) in which epilepsy may be defined as the occurrence of a single seizure in the presence of an "enduring alteration in the brain" that increases the likelihood of future seizures. This definition, however, is not universally accepted, particularly since the concept of what constitutes an "enduring alteration in the brain" is poorly defined. At present, the epidemiological data support the continued use of the definition of at least two seizures more than 24 hours apart. Once two seizures have occurred, the risk of a third seizure is high across all groups. The need for treatment is still based on an individualized risk/benefit analysis so that children with a self limited syndrome such as Rolandic epilepsy with rare brief seizures may not need treatment even though they meet the definition of epilepsy (Ambrosetti et al., 1990; O'Dell and Shinnar, 2001).

■ Conclusions

Well-designed prospective studies of the recurrence risk after a first unprovoked seizure in children and adults show recurrence risks in the 40-50% range. Risk factors for recurrence appear consistent across study populations, including children and adults. These risks include seizure etiology, with highest recurrence risk associated with remote symptomatic or idiopathic etiology, and EEG abnormalities of any type, though the impact of an abnormal EEG may be higher in children. The epidemiological data support continuing the definition of epilepsy as two or more unprovoked seizures more than 24 hours apart. It is now clear that treatment following a first unprovoked seizure, while reducing recurrence risk, does not alter prognosis and is therefore usually not indicated. Recent approaches to stratifying patients presenting with a first or second or third unprovoked seizure based on risk level may improve the approach to determining the optimal therapeutic course after a first or second seizure.

Supported in part by grant 1 RO1 NS26151 (S. Shinnar) from the National Institute fo Neurological Disorders and Stroke, NIH, Bethesda MD

References

Ambrosetto G, Tassinari CA. Antiepileptic drug treatment of benign childhood epilepsy with Rolandic spikes: Is it necessary? *Epilepsia* 1990; 31: 802-5.

Annegers JF, Shirts SB, Hauser WA, Kurland LT. Risk of recurrence after an initial unprovoked seizure. *Epilepsia* 1986; 27: 43-50.

Berg A, Shinnar S. The risk of seizure recurrence following a first unprovoked seizure: A quantitative review. *Neurology* 1991; 41: 965-72.

Berg AT et al. Testa FM, Levy SR, Shinnar S. Neuroimaging in children with newly diagnosed epilepsy: A community-based study. *Pediatrics* 2000; 106: 527-32.

Berg AT, Shinnar S, Levy SR, Testa FM, Smith-Rapaport S, Beckerman B. Early development of intractable epilepsy in children: A prospective study. *Neurology* 2001; 56: 1445-52.

Berg AT, Shinnar S, Levy SR, Testa FM, Smith-Rapaport S, Beckerman B, Ebrahimi N. Two-year remission and subsequent relapse in children with newly diagnosed epilepsy. *Epilepsia* 2001; 42: 1553-62.

Camfield PR, Camfield CS, Dooley JM, Tibbles JAR, Fung T, Garner B. Epilepsy after a first unprovoked seizure in childhood. *Neurology* 1985; 35: 1657-60.

Camfield P, Camfield C, Dooley J et al. A randomized study of carbamazepine *versus* no medication following a first unprovoked seizure in childhood. *Neurology* 1989; 39: 851-2.

Camfield P, Camfield C Epilepsy Can Be Diagnosed When the First Two Seizures Occur on the Same Day. *Epilepsia* 2000; 41 (9): 1230-3.

Commission on classification and terminology of the International League Against Epilepsy. Proposal for revised classification of epilepsies and epileptic syndromes. *Epilepsia* 1989; 30: 389-99.

Commission on epidemiology and prognosis, International League Against Epilepsy. Guidelines for epidemiologic studies on epilepsy. *Epilepsia* 1993; 34: 592-6.

Daoud AS, Ajloni S, El-Salem K, Horani K, Otoom S, Daradkeh T. Risk of seizure recurrence after a first unprovoked seizure: a prospective study among Jordanian children. *Seizure*. 2004; 13 (2): 99-103.

Das CP, Sawhney IM, Lal V, Prabhakar S. Risk of recurrence of seizures following single unprovoked idiopathic seizure. *Neurol India* 2000; 48: 357-60.

Elwes RDC, Chesterman P, Reynolds EH. Prognosis after a first untreated tonic-clonic seizure. *Lancet* 1985; 2: 752-3.

First Seizure Trial Group. Randomized clinical trial on the efficacy of antiepileptic drugs in reducing the risk of relapse after a first unprovoked tonic-clonic seizure. *Neurology* 1993; 43: 478-83.

Gilad R, Lampl Y, Gabbay U, Eshel Y, Sarova-Pinhas I. Early treatment of a single generalized tonic-clonic seizure to prevent recurrence. *Arch Neurol* 1996; 53 (11): 1149-52.

Groupe CAROLE (Coordination Active du Reseau Observatoire Longitudinal de l'Epilepsie. Traitement des crises épileptiques nouvellement diagnostiquées. Une experience française. *Revue Neurol (Paris)* 2001: 157 (12): 1500-12.

Haut SR, Legatt AD, O'Dell C, Moshé SL, Shinnar S. Seizure Lateralization During EEG Monitoring in Patients with Bilateral Foci: The Cluster Effect. *Epilepsia* 1997; 38 (8): 937-40.

Hui ACF, Tang A, Wong KS, Mok V, Kay R. Recurrence After a First Untreated Seizure in the Hong Kong Chinese Population. *Epilepsia* 2001; 42 (1): 94-7.

Hauser WA, Anderson VE, Loewenson RB, McRoberts SM. Seizure recurrence after a first unprovoked seizure. *N Engl J Med* 1982; 307: 522-8.

Hauser WA, Rich SS, Annegers JF, Anderson VE. Seizure recurrence after a 1st unprovoked seizure: an extended follow-up. *Neurology* 1990; 40: 1163-70.

Hauser WA, Rich SS, Lee JR, Annegers JF, Anderson VE. Risk of recurrent seizures after two unprovoked seizures. *N Engl J Med* 1998; 338: 429-34.

Hirtz DG, Ellenberg JH, Nelson KB. The risk of recurrence of nonfebrile seizures in children. *Neurology* 1984; 34: 637-41.

Hirtz D, Ashwal S, Berg A, Bettis D, Camfield C, Camfield P, Crumrine P, Elterman R, Schneider S, Shinnar S. Practice Parameter: Evaluating a first nonfebrile seizure in children: Report of the Quality Standards Subcommittee of the American Academy of Neurology, the Child Neurology Society and the American Epilepsy Society. *Neurology* 2000; 55: 616-23.

Hirtz D, Berg A, Bettis D, Camfield C, Camfield P, Crunrine C, Gaillard WD, Schneider S, Shinnar S. Practice Parameter: Treatment of the child with a first unprovoked seizure. Report of the QSS of the AAN and the Practice Committee of the CNS. *Neurology* 2003; 60: 166-75.

Hopkins A, Garman A, Clarke C. The first seizure in adult life: value of clinical features electroencephalography and computerized tomographic scanning in prediction of seizure recurrence. *Lancet* 1988; 1: 721-6.

Kim LG, Johnson TL, Marson AG, Chadwick DW. Prediction of risk of seizure recurrence after a single seizure and early epilepsy: further results from the MESS trial. *Lancet Neurol* 2006; 5 (4): 317-22.

Kho LK, Lawn ND, Dunne JW, Linto J. First seizure presentation: do multiple seizures within 24 hours predict recurrence? *Neurology*. 2006; 67 (6): 1047-9.

Lindsten H, Stenlund H, Forsgren L. Seizure recurrence in adults after a newly diagnosed unprovoked epileptic seizure. *Acta Neurologica Scandinavica* 2001; 104 (4): 202-7.

Marson A, Jacoby A, Johnson A, Kim L, Gamble C, Chadwick D, Medical Research Council MESS study Group. Immediate *versus* deferred antiepileptic drug treatment for early epilepsy and single seizures: a randomized controlled trial. *Lancet* 2005; 365: 2007-13.

Musicco M, Beghi E, Solari A, Viani F for the First Seizure Trial Group (FIRST Group). Treatment of first tonic-clonic seizure does not improve the prognosis of epilepsy. *Neurology* 1997; 49: 991-8.

O'Dell C, Shinnar S. Initiation and discontinuation of antiepileptic drugs. *Neurologic Clinics* 2001; 19: 289-311.

Pohlmann-Eden B, Beghi E, Camfield C, Camfield P. The first seizure and its management in adults and children. *BMJ* 2006; 332 (7537): 339-42.

Roger J, Bureau M, Dravet C, Genton P, Tassinari CA, Wolf P eds. *Epileptic syndromes in infancy, childhood and adolescence*. Third Edition. Paris: John-Libbey Eurotext, 2002.

Sander JW, Hart YM, Johnson AL, Shorvon SD. National General Practice Study of Epilepsy: newly diagnosed epileptic seizures in a general population. *Lancet* 1990; 336 (8726): 1267-71.

Schreiner A, Pohlmann-Eden B. Value of the early electroencephalogram after a first unprovoked seizure. *Clin Electroencephalogr* 2003; 34 (3): 140-4.

Shinnar S, Berg AT Moshe SL et al. The risk of recurrence following a first unprovoked seizure in childhood: a prospective study. *Pediatrics* 1990; 85: 1076-85.

Shinnar S, Berg AT, Ptachewich Y, Alemany M. Sleep state and the risk of seizure recurrence following a first unprovoked seizure in childhood *Neurology* 1993; 43: 701-6.

Shinnar S, Kang H, Berg AT, Goldensohn ES, Hauser WA, Moshe SL. EEG abnormalities in children with a first unprovoked seizure. *Epilepsia* 1994; 35: 471-6.

Shinnar S, Berg AT. Does antiepileptic drug therapy prevent the development of "chronic" epilepsy. *Epilepsia* 1996;37: 701-8.

Shinnar S, Berg AT, Moshe SL et al. The risk of seizure recurrence following a first unprovoked afebrile seizure in childhood: An extended follow-up. *Pediatrics* 1996; 98: 216-25.

Shinnar S, O'Dell C, Berg AT. Distribution of epilepsy syndromes in a cohort of children prospectively monitored from the time of their first unprovoked seizure. *Epilepsia* 1999; 40: 1378-83.

Shinnar S, Berg AT, O'Dell C, Newstein D, Moshe SL, Hauser WA. Predictors of multiple seizures in a cohort of children prospectively followed from the time of their first unprovoked seizure. *Ann Neurol* 2000; 48: 140-7.

Shinnar S, Berg AT, Moshe SL, Shinnar R. How long do new-onset seizures in children last? *Ann Neurol* 2001; 49: 659-64.

Stroink H, Brouwer OF, Arts WF, Geerts AT, Peters AC, van Donselaar CA. The first unprovoked seizure in childhood: a hospital based study of the accuracy of the diagnosis, rate of recurrence, and long term outcome after recurrence. Dutch study of epilepsy in childhood. *J Neurol Neurosurg Psychiatry* 1998; 64: 595-600.

van Donselaar CA, Geerts AT, Schimsheimer RJ. Idiopathic first seizure in adult life: Who should be treated? *BMJ* 1990; 302: 620-3.

van Donselaar CE, Schimsheimer RJ, Geerts AT, Declerck AC. Value of the electroencephalogram in adult patients with untreated idiopathic first seizures. *Arch Neurol* 1992; 49: 231-7.

van Donselaar CA, Brouwer OF, Geerts AT, Arts WF, Stroink H, Peters AC. Clinical course of untreated tonic-clonic seizures in childhood: prospective, hospital based study. *BMJ* 1997; 314: 401-4.

Wiebe S. An evidence based approach to the first unprovoked seizure. *Can J Neurol Sci.* 2002; 29 (2): 120-4.

Section III:
Epileptogenesis and disease progression: the example of febrile seizures

"Complex" febrile seizures and the epilepsy: information from an experimental model

Céline Dubé[1], Tallie Z. Baram[1,2]

Depts Anatomy & Neurobiology[1], Pediatrics[2], University of California at Irvine, Irvine, USA

The study of febrile seizures has been driven, in part, by the association of these seizures with the development of temporal lobe epilepsy. The clinical question of whether long or recurrent febrile seizures cause temporal lobe epilepsy has remained unresolved. To address this issue directly, the authors developed a model of prolonged (complex) febrile seizures in immature rat and mouse. This should allow mechanistic examination of the potential causal relationship of febrile seizures and limbic epilepsy. Although the model relied on hyperthermia, the authors found that the hyperthermia provoked the release of endogenous fever mediators including interleukin 1 beta, and thus resembled human febrile seizures. The seizures were found to evoke epilepsy in a third of affected animals, permitting analysis of the mechanisms of epileptogenesis. To date, alteration of specific ion channels, perhaps driven by genomic effects of fever-related cytokines, as well as changes in endocannabinoid signaling, are candidate mechanisms. Importantly, MRI imaging of animals subsequent to experimental febrile seizures may provide a biomarker for individuals who are at risk for developing temporal lobe epilepsy after prolonged febrile seizures.

■ The clinical questions: febrile seizures and temporal lobe epilepsy

Febrile seizures, seizures occurring during fever without an obvious central nervous system (CNS)-invasive infection, are the most common type of convulsions in infants and young children (reviewed in Stafstrom 2002). Generally, seizures with duration of less than 10 (Annegers *et al.*, 1987; Berg *et al.*, 1997) or 15 minutes (Nelson and Ellenberg, 1978) have little association, in epidemiological, prospective or retrospective studies, with subsequent temporal lobe epilepsy or cognitive deficits (Verity *et al.*, 1985, 1998; Berg and Shinnar, 1996a). However, the consequences of prolonged febrile seizures, a type of febrile seizures, are controversial (Annegers *et al.*, 1987; Berg and

Shinnar, 1996b). Specifically, retrospective studies link a history of prolonged febrile seizures, defined here as seizures longer than 10-15 minutes, and including febrile status epilepticus, to the development of temporal lobe epilepsy (TLE) (Cendes et al., 1993; French et al., 1993; Hamati-Haddad and Abou-Khalil, 1998; Theodore et al., 1999). This is in contrast to prospective studies, that fail to implicate prolonged febrile seizures as a strong determinant of epileptogenesis (see Shinnar, 2002 for review and the chapter by Camfield and Camfield in this book).

The conflicting evidence over the clinical outcome of prolonged febrile seizures, and the potential that they may promote epileptogenesis, has provided a rational for the creation of animal models of these seizures. Animal models permit direct examination of the potential consequences of these seizures and permit the use of a variety of investigational tools (anatomical, molecular, electrophysiological, and imaging) to test hypotheses about mechanisms by which febrile seizures might promote epileptogenesis.

This chapter described briefly a model of prolonged febrile seizures in immature rat and mouse, and the use of this model to ask three questions: *1. Do experimental prolonged seizures cause epilepsy? 2. What are the mechanisms of epileptogenesis? 3. Can a biomarker be developed to assess the risk of epileptogenesis after prolonged febrile seizures?*

■ Characteristics of a model of prolonged febrile seizures: fever, hyperthermia, age duration and outcome

Fever

Febrile seizures in humans are convulsions associated with fever. This suggests that animal models of febrile seizures should involve a controlled generation of fever in the experimental animals. However, whereas it is quite feasible to generate fever using pyrogens in mature rodents, the core temperature elevations that can be provoked by administration of lipopolysaccharides (LPS) and other systemic pyrogens, is limited to ~ 1° C in immature rats (Heida et al., 2003). This conundrum can be solved by using older animals (e.g., Morimoto et al., 1991). However, human febrile seizures occur only during a restricted developmental age (~ 3 months to ~ 5-6 years; Stafstrom, 2002). Alternatively, animals can be used during an age where brain (and hippocampal) development is equivalent to those of infants (Avishai-Eliner et al., 2002), and brain temperature elevated using alternative means.

The authors chose to use hyperthermia, evoked by a stream of warm air. Importantly, using genetically engineered mice, it was discovered that fever and hyperthermia utilize common mechanisms to elicit seizures: The pyrogenic cytokine Interleukin-1β (IL-1β) contributes to fever generation and, conversely, fever leads to IL-1 production within hippocampus (Takao et al., 1990; Ban et al., 1991; Cartmell et al.,1999; Gatti et al., 2002). These facts support the involvement of IL-1 in the mechanisms of both febrile and hyperthermic seizures. Indeed, Blake et al., 1994; Haveman et al., 1996 and the authors (Dubé et al., 2005) found that increasing brain temperature (hyperthermia) was sufficient to release IL-1 in the brain, without the need for other components of the febrile response. The authors demonstrated that mice that lacked the receptor for IL-1β required a much higher temperature to generate experimental "febrile" seizures, implicating the need for endogenous cytokine in these seizures (Dubé et al., 2005). Thus, the basis of the rodent model *(Figure 1)* is a controlled and rapid increase of brain temperature over 3-4 minutes; this leads to release of endogenous IL-1β, and to the generation of seizures.

Seizure characterization

Behaviorally, the initial seizure behaviors in both immature rats and mice consist of *sudden* immobility, *i.e.*, arrest of the hyperthermia-evoked running and other types of activity. The freezing seems to be associated with loss of responsiveness to the environment, and is followed rapidly by oral automatisms. It should be noted that this sequence is typical for human as well as animal seizures of limbic origin.

In rats, the freezing (Racine stage 0; Racine, 1972) is followed by oral automatisms (Racine stage 1) that, in turn, is often followed by clonic movements (Racine stage 3). Later in the seizures, generalization is evident not only from the clonic movements but also from tonic body flexion that may occur, perhaps suggesting propagation of the seizure to the brainstem. In mice, the seizure onset is also evident from sudden immobility, with reduced response to stimulation ("altered consciousness?"), that is often followed by facial automatisms, but rarely if at all by tonic body flexion. The EEG components of the seizures have been found in recordings from multiple brain sites in both immature rats and mice. Along with the "limbic" nature of the behaviors, bipolar electrode recordings from basal amygdala, dorsal hippocampus and frontoparietal cortex of freely moving pups (Baram et al., 1992, 1997; Dubé et al., 2000) suggested that the seizures involve, and likely commence, with EEG spike-trains in hippocampus and amygdala that coincided with the immobility and oral automatisms. Cortical EEG at that time was not changed or flattened (Dubé et al., 2000; Brewster et al., 2002). In limbic EEGs, the seizures consist of trains of spikes and spike-waves with progressively increasing amplitude in hippocampal and amygdala leads, with variable progression to the cortex. The EEG patterns in the mouse are quite similar.

Duration

The duration of the seizures is governed by the duration of the hyperthermia. In most of the "author" published work, seizure duration is ~ 22-25 minutes: consistent with long ("complex") human febrile seizures, but not with febrile status epilepticus.

It should be noted that a careful correlation of core and brain temperature was conducted by the authors, so that brain temperatures do not exceed ~ 42° C. This eliminates potential toxicity of high temperature in itself. To further exclude this possibility, the authors have also studied hyperthermic controls, where the hyperthermia was provoked to the same extent, but the seizures were blocked (Toth et al., 1998; Dubé et al., 2000, 2006).

Benign outcome and adaptability

In an additional similarity to the human situation, the febrile seizures in the model are free of mortality and major morbidity. There is virtually no dehydration (< 3% loss of body weight), and survival for months can be achieved. It should be noted that this

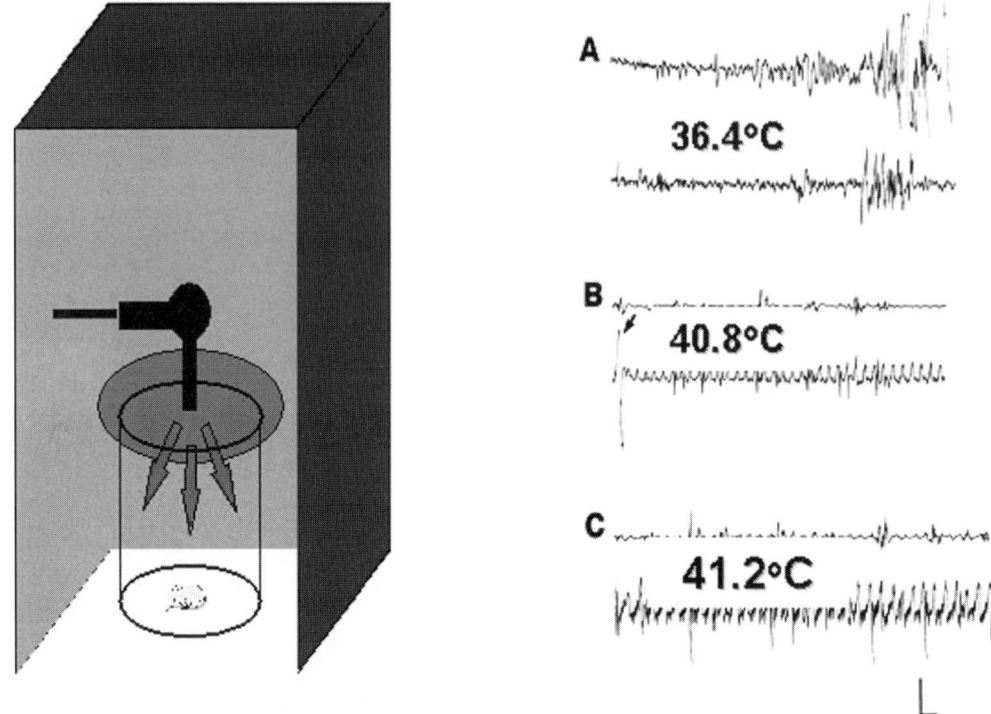

Figure 1. A schematized view of the set-up of the experimental model for long febrile seizures. Toth et al., 1998; Dubé et al., 2000, 2006.

general model has been now adopted by several other laboratories (Chang et al., 2003; Scantlebury et al., 2004; Heida et al., 2005; Lemmens et al., 2005; Kamal et al., 2006; Escayg et al., Wallace et al., personal communications)

■ Do experimental prolonged seizures cause epilepsy?

Initial studies by the authors involved daytime intermittent observation and EEG recording (Dubé et al., 2000), and did not demonstrate the onset of spontaneous seizures in rats that had experienced experimental febrile seizures. More recent repeated experiments, employing nocturnal simultaneous video-EEG recordings, discovered that epileptogenesis and the development of limbic epilepsy does occur in a fraction (~ a third) of rats that sustain experimental febrile seizures (Dubé et al., 2006). In essence, these studies considered the possibility that limbic epilepsy/seizures after prolonged febrile seizures might be behaviorally subtle, requiring behavior/EEG correlations to ascertain their presence. The studies compared adult rats (starting around 3 months of age) that had experienced experimental febrile seizures, with groups that had undergone hyperthermia but in whom seizures had been prevented (hyperthermic controls), as well as with normothermic controls. Seizures were defined conservatively as events that included both epileptiform hippocampal EEGs and behaviors. In rats that had sustained early-life experimental febrile seizures, 6/17 (35%) had spontaneous electro-clinical seizures.

These seizures consisted of sudden immobility and typical limbic automatisms that were coupled with polyspike/sharp-wave trains with increasing amplitude and slowing frequency on EEG. In addition, inter-ictal epileptiform discharges were recorded in 15 (88.2%) of this group. Neither the EEG (> 400 recorded hours) nor the behaviors of normothermic and hyperthermic control rats demonstrated any epileptiform abnormalities.

These findings, in an experimental model, indicate that prolonged febrile seizures per se, without any genetic or acquired predisposing factors, can convert a "normal" limbic circuit into an epileptic one. Therefore, the model should be very useful to study how this epileptogenic process takes place, and to identify molecular targets for intervention, as well as potential biomarkers for the disease process.

■ What are the mechanisms of epileptogenesis provoked by experimental prolonged febrile seizures?

A series of studies by the authors explored the possibility that experimental febrile seizures lead to epileptogenesis by provoking death of vulnerable neurons in hippocampus, amygdala and limbic cortices (Toth et al., 1998; Dubé et al., 2000; Baram et al., 2002; Bender et al., 2003a, 2004; Dubé et al., 2006). This notion was found not to be the case.

Whereas transient neuronal injury was elicited by these seizures, the involved neurons did not die (Toth et al., 1998). Neuronal counts in several brain regions did not suggest cell loss (Toth et al., 1998; Bender et al., 2003a, Dubé et al., 2006). Studies for apoptosis did not show increased cell death at any time point after the seizures (Toth et al., 1998), even when these were carried out for 60 minutes. In addition, neurogenesis, confirmed for other developmental seizures (Bender et al., 2003a), did not follow experimental febrile seizures (Bender et al., 2003a, but see Lemmens et al., 2005). Other expected structural changes, including mossy fiber sprouting, were also minimal after these seizures (Bender et al., 2003a), and did not explain the conversion of the hippocampal circuit into a hyper excitable one.

The seizure-evoked hippocampal hyperexcitability, defined *in vitro* by drastically reduced threshold to provocation of electrical status epilepticus, was evident already by seven days later, and persisted long term (Chen et al., 1999, 2001; Dubé et al., 2000). It is likely a result of profound molecular changes in hippocampal neurons. Whereas the repertoire and sequence of molecular changes evoked by experimental prolonged febrile seizures in this model have not yet been fully determined, persistent changes in the expression of specific ion channels likely play a role, as do alterations in endocannabinoid signaling.

Briefly, calcium (Ca^{2+}) entry was altered within hours following the seizures because of transient downregulation of GluR2 expression and the formation of Ca^{2+}-permeable AMPA receptors (Pellegrini-Giampietro et al., 1997; Richichi et al., 2006). Resulting activation of CaM Kinase II, as well as other calcium mediated mechanism influenced the expression of the hyperpolarization-activated cyclic nucleotide-gated cation (HCN) channels, starting already by 24-48 hours (Richichi et al., 2006).

Interestingly, HCN channel type 1 mRNA and protein levels were decreased whereas HCN2 channel gene expression was enhanced (Brewster et al., 2002). These mRNA levels were followed by a "molecular switch" of HCN1/HCN2 ratios also at the protein level (Brewster et al., 2005), and should promote hyperpolarization-evoked rebound neuronal firing (Chen et al., 2001; Santoro and Baram 2003), i.e., enhanced hippocampal excitability.

It is notable that expression of HCN channels is altered also in human hippocampi of patients with severe TLE, typically a history of early life seizures, and severe mesial temporal sclerosis (Bender et al., 2003b). These expression changes, consisting of *increased* HCN1 may potentially be neuroprotective (Bender et al., 2003b; Santoro and Baram, 2003). Additional persistent and important changes after experimental febrile seizures involve potentiation of endocannabinoid signaling, resulting from an increase in the number of presynaptic cannabinoid type 1 (CB-1) receptors. This, in turn, leads to increased retrograde inhibition of GABA release, promoting hyperexcitability (Chen et al., 2003).

Clearly, other important changes may take place in gene-expression programs within hippocampus of animals sustaining experimental prolonged febrile seizures. Many questions remain, about this process, including the fundamental puzzle of the long-lasting maintenance of pathological expression levels of HCN and CB-1.

■ Can a biomarker be developed to assess the risk of epileptogenesis after prolonged febrile seizures?

Reliable criteria or "markers" for progressive epileptogenesis and neuronal dysfunction are required in order to intervene in the epileptogenic process and abort the development of epilepsy and associated cognitive dysfunction. For the epileptogenic process commencing with prolonged febrile seizures and culminating in TLE in the immature rodent model, serial MRI was used to probe the possibility that altered MRI signal might be a biomarker for the epileptogenic process. In essence, a subset of animals were found to develop abnormal MRI signal within days of the seizures. In addition, as mentioned above, nocturnal video-EEG monitoring has indicated that a subgroup of adult animals that had experienced experimental prolonged FS early in life developed classical limbic seizures, with behavioral and EEG correlates. Ongoing research is testing the notion that **MRI lesions will serve as surrogate markers for epileptogenesis and/or hippocampal cognitive deficits**.

Specifically, to date, initially a 4 Tesla magnet, then a 7 Tesla magnet, with much improved signal to noise contrast and resolution, were used to examine if rats develop abnormal T2 signal after experimental prolonged febrile seizures. Rats were scanned before the seizures to obviate pre-existing abnormalities. A time course of the T2 signal changes is being constructed. To date, a subgroup of rats that had endured experimental febrile seizures has developed MRI T2 signal elevation changes in relevant limbic regions. In addition, the location of abnormal T2 signal in the model correlates well with that found in children with long febrile seizures: both involve hippocampal CA1 preferentially. The question of whether MRI changes are a surrogate marker for epileptogenesis, in both human and rat, has not yet been answered; in other words, it is not yet known whether the MRI signal changes are predictive of the development of epilepsy. These studies are ongoing.

References

Annegers JF, Hauser WA, Shirts SB, Kurland LT. Factors prognostic of unprovoked seizures after febrile convulsions. *N Engl J Med* 1987; 316: 493-8.

Avishai-Eliner S, Brunson KL, Sandman CA, Baram TZ. Stressed-out, or in (utero)? *Trends Neurosci* 2002; 25: 518-24.

Ban E, Milon G, Prudhomme N, Fillion G, Haour F. Receptors for interleukin-1 (alpha and beta) in mouse brain: mapping and neuronal localization in hippocampus. *Neuroscience* 1991; 43: 21-30.

Baram TZ, Hirsch E, Snead OC, Schultz L. Corticotropin-releasing hormone-induced seizures in infant rats originate in the amygdala. *Ann Neurol* 1992; 31: 488-94.

Baram TZ, Gerth A, Schultz L. Febrile seizures: an appropriate-aged model suitable for long-term studies. *Dev Brain Res* 1997; 98: 265-70.

Baram TZ, Eghbal-Ahmadi M, Bender RA. Is neuronal death required for seizure-induced epileptogenesis in the immature brain? *Prog Brain Res* 2002; 135: 365-75.

Bender RA, Dubé C, Gonzalez-Vega R, Mina EW, Baram TZ. Mossy fiber plasticity and enhanced hippocampal excitability, without hippocampal cell loss or altered neurogenesis, in an animal model of prolonged febrile seizures. *Hippocampus* 2003; 13: 399-412.

Bender RA, Soleymani SV, Brewster AL, Nguyen ST, Beck H, Mathern GW, Baram TZ. Enhanced expression of a specific hyperpolarization-activated cyclic nucleotide-gated cation channel (HCN) in surviving dentate gyrus granule cells of human and experimental epileptic hippocampus. *J Neurosci* 2003; 23: 6826-36.

Bender RA, Dubé C, Baram TZ. Febrile seizures and mechanisms of epileptogenesis: insights from an animal model. *Adv Exp Med Biol* 2004; 548: 213-25.

Berg AT, Shinnar S. Unprovoked seizures in children with febrile seizures: short-term outcome. *Neurology* 1996; 47: 562-8.

Berg AT, Shinnar S. Complex febrile seizures. *Epilepsia* 1996; 37: 126-33.

Berg AT, Shinnar S, Darefsky AS, Holford TR, Shapiro ED, Salomon ME et al. Predictors of recurrent febrile seizures. A prospective cohort study. *Arch Pediatr Adolesc Med* 1997; 151: 371-8.

Blake D, Bessey P, Karl I, Nunnally I, Hotchkiss R. Hyperthermia induces IL-1 alpha but does not decrease release of IL-1 alpha or TNF-alpha after endotoxin. *Lymphokine Cytokine Res* 1994; 13: 271-5.

Brewster A, Bender RA, Chen Y, Dubé C, Eghbal-Ahmadi M, Baram TZ. Developmental febrile seizures modulate hippocampal gene expression of hyperpolarization-activated channels in an isoform- and cell-specific manner. *J Neurosci* 2002; 22: 4591-9.

Brewster AL, Bernard JA, Gall CM, Baram TZ. Formation of heteromeric hyperpolarization-activated cyclic nucleotide-gated (HCN) channels in the hippocampus is regulated by developmental seizures. *Neurobiol Dis* 2005; 19: 200-7.

Cartmell T, Southgate T, Rees GS, Castro MG, Loweinstein PR, Luheshi GN. Interleukin-1 mediates a rapid inflammatory response after injection of adenoviral vectors into the brain. *J Neurosci* 1999; 19: 1517-23.

Cendes F, Andermann F, Dubeau F, Gloor P, Evans A, Jones-Gotman M et al. . Early childhood prolonged febrile convulsions, atrophy and sclerosis of mesial structures, and temporal lobe epilepsy: an MRI volumetric study. *Neurology* 1993; 43: 1083-7.

Chang YC, Huang AM, Kuo YM, Wang ST, Chang YY, Huang CC. Febrile seizures impair memory and cAMP response-element binding protein activation. *Ann Neurol* 2003; 54: 706-18.

Chen K, Baram TZ, Soltesz I. Febrile seizures in the developing brain result in persistent modification of neuronal excitability in limbic circuits. *Nat Med* 1999; 5: 888-94.

Chen K, Aradi I, Thon N, Eghbal-Ahmadi M, Baram TZ, Soltesz I. Persistently modified h-channels after complex febrile seizures convert the seizure-induced enhancement of inhibition to hyperexcitability. *Nat Med* 2001; 7: 331-7.

Chen K, Ratzliff A, Hilgenberg L, Gulyas A, Freund TF, Smith M, Dinh TP, Piomelli D, Mackie K, Soltesz I. Long-term plasticity of endocannabinoid signaling induced by developmental febrile seizures. *Neuron* 2003; 9: 599-611.

Dubé C, Chen K, Eghbal-Ahmadi M, Brunson KL, Soltesz I, Baram TZ. Prolonged febrile seizures in immature rat model enhance hippocampal excitability long-term. *Ann Neurol* 2000; 47: 336-44.

Dubé C, Vezzani A, Behrens M, Bartfai T, Baram TZ. Interleukin-1beta contributes to the generation of experimental febrile seizures. *Ann Neurol* 2005; 57: 152-5.

Dubé C, Richichi C, Bender RA, Chung G, Litt B, Baram TZ Temporal lobe epilepsy after experimental prolonged febrile seizures: prospective analysis. *Brain* 2206; 129: 911-22.

French JA, Williamson PD, Thadani VM, Darcey TM, Mattson RH, Spencer SS, Spencer DD Characteristics of medial temporal lobe epilepsy: I. Results of history and physical examination. *Ann Neurol* 1993; 34: 774-80.

Gatti S, Vezzani A, Bartfai T. Mechanisms of fever and febrile seizures: putative role of interleukin-1 system. In *Febrile Seizures*, TZ Baram, S Shinnar, ed. Academic Press, San Diego, 2002: 169-88.

Hamati-Haddad A, Abou-Khalil B. Epilepsy diagnosis and localization in patients with antecedent childhood febrile convulsions. *Neurology* 1998; 50: 917-22.

Haveman J, Geerdink AG, Rodermond HM. Cytokine production after whole body and localized hyperthermia. *Int J Hyperthermia* 2006; 12: 791-800.

Heida JG, Teskey GC, Pittman QJ. Experimental febrile convulsions in the rat and their effects on the development of kindling induced epilepsy in adulthood. *Soc Neurosci Abstr* 2003: 303-12.

Heida JG, Teskey GC, Pittman QJ. Febrile convulsions induced by the combination of lipopolysaccharide and low-dose kainic acid enhance seizure susceptibility, not epileptogenesis, in rats. *Epilepsia* 2005; 46: 1898-905.

Kamal A, Notenboom RG, de Graan PN, Ramakers GM. Persistent changes in action potential broadening and the slow afterhyperpolarization in rat CA1 pyramidal cells after febrile seizures. *Eur J Neurosci* 2006; 23: 2230-4.

Lemmens EM, Lubbers T, Schijns OE, Beuls EA, Hoogland G. Gender differences in febrile seizure-induced proliferation and survival in the rat dentate gyrus. *Epilepsia* 2005; 46: 1603-12.

Morimoto T, Nagao H, Sano N, Takahashi M, Matsuda H. Electroencephalographic study of rat hyperthermic seizures. *Epilepsia* 1991; 32: 289-93.

Nelson KB, Ellenberg JH. Prognosis in children with febrile seizures. *Pediatrics* 1978; 61: 720-7.

Pellegrini-Giampietro DE, Gorter JA, Bennett MV, Zukin RS. The GluR2 (GluR-B) hypothesis: Ca(2+)-permeable AMPA receptors in neurological disorders. *Trends Neurosci* 1997; 20: 464-70.

Racine RJ. Modification of seizure activity by electrical stimulation. II. Motor seizure. *Electroencephalogr Clin Neurophysiol* 1972; 32: 281-94.

Richichi C, Patel NA, Brewster AL, Bender RA, Baram TZ. (Long-lasting, activity-dependent plasticity of hcn channel isoform expression involves Ca^{2+}/calmodulin-dependent protein kinase (CaM kinase) II and, potentially, rest (nrsf)-mediated mechanisms. *Soc Neurosci Abstr* 2006: 334-7.

Santoro B, Baram TZ The multiple personalities of h-channels. *Trends Neurosci* 2003; 26: 550-4.

Scantlebury MH, Ouellet PL, Psarropoulou C, Carmant L. Freeze lesion-induced focal cortical dysplasia predisposes to atypical hyperthermic seizures in the immature rat. *Epilepsia* 2004; 45: 592-600.

Shinnar S. Do Febrile Seizures Lead to Temporal Lobe Epilepsy? Prospective and Epidemiological Studies. *In Febrile Seizures*, TZ Baram, S Shinnar, ed., Academic Press, San Diego, 2002: 87-102.

Stafstrom CE. The incidence and prevalence of febrile seizures. *In Febrile Seizures*, TZ Baram, S Shinnar, ed, Academic Press, San Diego, 2002: 1-25.

Takao T, Tracey DE, Mitchell WM, De Souza EB. Interleukin-1 receptors in mouse brain: Characterization and neuronal localization. *Endocrinology* 1990; 127: 3070-8.

Theodore WH, Bhatia S, Hatta J, Fazilat S, DeCarli C, Bookheimer SY, Gaillard WD. Hippocampal atrophy, epilepsy duration, and febrile seizures in patients with partial seizures. *Neurology* 1999; 52: 132-6.

Toth Z Yan XX, Haftoglou S, Ribak CE, Baram TZ. Seizure-induced neuronal injury: vulnerability to febrile seizures in an immature rat model. *J Neurosci* 18: 4285-94.

Verity CM, Butler NR, Golding J. Febrile convulsions in a national cohort followed up from birth. II – Medical history and intellectual ability at 5 years of age. *Br Med J* 1985; 290: 1311-5.

Verity CM, Greenwood R, Golding J Long-term intellectual and behavioral outcomes of children with febrile convulsions. *N Engl J Med* 1998; 338: 1723-8.

Febrile seizures as a risk factor for the development of epilepsy: human data

Peter Camfield, Carol Camfield

Department of Pediatrics, Dalhousie University and the IWK Health Centre, Halifax, Nova Scotia, Canada

About 4% of all people will have at least one febrile seizure during their lifetime (Stafstrom, 2002). It has been estimated that everyone faces an 8% risk during their lifetime of having a seizure of some kind, so febrile seizures make up half of the seizures that are experienced by humans (Hauser, 1975).

Febrile seizures have been variously defined but common to all definitions is that they occur at a young age, usually less than 5 years with an elevated body temperature but without evidence of direct brain infection. The National Institutes of Health Consensus Conference in 1981 defined a febrile seizure as "an event in infancy or childhood, usually occurring between 3 months and 5 years of age, associated with fever but without evidence of intracranial or defined cause. Seizures with fever in children who have suffered a previous non-febrile seizure are excluded." The ILAE Commission on Epidemiology and Prognosis came to a similar definition except that the lower age was pegged at 1 month and the child was not to have previous neonatal seizures. In all studies of first febrile seizures the peak incidence lies between 1 and 2 years of age and very few children have a febrile seizure before 6 months – so the lower age limit is not very important. Occasional children older than 5 years of age may have what seems clearly to be a febrile seizure, again not many (Webb, 1999). It is not clear how many children have an afebrile seizure and then seizures with fever. Presumably this exclusion tries to distinguish epilepsy unmasked by fever but systematic studies of this group of children do not exist and it may be that their seizures with fever should be considered to be febrile seizures.

To have a febrile seizure, a fever is required although the definition of fever has not been very consistent. Some authors have accepted any temperature $> 38°$ C and others $> 38.4°$ C but the method of measuring the temperature has not been spelled out.

There may be major discrepancies between various types of thermometers, especially digital thermometers and major differences between rectal, oral, tympanic and axillary temperatures. Typically the fever is high, often above 39 C.

The term "seizure" is not well-defined. Stephenson has argued strenuously that children with "atonic" febrile seizures have fever induced syncope – so a simple limp collapsing event during fever should be viewed as unlikely to be a seizure (Stephenson, 1990). Because of this observation, we have argued that unless there are tonic-clonic movements, the event should not be called a febrile seizure, recognizing of course that some febrile syncope can also be associated with clonic jerks. The entity of febrile myoclonus has not been clearly delineated in any of the basic epidemiological studies of febrile seizures (Rajakumar, 1996) and its relationship with epilepsy is unknown. Febrile myoclonus consists of repeated symmetrical myoclonic jerks during fever. The children are in the febrile seizure age range and the outcome seems to be completely benign.

Recently the issue of febrile seizure has been further complicated by the recognition of illness related seizures (Lee, 2004). A group of children, again in the febrile seizure age range, have been documented to have seizures in association with an infectious illness (often diarrhea) but without fever. Their subsequent clinical course and family histories are very similar to children with febrile seizures, although their rate of subsequent afebrile seizures is about double those with febrile seizures (~ 5% vs 2%). By comparison the rate of recurrence after an unprovoked, afebrile seizure is about 40-50%.

So as the relationship between febrile seizures and epilepsy is considered it is worthwhile to keep in mind that there are a number of children who have been diagnosed by physicians as having febrile seizures who have some other disorder. How many probably varies by the sophistication of the history taker.

It remains uncertain why one child has a febrile seizure while another does not. The strongest risk factor for a first febrile seizure is a close family relative with a febrile seizure(s) indicating a major genetic component (see section below on genetics) (Camfield, 2002). If there are first and second degree relatives with febrile seizures, the risk of febrile seizures is further increased. The pattern of inheritance may appear to be autosomal dominant or multifactorial. The accuracy of family histories for febrile seizures is likely not very good because the events may have occurred 20-40 years before the febrile seizure in the proband. Febrile seizure susceptibility genes have been mapped to at least 6 different chromosomal loci (Nakayama, 2006). The "syndrome" of GEFS+ (generalized epilepsy with febrile seizures plus) includes febrile seizures in most affected individuals and has been associated with more than 100 different mutations that affect at least 5 different ion channels and neurotransmitters (Audenaert, 2006).

The next strongest risk factor is any suggestion of other brain abnormalities as manifested by mental retardation, cerebral palsy or other disorders of cortical function. A third risk factor is not consistently reported. Some authors have noted that more frequent exposure to fever increases the risk, such as attendance at daycare. A high fever is, not surprisingly also a very frequent association.

In the Nova Scotia study about 3% of children in a regional population had two or more major risk factors for incidence febrile seizures (close family history of febrile seizures, slowed development, attendance at day care and delayed discharge from the neonatal unit) (Bethune, 1993). Thirty percent of this group developed febrile seizures. When there were no risk factors the risk of febrile seizures was only about 2.2%.

As noted above, febrile seizures are rare before 6 months of age. This may be due to either the degree of brain maturation needed to allow expression of the genetic febrile seizure tendency or to the rarity of high temperatures in children under 6 months of age. Obviously, there are many changes in brain maturation between ages 6 months and 5 years so there are many possible neural processes that may change to decrease the effect of fever. It also follows that there are children with febrile seizure susceptibility genes who do not acquire an illness with a sufficiently high fever during the age of susceptibility to provoke a febrile seizure.

There are two different ways of reviewing the relationship between febrile seizures and epilepsy. One is to start with children who have a febrile seizure and see who develops epilepsy. The other is to start with children or adults with epilepsy and look back to see who had febrile seizures. The two approaches give very different results although in both cases there is an association. When the first approach (looking forward) is used, very few turn out to have epilepsy but certain factors will at least point to those at highest risk. The second approach (looking back) finds that many people with epilepsy have had previous febrile seizures but the type of epilepsy or seizures is not closely related to the febrile seizures. For this paper epilepsy is defined as recurrent, unprovoked seizures – people with a single unprovoked seizure are not considered to have epilepsy.

■ Children with a febrile seizure who go on to develop epilepsy

If a child has a febrile seizure there is strong evidence of an increased risk of developing epilepsy compared with children without febrile seizures; however, the degree of increased risk is more meaningful in statistical terms than in clinical terms (Nelson, 1976; Annegers, 1987; Verity, 1991). Overall the risk of epilepsy developing by 7-10 years of age after a febrile seizure is about 2-4% compared with about a 1% chance in the population without febrile seizures. Given this low level of absolute risk, it is not surprising that all of the prospective cohort studies of febrile seizures have ended up with very few children with epilepsy. The NCPP study identified about 55,000 children before birth and followed them to 7 years of age (Nelson, 1976). Of 1706 children with at least one febrile seizure, only 34 (2%) developed epilepsy (2 or more unprovoked seizures with at least one seizure after 48 months of age). The Rochester study identified 709 children with at least one febrile seizure between 1935 and 1979 and subsequently 44 developed unprovoked seizures (Annegers, 1987). It is unclear how many in the Rochester study had just had a single unprovoked seizure and how many had epilepsy. The Rochester study noted a major distinction between those who were neurologically normal at the time of their first febrile seizure (7% risk of at least one unprovoked seizure by age 25 years) compared with those who were neurologically abnormal (mental retardation or cerebral palsy) prior to the febrile seizure (55% risk of epilepsy by 25 years). In the neurologically normal (n = 687), the risk of epilepsy seemed to increase with the length of follow up although the number of patients is small. By age 5 years 2% (9 patients) had developed unprovoked seizures, by age 10 years 4.5% (13 more patients), by age 15 years 5.5% (5 more patients) and by age 25 years 7% (5 more patients). This elegant study is still based on very few patients and may suffer methodologically from case ascertainment from medical records, some dating from a time when febrile seizures were not clearly recognized as a separate entity. Nonetheless, there is a strong suggestion that the febrile seizure susceptibility genes remain important over many years to determine epilepsy susceptibility.

For children with febrile seizures it is possible to define further risk factors for subsequent epilepsy. Risk factors that appear fairly consistent across studies are complex febrile seizures, neurological abnormalities and a family history of epilepsy (Hesdorffer, 2002). Sixty to seventy percent of febrile seizures are "simple" – the seizure is generalized, lasts < 15-30 minutes and occurs only once within a given illness. The lowest risk of epilepsy (about 2%) is for children with "simple" febrile seizures who are neurologically normal and have no family history of epilepsy. Thirty to forty percent of febrile seizures are "complicated" or "complex". The seizure is focal, prolonged (prolonged febrile seizures are often focal) or repeated with the illness. Each of these factors increases the risk of subsequent epilepsy by about 3-5%. Children with all 3 factors have about a 10-15% chance of subsequent epilepsy. While this is 10-15 times the risk in the general population it still means that nearly all children (85-90%) with a complex febrile seizure will not develop epilepsy.

The Rochester study addressed risk factors that predict the type of unprovoked seizures or epilepsy that follows febrile seizure, at least for those without neurological deficit (Annegers, 1987). Overall there were 32 patients who developed unprovoked seizures – 16 were judged to be partial and 16 to be generalized. Partial seizures were statistically associated with complex febrile seizures while generalized seizures were associated with ≥ 3 febrile seizures, positive family history and age of febrile seizures > 3 years of age. Other studies have not addressed these particularly provocative findings. In most cohort studies, it needs to be kept in mind that more than half of the children who develop epilepsy after a febrile seizure have had a simple febrile seizure!

Identifying a febrile seizure as complex is not necessarily easy. In a study of interobserver reliability three child neurologists judged 100 descriptions of febrile seizures to be focal or generalized (Berg, 1992). The Kappa statistic measures interobserver reliability and for focality was 0.58 which indicates moderate agreement. The child neurologists involved in this study all had a special interest in clinical research in epilepsy and presumably were quite expert. It is likely that all cohort studies of febrile seizures that have relied on less expert evidence have many errors of classification for the complex feature of generalized or focal.

The length of a febrile seizure is also not easy to judge. The information often comes from terrified parents who feared that their child was dying (Baumer, 1981). However, even in the emergency room it can be very difficult to decide if a febrile seizure has stopped. A group of Japanese investigators coined the term "epileptic twilight state"

(Yamamoto, 1996). They carried out EEG recordings in 14 children in an emergency room who had a febrile seizure but who had not recovered consciousness for 30 minutes. There was clinical uncertainty for these patients about whether the seizure had stopped because of ongoing features such as extensor posturing, increased limb tone, focal clonic movements or eye deviation. The EEG showed that the seizure had indeed stopped even though the clinical findings suggested that it was ongoing. Therefore defining the duration of a febrile seizure may be difficult. We suspect that the complex feature of repeated seizures within the same illness is the only complex feature that is fairly accurately reported.

The two other risk factors for the development of epilepsy are also not always easy to assess. Neurological deficits, especially mild mental retardation, are difficult to identify clinically in children less than 1-2 years of age. The accuracy of a family history of epilepsy or febrile seizures has not been critically assessed but is certainly not always accurate. The history of febrile seizures in relatives of an index case is usually based on family folklore or the incomplete information from a family guru. In Finland a prospective birth cohort (n = 1294) found that when the children were twelve years old, some parents had forgotten that their child had had a febrile seizure while other parents reported a previous febrile seizure when there apparently was not one (Sillanpaa, 2006, personal communication). These were parent reports for their own children, so it is likely that more errors are made for more extended family members.

We conclude that the assessment of risk factors for epilepsy after a first febrile seizure is an inexact science and great care should be taken with individual patients to avoid giving an inaccurate negative or positive prognosis.

■ Patients with epilepsy and preceding febrile seizures

Once a person has developed epilepsy it is interesting and instructive to examine the previous history of febrile seizures. Several population based studies have assessed this issue (Camfield, 1994; Berg, 1999).

In Nova Scotia we documented all incidence cases of childhood epilepsy (onset 1 month-16 years) with onset between 1977-1985. There were a total of 692 patients. We divided the patients into 3 broad categories – those with epilepsies characterized by partial or convulsive seizures (n = 511), those with secondary generalized epilepsies (n = 85) and those with epilepsies characterized by frequent absence seizures (n = 97). A history of febrile seizures prior to the onset of epilepsy was remarkably consistent across these three groups. In the partial and convulsive group 15% had preceding febrile seizures, in the SGE group 15% and in the absence group 17%. Our analysis of the partial and convulsive group has been the most comprehensive (Camfield, 1994). No epilepsy seizure type was particularly associated with a history of febrile seizures. Four broad categories of etiology were considered (cause unknown, idiopathic epilepsy syndrome, remote symptomatic and genetic, not otherwise specified). Febrile seizures were equally common across these four categories. Prolonged febrile seizures were not associated with specific seizure types but were strongly associated with eventual intractable epilepsy. The relationship between febrile status and mesial temporal lobe epilepsy is commented on further below. This study strongly suggested that from the perspective of children with established epilepsy, febrile seizure susceptibility genes are associated with most types of epilepsy and all kinds of causes for epilepsy – these genes appear to have a fundamental role in the seizure threshold of many patients with epilepsy.

Other studies have noted a very similar rate of preceding febrile seizures in children with epilepsy. In the NCPP study there were 386 children with at least one afebrile seizure – 13% had a preceding febrile seizure. In a regional epilepsy clinic in the former Yugoslavia, 20.3% of 846 children had preceding febrile seizures (Sofijanov, 1983). In the Connecticut community study 13.9% of 613 children with new onset epilepsy had a preceding febrile seizure (Berg, 1993). In this study there seemed to be fewer febrile seizures in children who later developed absence epilepsy, a difference from the Nova Scotia study that is not easily explained. The authors noted about an equal number of children with epilepsy had preceding simple febrile seizures and complex partial seizures. As in the Nova Scotia study the age of onset of epilepsy in children with febrile seizures was younger by 2-3 years on average than those without febrile seizures. This difference seemed to be related to complex febrile seizures.

In the Rochester study the relationship between epilepsy and previous febrile seizures was extended to consider people who developed epilepsy at any age (child or adult). Nineteen percent of those with generalized tonic-clonic seizures had preceding febrile seizures (Rocca, 1987a), 18% of those with partial complex seizures (Rocca, 1987b) and 21% of those with absence (Rocca, 1987c). Recently a study from Iran studied 92 adults (median age 18 years, range 14-43) with new onset epilepsy. In all cases the parents or siblings were interviewed in face to face interviews and overall 33.7% of the new onset epilepsy adults had a history of preceding febrile seizures with a stronger association with partial than generalized epilepsy syndromes (Mohebbi, 2004).

We conclude that at least 15% of all types of epilepsy that begin after the peak febrile seizure age are preceded by febrile seizures, at least up to age 25 years. Febrile seizures may precede epilepsy of many different causes.

■ Cause and effect

It would seem very unlikely that short febrile seizures cause damage to the brain that in turn causes epilepsy. There is little consistent relationship between the number of febrile seizures and subsequent epilepsy. There is no evidence of cognitive deficits after short (or long) febrile seizures (Ellenberg, 1978).

The relationship between prolonged febrile seizures, mesial temporal sclerosis and intractable temporal lobe epilepsy has been a source of endless controversy. Nonetheless there is a very consistent observation that adults with intractable temporal lobe epilepsy often have mesial temporal sclerosis linked with a history of a prolonged febrile seizure (Falconer, 1964). One might question the accuracy of recall for the length of a febrile seizure that occurred many years before. The importance of this relationship is that these patients seem to have a very good response to temporal lobectomy (Abou-Khalil, 1993).

The epidemiological and pathophysiological links are murky. From the Nova Scotia study we learned that the sequence of a prolonged febrile seizure followed by mesial temporal sclerosis and intractable temporal lobe epilepsy is rare – it occurs about once in 75,000 children (Camfield, 1994). From the Connecticut study it appears that nearly all children with mesial temporal sclerosis at the onset of their epilepsy do not have a history of febrile seizures of any kind, let alone prolonged febrile seizures (Berg, 1999). In Dravet syndrome there are frequent, very severe episodes of febrile status. In one longitudinal study of 14 children with Dravet syndrome 10 eventually developed MTS, although it was not present at the onset of the disorder (Siegler, 2005). On the other hand, there is abundant evidence from pathology studies that MTS is often associated with other developmental pathology – dual pathology (Ho 1998). There is also evidence that a very prolonged febrile seizure (more than 1.5 hours) may be associated with bilateral or unilateral hippocampal swelling (Scott, 2003, VanLandingham 1998). So the cause of this important relationship is not always clear. It is possible that some case of MTS are caused by only by febrile status and in others temporal lobe pathology creates a special vulnerability for prolonged febrile seizures.

The Special Issue of GEFS+ and Dravet Syndrome

GEFS+ (generalized epilepsy with febrile seizures plus) is an autosomal dominant disorder, most often the result of an inherited abnormality in the SCN1A gene; however a variety of other gene problems have been identified including defects in SCN1B and defects in GABA receptor genes (Scheffer 1997). The disorder has high penetrance and about 1/3 of affected patients only have febrile seizures, although the febrile seizures may persist beyond the usual age. One third has a generalized but relatively benign epilepsy that resolves in adolescence and one-third has other forms of epilepsy, particularly idiopathic epilepsies. Dravet Syndrome is caused most often by a mutation in the SCN1A gene but the mutations are more severe truncating or missense mutations than in GEFS+. To date more than 100 different mutations have been found in Dravet patients (Audenaert, 2006). Rarely a Dravet patient appears in a GEFS+ kindred. A search for SCN1A mutations in other patients without GEFS+ but just "ordinary" febrile seizures has not been fruitful but at least 6 other linkages have been noted with "ordinary" febrile seizures. We conclude that it is unlikely that SCN1A mutations cause many of the cases of "pure" febrile seizures.

Speculation

Some AEDs are effective at preventing febrile seizures and others are not, an observation that may give some insight into the mechanisms of febrile seizures (Camfield, 1995). The most effective drugs for prevention of febrile seizures are those that interact with or enhance GABA effects – phenobarbital, a variety of benzodiazepines and valproic acid. Ineffective drugs are those that interact with sodium channels, especially CBZ and PHT. The syndrome of GEFS+ has febrile seizures as its most important component with sodium channel disorders as the most frequent cause. We propose that the genetic propensity to febrile seizures is most often a relative lack of inhibition with diminished GABAergic effect in the brain although rarely excessive excitatory transmission may overwhelm a normal GABAergic reserve.

Some of the susceptibility to seizures outlasts the febrile seizure age and eventually some children with febrile seizures develop spontaneously occurring, unprovoked seizures or epilepsy. It is interesting that the type of epilepsy and the presumed cause of the epilepsy does not matter – febrile seizures are the harbinger of many epilepsy syndromes with many different causes.

It is presumed that everyone can have a seizure if the wrong thing happens. The drug methohexital will induce seizures in people with epilepsy although the dose varies greatly from one person to another. We all presumably have a seizure threshold. Not everyone with a given cerebral lesion will have a seizure – for example some people with a cerebral glioma will have seizures while others with the same tumor do not. Given the high prevalence of febrile seizures in people with epilepsy it appears that the febrile susceptibility genes are strong determinants of that seizure threshold.

References

Abou-Khalil B, Andermann E, Andermann F, Olivier A, Quesney LF. Temporal lobe epilepsy after prolonged febrile convulsion: excellent outcome after surgical treatment. *Epilepsia* 1993; 34: 878-83.

Audenaert D, Van Broeckhoven C, De Jonghe P. Genes and loci involved in febrile seizures and related epilepsy syndromes. *Human mutation* 2006; 27: 391-401.

Annegers JF, Hauser WA, Shirts SB, Kurland LT. Factors prognostic of unprovoked seizures after febrile convulsions. *N Engl J Med* 1987; 316: 494-8.

Baumer JH, David TJ, Valentine SJ, *et al.* Many parents think their child is dying when having a first febrile convulsion. *Dev Med Child Neurol* 1981; 23: 462-4.

Berg AT, Steinschneider M, Kang H, Shinnar S. Classification of complex features of febrile seizures: interrater agreement. *Epilepsia* 1992; 33: 661-6.

Berg AT, Shinnar S, Levy S, Testa FM. Childhood-onset epilepsy with and without preceding febrile seizures. *Neurology* 1999; 53: 1742-8.

Bethune P, Gordon KG, Dooley JM, Camfield CS, Camfield PR. Which child will have a febrile seizure? *Am J Dis Child* 1993; 147: 35-9.

Camfield PR, Camfield CS, Gordon K, Dooley JM. What types of epilepsy are preceded by febrile seizures? A population based study of children. *Dev Med Child Neurol* 1994; 36: 887-92.

Camfield PR, Camfield CS, Gordon K, Dooley JM. Prevention of recurrent febrile seizures. *J Pediatr* 1995; 126: 929-30.

Camfield PR, Camfield CS, Gordon K. *Antecedents and risk factors for febrile seizures in Febrile Seizures*, eds Baram TZ, Shinnar S. Academic Press, London 2002: 27-35.

Ellenberg JH, Nelson KB. Febrile seizures and later intellectual performance. *Arch Neurol* 1978; 35: 17-21.

Falconer MA, Serafetinides EA, Corsellis JA. Etiology and pathogenesis of temporal lobe epilepsy. *Arch Neurol* 1964; 10: 233-48.

Hauser WA, Kurland LT. The epidemiology of epilepsy in Rochester, Minnesota, 1935 through 1967. *Epilepsia* 1975; 16: 1-66.

Hesdorffer DC, Hauser WA. *Febrile seizures and the risk of epilepsy in Febrile Seizures*, eds Baram TZ, Shinnar S. Academic Press, London 2002: 63-74.

Ho SS, Kuzniecky RI, Gilliam F, Faught E, Morawetz R. Temporal lobe developmental malformations and epilepsy: Dual pathology and bilateral hippocampal abnormalities. *Neurology* 1998; 50: 748-54.

Lee W, Ong H. Afebrile seizures associated with minor infections: Comparison with febrile seizures and unprovoked seizures *Pediatr Neurol* 2004; 31: 157-64.

Mohebbi MR, Navipour R, Seyedkazemi M, Zamanian H, Khamseh P. Adult-onset epilepsy and history of childhood febrile seizures: a retrospective study. *Neurol India* 2004; 52: 463-5.

Nakayama J, Arinami T. Molecular genetics of febrile seizures. *Epi Res* 2006; 70, suppl 1: s190-8.

Nelson KB, Ellenberg JH. Predictors of epilepsy in children who have experienced febrile seizures. *N Engl J Med* 1976; 295: 1029-33.

Rajakumar K, Bodensteiner JB. Febrile myoclonus: A survey of pediatric neurologists. *Clinical Pediatrics* 1996; 22: 331-2.

Rocca WA, Sharbrough FW, Hauser WA, Annegers JF, Schoenberg BS (1987a) Risk factors for generalized tonic-clonic seizures: a population-based case control study in Rochester, Minnesota. *Neurology* 1987; 37: 1315-22.

Rocca WA, Sharbrough FW, Hauser WA, Annengers JF, Schoenberg BS (1987b). Risk factors for complex partial seizures: a population-based case-control study. *Ann Neurol* 1987; 21: 22-31.

Rocca WA, Sharbrough FW, Hauser WA, Annegers JF, Schoenberg BS (1987c). Risk factors for absence seizures: a population-based case-control study in Rochester, Minnesota. *Neurology* 37: 1309-14.

Scheffer IE, Berkovic SF. Generalized epilepsy with febrile seizures +: a genetic disorder with heterogeneous clinical phenotypes. *Brain* 1997; 120: 479-90.

Scott RC, King MD, Gadian DG, Neville BG, Connelly A. Hippocampal abnormalities after prolonged febrile convulsion: a longitudinal MRI study. *Brain* 2003; 126: 2551-7.

Siegler Z, Barsi P, Neuwirth M, Jerney J, Kassay M, Janszky J, Paraicz E, Hegyi M, Fogarasi. Hippocampal sclerosis in severe myoclonic epilepsy in infancy: a retrospective MRI study. *Epilepsia* 2005; 46: 704-8.

Sofijanov N, Sadikario A, Dukovski, Kuturec M. Febrile convulsions and later development of epilepsy. *Am J Dis Child* 1983; 137: 123-6.

Stafstrom CE. *The Incidence and Prevalence of Febrile Seizures in Febrile Seizures*, eds Baram TZ, Shinnar S. Academic Press, London, 2002: 1-25.

Stevenson JB. *Fits and faints*. Oxford: MacKeith Press, 1990.

VanLandingham KE, Heinz ER, Cavazos JE, Lewis DV (1998): Magnetic resonance imaging evidence of hippocampal injury after prolonged focal febrile convulsions. *Ann Neurol* 43: 413-26.

Verity CM, Golding J. Risk of epilepsy after febrile convulsions: a national cohort study. *BMJ* 1991; 303: 1373-6.

Webb DW, Jones RR, Manzur AY, Farrell K. Retrospective study of late febrile seizures. *Pediatr Neurol* 1999; 20: 270-3.

Yamamoto N. Prolonged non-epileptic twilight state with convulsive manifestations after febrile convulsions: a clinical and electrographic study. *Epilepsia* 1996; 37: 31-5.

Section IV:
Novel approaches of medical risk factors for unprovoked seizures and cryptogenic epilepsy

Comorbidity of epilepsy and neuropsychiatric disorders: epidemiological considerations

Dale C. Hesdorffer

Gertrude H. Sergievsky Center and the Department of Epidemiology, Columbia University, New York, USA

Comorbidity is defined as the co-occurrence of two supposedly separate conditions at above chance levels (Rutter, 1994). This chapter considers the comorbidity of epilepsy with major depression, bipolar disorder, suicidality, generalized anxiety disorder, and migraine. Several reasons that two conditions may occur together at levels exceeding chance (*Table I*) are described below and examples are given for clarification.

Comorbidity may occur because one condition causes another condition (*Table I*). For example, diabetes may cause retinopathy. One possible explanation of the comorbidity of epilepsy and depression observed in cross-sectional studies is that factors associated with having epilepsy (*e.g.*, stigma, stress) may lead to depression, either by themselves or as an environmental risk factor acting in the presence of a genetic susceptibility to depression (Caspi, 2003) as recently shown in post-stroke depression (Ramasubbu, 2006).

Comorbid conditions may be due to a common risk factor (*Table I*). An example described by Rutter (1994) is that lung cancer, coronary artery disease and emphysema all occur together more than would be expected by chance, but they are also all influenced by smoking. An intervention to reduce the occurrence of coronary artery disease will, therefore, have no effect on the occurrence of lung cancer, unless it involves smoking. Shared genetic factors offer a similar explanation for comorbidity as shared environmental risk factors. An example of this is the shared genetic susceptibility to Attention Deficit Hyperactivity Disorder (ADHD) and reading disability, which may explain at least part of the observed comorbidity of these conditions.

Two conditions may be comorbid if they share an underlying characteristic that is part of the diagnosis of both conditions (*Table I*). This is particularly common in studies of the comorbidity of different psychiatric conditions (Lilienfeld et al., 1994) where a shared underlying construct may be common to two concurrent conditions.

Table I. Possible explanations for the comorbidity of two conditions

Explanations	Examples
1. One condition causes the other	Diabetes → Retinopathy
2. A common risk factor	Smoking → Lung cancer and coronary artery disease and emphysema Shared genetic etiology → ADHD and Reading disability
3. Assessment of the same latent entity	Social anxiety → Avoidant personality disorder and social phobia
4. Covariation between error components in measuring two conditions	Raters (*e.g.*, parents vs teachers for ADHD) have biases or differ in their threshold for endorsing behaviors
5. Bias in hospital-based studies	Berkson's bias: A mathematical phenomenon based upon the increased probability of hospitalization for individuals with two conditions compared to the probability for individuals with either condition alone Clinical selection bias: Increases the probability of seeking treatment for one condition because another condition is also present

An example of this is the comorbidity of avoidant personality disorder and social phobia, which differ based upon the severity of underlying social anxiety, a trait common to both conditions.

Study methodology and bias may lead to the observation that two conditions are comorbid (*Table I*, explanations 3 and 4). For example, the covariation between error components may account for comorbidity, particularly in psychiatry. This may arise due to differences in the threshold for endorsing behaviors by parents compared to teachers in the case of ADHD rather than to common pathophysiology or shared risk factors. It is well-known that hospital-based studies of comorbidity can be biased. For example, Berkson's bias is a mathematical phenomenon that stipulates that the likelihood of hospitalization for one condition is greater when a second condition is also present than for either condition alone. Clinical selection bias can also account for comorbidity and is the ascertainment of cases with the comorbid condition under study to an extent greater than present in the community, because there is an increased probability of seeking care for one condition when another condition is also present. These biases may affect cross-sectional studies of comorbidity in epilepsy in particular.

Thus, observing the presence of comorbidity does not itself implicate any one specific mechanism but rather suggests that different explanations for the observation should be explored and perhaps new studies undertaken to understand the reason for the observed co-occurrence of two or more disorders.

Study design considerations: incident *versus* prevalent cohorts

We would like to be able to observe the natural history of epilepsy, but in reality, we are able to observe only the medical history. Once the patient enters clinical phase of epilepsy with signs and symptoms, medical attention is sought and the diagnosis is made. The moment of diagnosis is equivalent to the inception of incident (new) epilepsy. The cases that are identified after the diagnosis is made are prevalent case or survivors with epilepsy (*i.e.*, new and old cases).

A cohort of incident cases of epilepsy is different from a cohort of prevalent cases of epilepsy. In a comparison of an incident and a prevalent cohort of epilepsy assembled from the same source population in Rochester, Minnesota, during the same time period, there were many differences between the incident cohort and the prevalent cohort. There were: more incident than prevalent cases among the children and the elderly; more males than females in the incident than in the prevalent cohort; more cases with remote symptomatic seizures, especially cases with cerebrovascular disease, among incident than prevalent cases; and more generalized-onset than partial-onset among incident cases compared with prevalent cases. Each of these variables has a prognostic value that may be associated with comorbidities in epilepsy. One additional point concerning the case mix in an incident cohort with epilepsy deserves discussion. A diagnosis of epilepsy is made after the patient sees a physician due to at least two unprovoked seizures. It is much easier to recognize two generalized tonic-clonic seizures than two absence or two complex partial seizures, and patients with these latter seizure types tend to be diagnosed later in the course of their epilepsy. Thus, the inception of incident cases of epilepsy is probably not homogeneous, but depends upon characteristics of the seizures. Incident cohorts are, therefore, heterogeneous for the number of seizures preceding diagnosis and the duration of epilepsy prior to diagnosis.

Different types of cohorts can be assembled for studies of comorbidity, depending on the source of cases. Most published studies are based upon clinical series collected in a neurology department or in tertiary centers that specialize in the diagnosis and treatment of epilepsy. There are also some reports from cohorts of institutionalized patients in studies of comorbidity of depression and epilepsy. These types of settings are more likely to include severe cases with respect to seizure frequency, duration of epilepsy, and resistance to antiepileptic drug therapy. Thus, it can be seen that the selection of cases based on a characteristic of the epilepsy (*e.g.*, severity), which may lead people to seek care at a specialty clinic, might affect the results of the study if the characteristic is related to the comorbid condition under study. This problem was minimized in a study of the comorbidity of prevalent epilepsy and depression (Behgi, 2002) by studying a cohort with prevalent idiopathic/cryptogenic epilepsy that had been diagnosed at the tertiary care center. However, population-based studies remain the cleanest way to avoid any selection bias that could be present in the other series.

From an epidemiologic standpoint, the frequency of epilepsy and comorbid conditions of interest must be considered when designing studies to examine their co-occurrence. While incidence provides the most useful information in evaluating the joint occurrence of disease, there are few incidence studies of epilepsy and psychiatric disorders or epilepsy and migraine. Additionally, studies that allow evaluation of the joint probabilities of epilepsy and other conditions and also allow one to distinguish time order are rare in comparison to cross-sectional studies of these associations. Below is a discussion of the prevalence and the incidence of epilepsy. The frequency of each comorbid condition considered in this chapter is discussed in sections relating to the association of that condition with epilepsy. Except for bipolar disorder, epilepsy is considerably rarer than the other condition discussed. Thus, to maximize statistical power, incident studies must begin with epilepsy and then look for the more common condition.

Prevalence is a measure of the number of cases of a disease existent in the population at a particular point in time. The prevalence of *epilepsy (defined as (recurrent unprovoked seizures)* shows wide variation across studies, but generally ranges from 4 to 10 per 1,000 population (Hauser, 1991; Cowan, 1989; Placencia, 1994). This two- to three-fold variation is related in part to varying definitions, but it also is related to true differences in frequency across populations. The prevalence of epilepsy generally is higher in developing countries than in industrialized nations. In industrialized countries, prevalence tends to increase with advancing age, reaching a peak in the oldest age groups. In contrast, prevalence in developing countries is highest in young adults. prevalence cases are characterized by chronicity and by survival from diagnosis; thus, they are highly selected. Population-based prevalence cases are akin to cases seen in general medical or neurological clinics. They generally have much less severe disease than cases seen at tertiary referral centers. This difference in severity must be taken into account when considering reports of comorbidity of various conditions with epilepsy, because most reports are generated from tertiary referral centers.

There are only a few total population incidence studies of epilepsy. The incidence of epilepsy in industrialized countries is about 50 per 100,000 population per year (Olafsson, 2005; Hauser 1993). The incidence in developing countries probably is double this rate (Placencia, 1994; Lavados, 1992). Regardless of geographic area, there is an excess incidence in males, and only about 35% of cases have a clearly identified antecedent. In industrialized countries, incidence is high in children up to 1 year and in the elderly. This contrasts with developing countries, where incidence generally peaks in childhood and few new-onset cases are identified in adults after the age of 50 years.

■ Associations between epilepsy and psychiatric disorders

In industrialized countries, diagnosis of a major psychiatric illness of some type can be expected in at least 50% to 60% of the population during their lifetime (lifetime prevalence) (Anthony, 1995). Substance abuse or dependence (alcohol in 15% to 25% of the population or tobacco in about 30% of the population) accounts for a large proportion of cases, but a substantial proportion of the population at some time can be expected to be diagnosed with other major disorders, including psychosis (Anthony, 1994).

A number of studies have evaluated the frequency of psychiatric disorders in people with prevalent epilepsy. These reports are generally cross-sectional, from referral centers, fail to take into account the time order of the two conditions, and do not have

Attention deficit hyperactivity disorder (ADHD)

ADHD occurs in 3-5% of children (Kaplan 1991) and is characterized by inattention and/or hyperactivity-impulsivity occurring with greater frequency or severity than is usual for the person's development (Diagnostic and statistical manual fourth edition (DSM-IV) 1997). Symptoms begin before 7 years of age, occur at home *and* at school or work, cause impairment of developmentally appropriate functioning, and are not due to another mental disorder (DSM-IV 1997). ADHD also occurs in adults with onset of symptoms in childhood. A population-based study in the Netherlands of 1,813 adults, age 18-75 years, reported an ADHD prevalence of 1.0% (95% CI = 0.6-1.6%) (Kooij, 2005). This study and another (Biederman, 2004) have supported the validity of the adult ADHD diagnosis. Family studies of ADHD consistently support a strong familial component. In the majority of family studies, there is a 2- to 8-fold increased risk of ADHD in parents and siblings of children with ADHD (Biederman, 1990; Faraohne, 1992; Pauls, 1983). Similarly, among families of adults with ADHD, the risk of ADHD is high in children (Biederman, 1995).

Clinically, there is a perception that ADHD is more common among children with epilepsy, due to the seizure disorder or its treatment (Lindsay, 1984; Hempel, 1995). In studies of children with prevalent epilepsy, 28.1% to 39% had "hyperactivity-impulsivity" (Carlton-Ford, 1995; McDermott, 1995), 42.4% had problems with attention (Holdsworth, 1991), and 13.9% had ADHD (Williams, 1998). This is in excess of the 5% prevalence of ADHD in the general population (Kaplan, 1991). Large surveys of the general population (Carlton-Ford, 1995; McDermott, 1995) confirm associations seen in smaller studies of prevalent epilepsy. In the 1988 National Health Interview study (Carlton-Ford, 1995; McDermott, 1995), hyperactivity assessed by the Behavior Problem Index was 5.7-fold more prevalent among 121 children with epilepsy (28.1%), aged 5 to 17 years, compared to 3,950 controls (4.9%) (McDermott, 1995). "Highly impulsive behavior" assessed by four questions occurred among 39% of 118 children with a history of epilepsy, aged 6 to 17 years, compared to 11% of 11,042 children without a history of epilepsy (Carlton-Ford, 1995). These population-based cross-sectional studies confirm the association between ADHD and prevalent epilepsy, but they are unable to address potential causes of the comorbidity.

When time order is examined as one method of understanding more about the comorbidity of ADHD and epilepsy, studies show that ADHD is associated with increased risk for *developing* epilepsy. This has been revealed in case-control studies of children with epilepsy (Austin, 2001; Dunn, 1997; Hesdorffer, 2004) and in cohort studies of select populations of children with ADHD (Hughes, 2000; Williams, 2001; Hemmer, 2001; Holtman, 2003). In two case-control studies of children with incident unprovoked seizure (Austin, 2001; Dunn, 1997), behavioral disturbances *before* the onset of first seizure were more frequent than among controls. In the later study of 148 children with first unprovoked seizure and 89 seizure-free sibling controls, attention problems as assessed by the Child Behavior Checklist were 2.4-fold more common prior to identification of the first seizure (8.1%) than in controls (3.4%) (Austin, 2001). This has been replicated in a population-based case-control study conducted among Icelandic children (Hesdorffer, 2004), in which children with incident unprovoked seizure were 2.5-fold more likely than age- and gender-matched controls to have a history of ADHD (95% CI = 1.1-5.5), meeting DSM-IV cri teri a *prior* to seizure onset. Interestingly, the association was restricted to ADHD-predominantly inattentive type (OR = 3.7; 95% CI = 1.1-13).

One possible explanation for this finding is that some symptoms of ADHD- predominantly inattentive type overlap with symptoms that might be observed in absence and complex partial seizures. In the Icelandic study (Hesdorffer 2004), there were 8 children with absence seizures: none met criteria for ADHD- predominantly inattentive type. Of the 37 children with complex partial seizures, 3 met criteria for ADHD- predominantly inattentive type. Excluding these cases and their controls did not change the results, suggesting that overlapping symptoms does not explain the comorbidity.

When the occurrence of new onset seizures is examined in selected samples with ADHD (Hughes, 2000; Williams, 2001; Holtman, 2003), the percentage of children who develop unprovoked seizures (0.2% to 2%) is greater than the expected rate in the general population, because the average annual incidence of seizures is approximately 0.0470 per year in children aged 5 to 16 years (Hauser, 1993). Thus, there is an increased risk for *developing* unprovoked seizures in children with ADHD, and the reported increased risk is smaller in case-control studies than in cohort studies. However the cohort studies were limited by small numbers of ensuing unprovoked seizures during short follow-up periods in selected clinical populations of children with ADHD.

A recent study of 51 children age 8-18 with epilepsy of idiopathic etiology diagnosed within the past 12 months examined the association between ADHD and a previous history of academic problems (Jones, 2006); a control group was also included. Academic problems were defined as either special education, special assistance in reading and math, mandatory summer school, tutors, or grade retention. ADHD was diagnosed in 31% of children with new onset epilepsy compared to about 6% of control children. ADHD- predominantly inattentive type accounted for more than 50% of ADHD in children with epilepsy. Compared to children without prior academic problems, children with academic problems had higher rates of externalizing disorders (62.5% vs 11.4%, p < .001), including ADHD (26.4% vs 10%) and conduct disorders (12.5% vs 0.0%, p < .05). A majority of the children with academic problems (62.5%) exhibited psychiatric comorbidity prior to the first recognized seizure. Additionally, children with epilepsy and ADHD had a larger frontal lobe volume (475 cm^3) on MRI compared to children with epilepsy and no ADHD (456 cm^3) and to control children (463 cm^3).

Collectively, these studies show that epilepsy and unprovoked seizures are comorbid and that ADHD, particularly the inattentive type, is associated with an increased risk for new onset epilepsy in children. The association does not appear to be explained by misclassification of ADHD in children with epilepsy due to seizure types that have similar symptoms to ADHD- predominantly inattentive type (Hesdorffer, 2004).

Nor does the comorbidity appear to be explained by parental over-reporting of ADHD symptoms in children diagnosed with epilepsy, because the association appears to be limited to a subtype of ADHD. There is some suggestion that epilepsy and ADHD share underlying brain pathology (Jones, 2006), which may account for the earlier reported onset of ADHD in cases than in controls in the Iceland study (Hesdorffer, 2004). Because the association between ADHD and epilepsy has been found in population-based studies as well as in studies conducted in more selected populations, biases inherent in hospital-based studies are an unlikely explanation for the comorbidity. Neither does it appear that ADHD causes seizures directly or vise versa. Further studies are needed to elucidate whether common underlying risk factors or shared genetic etiology contribute to the comorbidity of epilepsy and ADHD.

Major depression

Major depression is a common psychiatric disorder associated with marked disability and excess mortality. It is defined as a period of at least 2 weeks with depressed mood or loss of interest or pleasure in almost all activities, associated with other symptoms (*e.g.*, psychomotor agitation or retardation), and with functional impairment. Community-based studies suggest a point prevalence of depression of 2% to 4%, although estimates are higher in studies of selected populations (Anthony, 1995; Murphy, 2000a; Ohavon, 1999; Blazer, 1994). Prevalence is higher in females, and point prevalence is highest in the adult population. Prevalence increases as one goes from community to primary care settings to inpatients, a phenomenon of potential importance in studies of major depression and epilepsy. The lifetime prevalence of major depression approaches 20% in some studies and is higher in females (Wittchen, 1994; Kessler, 2005a).

Incidence based on first episode or first treatment for major depression varies markedly among studies, but is consistently higher in females (Newman, 1998; Murphy, 2000b; Rorsman, 1990). Incidence has been reported to be 1 to 2 per 1,000 per year in males and 3 to 5 per 1,000 in females. In the epidemiologic catchment area study, an incidence of 2% per year was reported. This is similar to that recently reported in Finland (Lehtinen, 2005). In Sweden (Rorsman, 1990), cumulative incidence of major depresssion to age 70 years was 27% in males and 46% in females. In studies from the United States, cumulative incidence was reported to be about 17% (Kessler, 2005a).

A number of studies indicate that major depression is co-morbid with epilepsy, but many of these studies have methodological problems. Most are cross-sectional (see for example, Cramer, 2004; O'Donoghue, 1999; Boylan, 2004; Jacoby, 1996; Dominian, 1963; Beghi, 2002) and find that depression occurs more often than expected among people with epilepsy. Some are conducted in select populations from epilepsy centers with resulting over-representation of complex partial seizures refractory to medication and none use instruments from which DSM diagnoses of depression can be made. In these studies, about 20% of people with prevalent epilepsy are classified as having a moderate to severe number of depressive symptoms. Slightly smaller percentages (10%-24%) have a moderate or severe number of depressive symptoms in community surveys (Cramer, 2004; O'Donoghue, 1999) than in an epilepsy monitoring unit (29.7%) (Boylan, 2004), reflecting either selection factors or real differences by seizure severity. Real differences by seizure severity is the more likely explanation as two community surveys of patients with prevalent epilepsy from the British general practice system showed a positive correlation between seizure frequency and prevalence of depressive symptoms (Jacoby, 1996; O'Donoghue, 1999). In these studies, a moderate to severe number of depressive symptoms occurred in 4%-20% of cases in remission, 10%-39% in those with less than one seizure per month, and 21%-55% of those with one or more seizures per month. Two explanations for this finding seem plausible: 1. depression is a reaction to having seizures due to the uncertain timing of seizures and associated stigma; or 2. the pathology that leads to frequent seizures in epilepsy is also associated with depression.

Based upon these and other cross-sectional studies, many clinical epileptologists believe that the co-occurrence of depression and epilepsy is limited to individuals with epilepsy involving the limbic system. This impression may have originated with biased samples from studies restricted to patients at specialized epilepsy centers, which contain an excess of patients with complex partial seizures, because they are more likely to be intractable than other types of epilepsy. However, one cross-sectional study (Beghi, 2002) based at a tertiary referral center, minimized selection bias associated with referral of the most severe epilepsy case to tertiary centers, by restricting the analysis to patients with prevalent idiopathic/cryptogenic epilepsy who were initially diagnosed at that center. In that study, 60% of patients had generalized seizures and 63% were without seizures for 12 months or more, suggesting that this is a less severe population with epilepsy than the total population seen at tertiary referral centers. Compared with blood donors, people with epilepsy were 11.3-fold (95% CI = 1.4-247.8) more likely to have moderate to severe depression with no difference by seizure type. Thus, associations between prevalent epilepsy and depression are not confined to prevalent complex partial seizures or to individuals with the most frequent seizures. This study cannot address whether factors like stigma lead to the development of depression in people with epilepsy.

Studies suggest that a history of major depression is associated with an increased risk for *developing* unprovoked seizures, suggesting a common underlying susceptibility. The possibility that depression might precede epilepsy was originally suggested by Dominian (1963) who observed that 16% of 51 patients with late-onset prevalent epilepsy had a history of depression before the initial seizure.

In a hospital-based retrospective cohort study, Nilsson et al. (2003) found an increased risk for developing epilepsy over a 10-year period in 13,748 patients hospitalized for major depression or bipolar disorder compared to 81,380 controls hospitalized for osteoarthritis and 69,149 controls hospitalized for diabetes. These authors found that adjustment for alcohol or drug "abuse" diminished the magnitude of the increased risk for epilepsy in individuals hospitalized for depression. Generalizability of these findings is limited by the use of hospitalized depression, because fewer than half of people who meet criteria for major depression seek medical care, and even fewer are hospitalized (Olfson, 2005; Kessler, 1999). Clinical selection bias could also account for the impact of substance abuse on the association between epilepsy and major depression in this study.

Population-based case-control studies also consistently demonstrate that a history of depression is associated with an increased risk for developing an isolated unprovoked seizure or newly diagnosed epilepsy. In the first of these studies conducted by Forsgren and Nystrom (1990), a history of depression was associated with a 7-fold increased risk of developing unprovoked seizure ($p = 0.03$) in Swedish adults. When analyses were restricted to cases with a "localized onset" seizure, depression was 17 times more common among cases than among controls ($p = 0.002$). Because patients responded to the questionnaire 4 to 6 weeks after the diagnosis of their first seizure, it is possible that responses were not limited to depression preceding the first diagnosis of epilepsy.

Two other studies have found that a history of depression, diagnosed according to DSM criteria, increased the risk of developing unprovoked seizure. Among older adults residing in Rochester, Minnesota (Hesdorffer, 2000), a history of major depression was associated with a 6-fold increased risk of developing a first idiopathic/cryptogenic unprovoked seizure (95% CI = 1.56-22). After adjusting for medical therapies for depression, including electroconvulsive shock therapy, antidepressants, and antipsychotics, major depression was 3.7 fold more common (95% CI = 0.8-17) before the case's seizure came to medical attention than among controls. This increased risk was most prominent among cases with partial-onset seizures. Among cases, major depression occurred closer to the index date than for controls, suggesting that pathophysiology leading to depression may lower seizure threshold in older adults.

In an Icelandic population-based case-control study (Hesdorffer, 2006) of 324 children and adults aged 10 years and older with first unprovoked seizure or newly diagnosed epilepsy and 647 age and gender matched controls, a history of major depression diagnosed according to DSM-IV criteria was associated with a 1.7-fold increased risk for developing epilepsy (95% CI = 1.1-2.7). This increased risk was also present in the subgroup with idiopathic/cryptogenic seizures (OR = 1.9, 95% CI = 1.1-3.3), even after adjustment for cumulative alcohol consumption.

Significant strengths of these population-based case-control studies are that: they were limited to incident unprovoked seizure and incident epilepsy, and are therefore able to address the time order of the association by examining a history of major depression before the first unprovoked seizure; controls were drawn from the population; major depression was diagnosed according to DSM criteria, using standardized instruments; and the association was evaluated separately in the subgroup with idiopathic/cryptogenic unprovoked seizure, thus eliminating causes of seizures (e.g., stroke, head injury) that are themselves associated with depression. Adjustment for alcohol consumption in the Icelandic study did not alter the association between major depression and epilepsy, ruling out one possible shared environmental risk factor.

Associations between depression and epilepsy may be caused by disturbances in neurotransmitter function common to depression, suicide attempt and seizures as has been suggested by a recent cohort study examining seizures as adverse events in FDA randomized clinical trials of SSRIs and SNRIs conducted between 1985 and 2004 (Alper, 2007). In this analysis, the risk for seizures in the placebo group with major depression was 19-fold that expected in the general population.

Possible explanation for the comorbidity of major depression and epilepsy

The above studies support the possibility that there may be a shared underlying susceptibility to depression and unprovoked seizure that is environmental, genetic or an interaction between environment and genetics. An alternative explanation is that therapies (antidepressants, electroconvulsive shock therapy, and antipsychotics) taken for major depression increase the risk for unprovoked seizure. While we review this possibility below, the time elapsed between the age at onset of depression and the age at onset of epilepsy argue against a direct effect of antidepressants or antipsychotics on the development of unprovoked seizures.

Antidepressant use has been reported to be associated with seizures (Messing, 1984; Devinisky, 1983; Pisani, 2002), but these reports are anecdotal, the risk is less than 1% in the general population (Pisani, 2002), and the underlying disorder is not taken into account. In animal studies, low doses of imipramine or amitriptyline raise the seizure threshold of mice; high doses of imipramine induce clonic seizures (Zaccara, 1990). Several tricyclic antidepressants increase spike activity of perfused guinea pig hippocampal slices in a dose-dependent fashion that differs for each tricyclic antidepressant tested (Luchins, 1994). In human populations, the Boston Collaborative Drug Surveillance Program reported no seizures in association with antidepressant use (Anonymous, 1972). However, given the incidence of epilepsy, at least one case would have been expected in the Boston study. Additionally, Greenblatt et al. (1964) reported no seizures during a randomized clinical trial comparing imipramine, phenelzine, isocarboxazid, ECT, and placebo for treatment of depression. While animal studies and clinical series are informative about the relationship between antidepressants and provoked or acute symptomatic seizures, they provide no longitudinal data to test possible associations between these drugs and epilepsy. In the one epidemiological study to examine the association between antidepressants and unprovoked seizures, the risk associated with antidepressants (OR for tricyclic antidepressants = 2.2, 95% CI = 1.1-4.5 before adjustment and OR = 1.6, 95% CI = 0.8-3.5 after adjustment for major depression and other medical therapies) could be explained almost entirely by major depression (Hesdorffer, 2000). The wide-spread use of antidepressants (Pincus, 1998), which has been increasing over time, argues against a meaningful seizure-inducing effect of these drugs, because a parallel increase in the incidence of unprovoked seizures has not been observed (Forsgren, 2005). Finally, in a reanalysis of FDA randomized clinical trials of SSRIs and SNRIs conducted between 1985 and 200, Alper et al (2007) found a protective effect on the risk for seizures in the treated group compared to the placebo group, suggesting that SSRIs and SNRIs lower the risk for seizures 52 percent (95% CI = 39% to 64%), suggesting that SSRIs and SNRIs are not epileptogenic. Thus, seizures induced by antidepressants are an unlikely explanation of the comorbidity of major depression and epilepsy.

Neuroleptics are associated with an increased risk of seizures (Zaccara, 1990). In one study of 859 patients treated with phenothiazines, 1.2% developed seizures (Logothetis, 1967). Incidence was dose dependent: 9% developed seizures high-dose phenothiazines compared to 0.5% on low-dose phenothiazines. Clozapine has also been associated with the occurrence of seizures (Haller, 1990). Most seizures occurred when therapy began or when the dose of phenothiazine was increased. The Boston Collaborative Drug Surveillance Study found a low risk (0.12%) of seizures due to neuroleptic drugs (Messing, 1984). These data again provide no information regarding the association between these agents and the development of *unprovoked* seizures or epilepsy. In the Rochester case-control of older adults with idiopathic/cryptogenic seizures, phenothiazine use was not associated with unprovoked seizure (OR = 1.3, 95% CI = 0.8 to 2.2) in multivariate analysis, making these drugs an unlikely reason for the observed comorbidity of epilepsy and major depression.

Animal and human studies support both the antiepileptic (Sackeim, 1983; Essig, 1961; Essig, 1966) and the convulsant (Adams, 1990; Racine, 1978) capabilities of electroconvulsive shock therapy (ECT). Whereas recent literature suggests that ECT can be utilized safely in patients with depression and epilepsy, two published studies report an increased risk of unprovoked seizure following ECT (Blackwood, 1980; Devinsky and Duchowny, 1983). Among 166 patients under the age of 70 years who had undergone at least one ECT course 1.8% experienced a first unprovoked seizure over a mean of 18 months of follow-up, an incidence more than 36 times the expected incidence. Devinsky and Duchowny (1983) reviewed all published cases of spontaneous seizures following ECT. The average annual incidence of seizures after ECT was 114 per 100,000, almost three times greater than the incidence of unprovoked seizures among adults in Rochester, Minnesota (Hauser, 1993). In the Rochester case-control study of older adults with new-onset idiopathic/cryptogenic unprovoked seizure (Hesdorffer, 2000), cases were 1.5 times more likely than controls to have received ECT (95% CI = 0.3-7.5), after adjusting for major depression and other medical therapies for depression. Thus, ECT probably does not explain the comorbidity of epilepsy and major depression.

The role of potentially shared environmental risk factors for idiopathic/cryptogenic epilepsy and major depression, other than alcohol consumption, has not been evaluated and could explain the comorbidity of major depression and epilepsy. The use of illicit drugs, mostly cocaine and heroin use, have been identified as risk factors for epilepsy (Ng, 1990). Additionally, substance abuse as defined in the DSM has been associated with an increased risk for major depression (Bakken, 2003). The DSM definition of substance abuse has not been applied in studies of newly diagnosed epilepsy, but based upon information on drug use, one would expect an association. Head injury, stroke, Parkinson's disease, multiple sclerosis, and Alzheimer's disease are shared risk factors for major depression and for epilepsy, but the comorbidity of major depression and epilepsy persists in the group with idiopathic/cryptogenic epilepsy, making these shared risk factors an unlikely explanation for the observed comorbidity. Other risk factors for depression have not been evaluated as potential risk factors for epilepsy, including maternal deprivation, childhood physical maltreatment, stressful life events with attendant conflict and violence (Caspi and Moffitt, 2006). These factors may be important because stressful events cause a rapid release of corticotrophin (Pich, 1995) and high levels of corticotrophin are convulsant in the rat (Baram and Schultz, 1991), making stressful life events of potential interest as a risk factor for developing seizures.

The potential role of genetics in the comorbidity of epilepsy and psychiatric disorders has been explored in a small family study. This study suggested that the risk of psychiatric disorders is increased in first-degree relatives of probands with prevalent juvenile myoclonic epilepsy (JME, an idiopathic epilepsy syndrome) compared with the first-degree relatives of control probands with "acquired" epilepsy (Murray, 1994). Among the probands, psychiatric diagnoses were present in 30% with JME (71% were major depression) and in 31% with "acquired" epilepsy (75% were major depression). Family members of JME probands without psychiatric diagnosis were 3.6 times more likely to have a psychiatric diagnosis than family members of comparison probands without a psychiatric diagnosis (p < 0.05). Anxiety with or without depression predominated in the family members of JME probands without a psychiatric diagnosis. These results support the potential for a common underlying genetic susceptibility to epilepsy and psychiatric disorders in families. However, there were methodological problems: the instrument used to diagnosis psychiatric disorders has low sensitivity (Kendler, 1995; Andreasen, 1977); major depression was not separately studied or analyzed; and no attempt was made to limit analyses to psychiatric disorders that occurred in family members before the proband's epilepsy was diagnosed in order to eliminate psychiatric disorders arising as a consequence of the stress of having a family member with epilepsy. Other family studies are needed to further evaluate the potential genetic contribution to the comorbidity of major depression and epilepsy.

Bipolar disorder

Compared to the prevalence and the incidence of major depression, bipolar disorder is rare. The prevalence of bipolar disorder ranges from 0.2% to 1.1% in a one year period (Pini, 2005) with a lifetime prevalence of 1.5% to 2.0% (Pini, 2005). The incidence of bipolar disorder peaks in 21-25 year olds at 16.4 per 100,000 population (Kennedy, 2005).

Because both bipolar disorder and epilepsy are relatively rare, studies of the association between these disorders require large cohorts in order to have adequate statistical power. In a study of older adults in Rochester, Minnesota one case met DSM-III-R criteria for mania prior to the onset of epilepsy; no controls were affected (Hesdorffer, 2000). In the recent population-based Icelandic study (Hesdorffer, 2006), bipolar disorder was associated with a 5-fold increased risk for developing epilepsy that was not statistically significant.

Suicidal behavior

The distribution of suicidality in the population is pyramidal with suicidal ideation more common than suicide attempt, which is, in turn, more common than completed suicide (Kessler, 2005b). For each completed suicide, there are 25 attempts (Steljes, 2005). In the United States, the rate of completed suicide is 12.0/100,000 (Li, 2001) with a marked predominance in males (McIntosh, 1986). In contrast, the lifetime prevalence of suicide attempt is 0.6% to 4.9% overall (Kessler, 2005b; Oquendo, 2004; Weissman, 1999) with a female preponderance. The 12-month prevalence of suicidal ideation is even greater, 2.8% to 21.8% (Kessler, 2005b; Weissman, 1999) with a weak female predominance.

There is considerable comorbidity between a number of other psychiatric disorders and suicidal tendancies. These comorbidities may provide clues to endophenotypes that are useful to examine to further explain the comorbidity between epilepsy and suicidality. Among people with major depression, the prevalence of suicidal ideation is 4.4% (Kessler, 2005b) and the prevalence of suicide attempt is 20.5% to 34.7% in people with a lifetime history of major depression (Kessler, 2005b; Oquendo, 2004). Additionally, suicidality is a symptom of major depression. Impulse control disorders are associated with a 28.5% prevalence of suicidal ideation and a 33.1% prevalence of suicide attempt (Kessler, 2005b), due mostly to ADHD and to oppositional-defiant disorder. Substance use disorders are associated with a 19.4% to 30.3% prevalence of suicidal ideation and a 26.1% to 49.5% prevalence of suicide attempt (Kessler, 2005b), due mostly to alcohol abuse or dependence. Finally anxiety disorders are associated with a 60.6% to 62.8% prevalence of suicidal ideation and a 70.4% to 70.6% prevalence of suicide attempt (Kessler, 2005b), again due mostly to alcohol abuse or dependence.

The association between suicide and epilepsy was first described by Pudhomme (1941). Originally, it was thought that people with epilepsy became suicidal due to their seizure disorder. This belief was later supported by studies showing that completed suicide occurs more often than expected in people with epilepsy than in the general population (Jones, 2003; Nilsson, 1997; Rafnsson, 2001; Barraclough, 1987; Henriksen, 1970). Standardized mortality ratios for suicide in people with epilepsy range from 3.5 (Nilsson, 1997) to 5.0 (Rafnsson, 2001), and the proportionate mortality ratio ranges from 0.7% (Barraclough, 1987) to 20% (Henriksen, 1970) when studies with at least 100 deaths are examined. Although the long held explanation for this finding was that depression leads to suicide in people with epilepsy, in part because their epilepsy makes them severely depressed, recent findings suggest that this explanation is unlikely. Rather it appears that suicidality can precede the development of a first unprovoked seizure. In the Icelandic population-based study (Hesdorffer, 2006), suicide attempt was associated with a 3.5-fold increased risk for *developing* epilepsy (95% CI = 1.5-8.6), after adjusting for major depression, bipolar disorder, and cumulative alcohol intake. Thus, parallel to the results of studies concerning major depression and epilepsy, suicidal behaviors *precede* the occurrence of a first unprovoked seizure. Because others have shown that suicide attempt increases the risk of later completed suicide (Suominen, 2004), the increased risk for completed suicide in people with epilepsy may reflect the recurrence of premorbid suicidal behavior rather than epilepsy leading to major depression and completed suicide. These results further suggest a common underlying susceptibility to epilepsy and suicidal behavior that is independent of major depression and bipolar disorder. Suicidality is comorbid with many psychiatric disorders, particularly impulse control, substance abuse and depressive disorders. Impulsivity, a trait that is strongly associated with suicidality (Mann, 2003), has not been studied in epilepsy and may further refine the epilepsy-suicidality phenotype.

Generalized anxiety disorder

In the National Comorbidity survey replication, the lifetime prevalence of generalized anxiety disorder was 6.1% (Kessler, 2005c); prevalence was 2.9% in the past 12 months and 1.8% in the past month. In European studies, the lifetime prevalence of generalized anxiety ranges from 0.1% to 6.4% (Lieb, 2005), with prevalence in the past 12 months, ranging from 0.1% to 2.1% and point prevalence ranging from 0.2% to 3.1%. The age at onset of generalized anxiety disorder is mostly between the early teens and the early thirties. Generalized anxiety disorder is comorbid with most other anxiety disorders (Lieb, 2005), mood disorders (Lieb, 2005), substance disorders (Lieb, 2005, and impulse-control disorders (Lieb, 2005). Additionally, post traumatic stress disorder, a subset of anxiety disorders, is associated with suicidal ideation and suicide attempts (Sareen, 2005).

Studies of the comorbidity of epilepsy and anxiety have all been cross-sectional. In studies of adults with prevalent epilepsy, anxiety and depression are the most common psychiatric disorders (for example, Jacoby, 1996). Until recently, most studies of anxiety in children with epilepsy have failed to include a control group against which to compare the frequency of anxiety disorders and some were conducted in chronic epilepsy (Ettinger, 1998; Caplan, 2005). Nonetheless, these studies report a high prevalence of anxiety in prevalent childhood epilepsy, ranging from 13% to 48.5% (Ettinger, 1998; Caplan, 2005; Williams, 2003; Caplan, 1998; Ott, 2001; Alwash, 2000). When comparison groups are included, anxiety with depression is more common in children with epilepsy than in normal children (Caplan, 2005; Oguz, 2002). It is possible that the presence of anxiety may further refine the epilepsy-major depression phenotype and further studies of anxiety preceding a first unprovoked seizure are needed to examine this issue and rule out the possibility that having epilepsy causes anxiety.

■ Associations between epilepsy and migraine

Migraine, a chronic disorder characterized by recurrent episodes of headache and associated symptoms, is co-morbid with epilepsy, with major depression and with suicidality. In the International Headache Society (IHS) definition (2004), migraine is further classified as migraine with aura (MA) and migraine without aura (MO). The lifetime prevalence of migraine is 14.7% in a health plan (Patel, 2004) with a female preponderance. The lifetime prevalence of migraine with aura (MA) was 7.9% in a Danish general population sample (Russell, 1996). Genetic and environmental factors contribute to the development of migraine in families (Stewart, 1997). Some have suggested that MA and migraine without aura (MO) are different disease entities (Russell, 1996; Goadsby, 2001), an assertion supported by familial aggregation and twin studies (Ulrich, 1999; Russell and Olesen, 1995). Additionally, a stronger genetic component has been found for MA than for MO (Russell and Olesen, 1995).

Cross-sectional studies show that migraine is associated with specific childhood epilepsy syndromes (Andermann and Zifkin, 1998; Giroud, 1989), such as Childhood Epilepsy with Occipital Paroxysms and Benign Childhood Epilepsy with Centrotemporal Spikes. The co-occurrence of migraine and epilepsy is more common in females (Ottman and Lipton, 1994; Leniger, 2003). Patients with MA are 1.6 times more likely to have epilepsy than those with only migraine (p = 0.02; Leniger, 2003). The association between epilepsy and migraine is bidirectional. The risk for new-onset migraine is increased 2.4-fold (95% CI = 2.02-2.89) in people with a history of epilepsy (Ottman and Lipton, 1994). The risk for a first unprovoked seizure is increased 3.7-fold (95% CI = 1.6-8.3) in children with a history of migraine, due to MA (OR = 8.2; 95% CI = 2.3-28.9) (Ludvigsson, 2006). Additionally, the prognosis of epilepsy is worse in the presence of migraine (Velioglu, 2005).

Analogous to studies of epilepsy *(Figure 1)*, migraine is also associated with both major depression and with suicide attempt (Breslau, 1991; Breslau, 1994; Breslau, 2000; Fasmer and Oedegaard, 2001; Lipton, 2000). The association between major depression and migraine is bidirectional and is strongest for MA (Breslau, 2000). Suicide attempt is also more common in migraine compared to controls, and the association is strongest for MA, even after adjusting for depression (Breslau, 1991). Interestingly, the one study of the familial co-aggregation of major depression and migraine was negative (Merikangas, 1988).

These overlapping relationships between migraine, major depression, suicidality and epilepsy *(Figure 1)* suggest that either migraine is a confounder of the relationship between major depression, suicidality and epilepsy or that there is a differential effect of depression or suicidality in the presence compared to the absence of migraine. We examined our Icelandic data and found that migraine is not a confounder of the relationship between major depression, suicidality and epilepsy (Hesdorffer, in press). We then examined whether the co-occurrence of MA with either major depression or with suicide attempt increases the risk for developing unprovoked seizure more than these conditions alone. This hypothesis was examined in the Icelandic population-based case-control study among 324 individuals aged 10 and older with newly diagnosed unprovoked seizures 647 matched controls. Major depression with MA increased the risk for unprovoked seizures more than either condition alone (major depression and MA, OR = 4.6; major depression only, OR = 1.4; MA only, OR = 2.5). The same was seen for suicide attempt with MA (suicide attempt and MA, OR = 7.9; suicide attempt only, OR = 4.7; MA only, OR = 2.4). Number of conditions showed a linear relationship to seizure risk (OR = 2.0 with any one condition, OR = 4.9 with any two conditions, and OR = 6.7 with all three conditions); this linear trend was statistically significant. These findings may reflect a new condition cluster defined by MA, major depression, suicide attempt and unprovoked seizures.

When migraine and epilepsy are examined and the other comorbid conditions ignored, shared genetic factors are not the explanation for the co-morbidity of migraine and epilepsy in the one study to examine this (Ottman and Lipton, 1996). Two possible methodological factors may explain this. First, the control group consisted of families of people with symptomatic seizures. To the extent that genetic factors linking susceptibility to migraine and to seizures exist regardless of seizure etiology, this control group would sharply attenuate the association. Second, shared genetic factors were studied in a select population of people with prevalent epilepsy who participate in voluntary organizations and are more likely to represent people with refractory partial seizures than a general population sample of people with prevalent epilepsy. If migraine and epilepsy are more likely to occur together in families with generalized forms of epilepsy, then this study was unlikely to detect familial aggregation of these disorders.

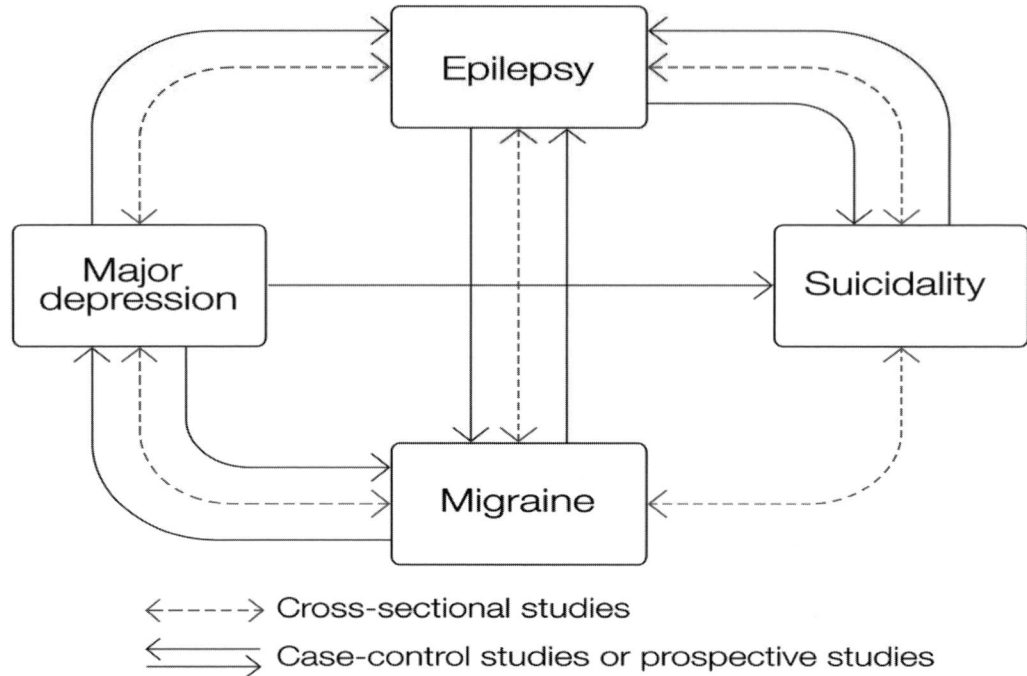

Figure 1. Relationships between epilepsy, major depression, suicidality, and migraine.

▪ Possible biologic explanations for the comorbidity of epilepsy, major depression, suicidality and perhaps migraine

Serotonergic dysfunction may be as a possible pathogenic pathway, explaining the comorbidity of epilepsy and major depression and epilepsy and suicidality. The potential role of serotonin (5HT) in migraine is not well described. Decreased concentrations of 5HT in the synaptic cleft play an epileptogenic role in both animal and human studies of epilepsy (Jakus, 2003; Watanabe, 1998), and are also associated with major depression (Delgado, 1994; Owens and Nemeroff, 1994) and with suicidality (Arango, 1990; Arango, 2001; Boldrini, 2005) Positron emission tomography (PET) studies in major depression and in prevalent epilepsy (mostly temporal lobe epilepsy) suggest dysfunction of $5HT_{1A}$ receptors. These receptors are found presynaptically in the raphe nuclei, inhibiting release of 5HT into the synaptic cleft (Sotelo, 1990; Riad, 1992), and postsynaptically where they mediate effects of 5HT (Jacobs and Azmitia, 1992). In genetically epilepsy prone rats (GEPR), the anticonvulsant effect of fluoxetine (Watanabe, 1998) is enhanced through administration of $5HT_{1A}$ antagonists (Browning, 1997). In rats, depletion of 5HT decreases seizure threshold (Statnick, 1996) through $5HT_{1A}$ activation (Lu and Gean, 1998) and administration of tryptophan, the 5HT precursor, increases seizure threshold (Watanabe, 1998). Additionally, citalopram, an SSRI, has been shown to decrease median seizure frequency 55.6% in non-depressed patients with poorly controlled epilepsy (Favale,

2003). Taken together these studies suggest that 5HT is anticonvulsant, an effect possibly mediated by $5HT_{1A}$ autoreceptors in the raphe nuclei. The role of serotonergic dysfunction is well described in major depression (Delgado, 1994; Owens and Nemeroff, 1994) and in suicide (Mann JJ, 2003). In people with a history of major depression, depleting the 5HT precursor, tryptophan, precipitates a redevelopment of depressive symptoms (Moreno, 2000). Additionally, SSRIs initially desensitize $5HT_{1A}$ autoreceptors in the raphe nuclei, explaining the delayed response to SSRI treatment (de Montigny, 1990), and later the 5HT transporter downregulates (Benmansour, 1999), increasing 5HT in the synaptic cleft.

Increased $5HT_{1A}$ binding in the raphe, with associated decreased 5HT in the synaptic cleft, may be a common pathway to the *development* of depression, suicidality and epilepsy. This model might explain the comorbidity of epilepsy with both major depression and suicidality. Other possible candidates, underlying the co-aggregation of epilepsy, suicidality and major depression, include corticotrophin-releasing factor (Coryell and Schlesser, 2001; Yehuda, 1996; Wang, 2001; Baram and Schultz, 1991), norepinephrine (Mann, 2003; Cameron, 2004; Jobe and Browning, 2005) and γ-aminobutyric acid (GABA) (Sanacora, 2004; Choudary, 2005; Simister, 2003; Merali, 2004). While magnetic resonance spectroscopy (MRS) studies of GABA in prevalent epilepsy and in depression show decreased GABA, there is evidence to suggest that, at least in depression, reduced GABA levels may occur secondary to 5HT dysfunction. In one randomized cross-over study in healthy volunteers (Bhagwagar, 2004), brain GABA levels rose 35% when 5HT availability was increased by treatment with a selective serotonin reuptake inhibitor (SSRI), suggesting that reduced GABA levels may be a marker of current depression and not a marker of the tendency to develop depression. None of these models successfully address the role of migraine in the cluster of comorbidity described in *figure 1*.

References

Adams RE. Does kindling model anything clinically relevant? *Biol Psychiatry* 1990; 27: 249-79.

Alper K, Schwartz KA, Kolts RL, Khan A. Seizure Incidence in Psychopharmacological Clinical Trials: An Analysis of Food and Drug Administration (FDA) Summary Basis of Approval Reports. *Biol Psychiatry* 2007 (in press and available on line).

Alwash R, Hussein M, Matloub F. Symptoms of anxiety and depression among adolescents and seizures in Irbid, Northern Jordan. *Seizure* 2000; 9: 412-6.

Andermann F, Zifkin B. The benign occipital epilepsies of childhood: An overview of the idiopathic syndromes and of the relationship to migraine. *Epilepsia* 1998: 39 (suppl 4): S9-S23.

Andreasen NC, Endicott J, Spitzer RL, Winokur G. The family history method using diagnostic criteria. Reliability and validity. *Arch Gen Psychiatry* 1977; 34 (10): 1229-35.

Anonymous. Drug-induced convulsions: Report from Boston Collaborative Drug Surveillance Program. *Lancet* 1972; 2: 677-9.

Anthony JC, Eaton WW, Henderson AS. Psychiatric epidemiology. *Epidemiol Rev* 1995; 17: 240-2.

Anthony JC, Warner LA, Kessler RC. Comparative epidemiology of dependence on tobacco, alcohol, controlled substances, and inhalants: basic findings from the National Comorbidity Survey. *Exp Clin Psychopharmacol* 1994; 2: 244-68.

Arango V, Ernsberger P, Marzuk PM, Chen JS, Tierney H, Stanley M, Reis DJ, Mann JJ. Autoradiographic demonstration of increased 5HT$_2$ and β-adrenergic receptor binding sites in the brain of suicide victims. *Arch Gen Psychiatry* 1990; 47: 1038-47.

Arango V, Underwood MD, Boldrini M, Tamir H, Kassir SA, Hsiung S, Chen JJX, Mann JJ. Serotonin 1A receptors, serotonin transporter binding, and serotonin transporter mRNA expression in the brainstem of depressed suicide victims. *Neuropsychopharm* 2001; 25: 892-903.

Austin JK, Harezlak J, Dunn DW, Huster GA, Rose DF, Ambrosius WT. Behavior problems in children before first recognized seizure. *Pediatrics* 2001; 107: 115-22.

Bakken K, Landheim AS, Vaglum P. Primary and secondary substance misusers: do they differ in substance-induced and substance-independent mental disorders? *Alcohol & Alcoholism* 2003; 38 (1): 54-9.

Baram TZ, Schultz L. Corticotropin-releasing hormone is a rapid and potent convulsant in the infant rat. *Dev Brain Res* 1991; 61: 97-101.

Barraclough BM. The suicide rate of epilepsy. *Acta Psychiatr Scand* 1987; 76: 339-45.

Beghi E, Spagnoli P, Airoldi L, Fiordelli E, Appollonio I, Bogliun G, Zardi A, Paleari F, Gamba P, Frattola L, Da Prada L. Emotional and affective disturbances in patients with epilepsy. *Epilepsy Behav* 2002; 3 (3): 255-61.

Benmansour S, Cecchi M, Morilak DA, Gerhardt GA, Javors MA, Gould GG, Frazer A. Effects of chronic antidepressant treatments on serotonin transporter function, density, and mRNA level. *JNeurosci* 1999; 19 (23): 10494-501.

Bhagwagar Z, Wylezinska M, Taylor M, Jezzard P, Matthews PM, Cowen PJ. Increased brain GABA concentrations following acute administration of a selective serotonin reuptake inhibitor. *Am JPsychiatry* 2004; 161 (2): 368-70.

Biederman J, Faraone SV, Keenan K, Knee D, Tsuang MT. Family-genetic and psychosocial risk factors in DSM-III attention deficit disorder. *J Am Acad Child Adolesc Psychiatry* 1990; 29: 526-33.

Biederman J, Faraone SV, Mick E, Spencer T, Wilens T, Keily K. High risk for attention deficit hyperactivity disorder among children of parents with childhood onset of the disorder: A pilot study. *Am JPsychiatry* 1995; 152: 431-5.

Biederman J, Faraone SV, Monuteaux M, Spencer T, Wilens T, Bober M. Genetic effects of attention deficit hyperactivity disorder in adults, revisited. *BiolPsychiatry* 2004; 55: 692-700.

Blackwood DH, Cull RE, Freeman CPL, Evans JI, Mawdsley C. A study of the incidence of epilepsy following ECT. *J Neurol Neurosurg Psychiatry* 1980; 43: 1098-102.

Blazer DG, Kessler RC, McGonagle KA, Swartz CS. The prevalence and distribution of major depression in a national community sample: the National Comorbidity Survey. *Am J Psychiatry* 1994; 151: 979-86.

Boldrini M, Underwood MD, Mann JJ, Arango V. More tryptophan hydroxylase in the brainstem dorsal raphe nucleus in depressed suicides. *Brain Res* 2005; 1041: 19-28.

Boylan Ls, Flint LA, Labovitz DL, Jackson SC, Starner K, Devinsky O. Depression but not seizure frequency predicts quality of life in treatment-resistant epilepsy. *Neurology* 2004; 62: 617-23.

Breslau N, Davis GC, Andreski P. Migraine, psychiatric disorders, and suicide attempts: an epidemiologic study of young adults. *Psychiatry Res* 1991; 37 (1): 11-23.

Breslau N, Davis GC, Schultz LR, Peterson EL. Migraine and major depression. *Headache* 1994; 34: S17-S26.

Breslau N, Schultz LR, Stewart WF, Lipton RB, Lucia VC, Welch KM. Headache and major depression: is the association specific to migraine? *Neurology* 2000; 54 (2): 308-13.

Browning RA, Wood AV, Merrill MA, Dailey JW, Jobe PC. Enhancement of the anticonvulsant effect of fluoxetine following blockade of 5-HT1A receptors. *Eur J Pharmacol* 1997; 336 (1): 1-6.

Cameron OG, Abelson JL, Young EA. Anxious and depressive disorders and their comorbidity: effect on central nervous system noradrenergic function. *Biol Psychiatry* 2004; 56: 875-83.

Caplan R, Arbelle S, Magharious W, Guthrie D, Komo S, Shields WD, Chayasirisobhon S, Hansen R. Psychopathology in pediatric complex partial and generalized epilepsy. *Dev Med Child Neurol* 1998; 40: 805-11.

Caplan R, Siddarth P, Gurbani S, Hanson R, Sankar R, Shields WD. Depression and anxiety disorders in pediatric epilepsy. *Epilepsia* 2005; 46: 720-30.

Carlton-Ford S, Miller R, Brown M, Nealeigh N, Jennings S. Epilepsy and children's social and psychological adjustment. *J Health Soc Behav* 1995; 36: 285-301.

Caspi A, Sugden K, Moffitt TE, Taylor A, Craig IW, Harrington H, McClay J, Mill J, Martin J, Braithwaite A, Poulton P. Influence of life stress on depression: moderation by a polymorphism in the 5-HTT gene. *Science* 2003; 301 (5631): 386-9.

Caspi A, Moffitt TE. Gene-environment interactions in psychiatry: Joining forces with neuroscience. *Nature Reviews* 2006; 7: 583-9.

Choudary PV, Molnar M, Evans SJ, Tomita H, Li JZ, Vawter MP, Myers RM, Bunney WE Jr, Akil H, Watson SJ, Jones EG. Altered cortical glutamatergic and GABAergic signal transmission with glial involvement in depression. *Proc Nat Acad Sci* 2005; 102: 15653-8.

Coryell W, Winokur G, Shea T, Maser JD, Endicott J, Akiskal HS. The long-term stability of depressive subtypes. *Am J Psychiatry* 1994; 151: 199-204.

Coryell W, Schlesser M. The dexamethasone suppression test and suicide predictions. *Am J Psychiatry* 2001; 158; 748-53.

Cowan LD, Leviton A, Bodensteiner JB, Doherty L. Problems in estimating the prevalence of epilepsy in children: the yield from different sources of information. *P aediatr Per inat Epidemiol* 1989; 3: 386-401.

Cramer JA, Blum D. Fanning K, Reed M for the Epilepsy Impact Project. The impact of comorbid depression on health resource utilization in a community sample of people with epilepsy. *Epilepsy Behav* 2004: 337-42.

Delgado PL, Price LH, Miller HL, et al. Serotonin and the neurobiology of depression. Effects of tryptophan depletion in drug-free depressed patients. *Arch Gen Psychiatry* 1994; 51 (11): 865-74.

de Montigny C, Chaput Y, Blier P. Modification of serotonergic neuron properties by long-term treatment with serotonin reuptake blockers. *J Clin Psychiatry* 1990; 51 (suppl B): 4-8.

Devinisky O, Duchowny MS. Seizures after convulsive therapy: A retrospective case survey. *Neurology* 1983; 33: 921-5.

Diagnostic and statistical manual of mental disorders (fourth edition). Washington, D.C.: American Psychiatric Association, 1997.

Dominian MA, Serafetinides EA, Dewhurst M. A follow-up study of late-onset epilepsy: II. Psychiatric and social findings. *Br Med J* 1963; 1: 431-5.

Dunn DW, Austin JK, Huster GA. Behavior problems in children with new-onset epilepsy. *Seizure* 1997; 6: 283-7.

Essig CF, Groce ME, Williamson EL. Reversible elevation of electroconvulsive threshold and occurrence of spontaneous convulsions upon repeated stimulation of the cat brain. *Exp Neurol* 1961; 4: 37-47.

Essig CF, Flanary HG. The importance of the convulsion in the occurrence and rate of development of electroconvulsive threshold elevation. *Exp Neurol* 1966; 14: 448-52.

Ettinger AB, Weisbrot DM, Nolan EE, Gadow KD, Vitale SA, Andriola MR, Lenn NJ, Novak GP, Hermann BP. Symptoms of depression and anxiety in pediatric epilepsy patients. *Epilepsia* 1998; 39: 595-9.

Faraone S, Biederman J, Chen WH, Krifcher B, Keenan K, Moore C. Segregation analysis of attention deficit hyperactivity disorder: Evidence for single gene transmission. *Psychiatr Genet* 1992; 2: 257-75.

Fasmer OB, Oedegaard KJ. Clinical characteristics of patients with major affective disorders and comorbid migraine. *World J Biol Psychiatry* 2001; 2 (3): 149-55.

Favale E, Audenino D, Cocito L, Albano C. The anticonvulsant effect of citalopram as an indirect evidence of serotonergic impairment in human epileptogenesis. *Seizure* 2003; 12 (5): 316-8.

Forsgren L, Nystrom L. An incident case-referent study of epileptic seizures in adults. *Epilepsy Res* 1990; 6: 66-81.

Forsgren L, Beghi E, Öun A, Sillanpää M. The epidemiology of epilepsy in Europe – a systematic review. *Eur JNeurology* 2005; 12: 245-53.

Giroud M, Couillault G, Arnould S, Dauvergne M, Dumas R, Nivelon JL: Epilepsie à paroxysmes rolandiques et migraine, une association non fortuite. Résultats d'une étude contrôlée. *Pédiatrie* 1989; 44: 659-64.

Goadsby PJ. Migraine, aura and cortical spreading depression: Why are we still talking about it? *Ann Neurol* 2001; 49 (1): 4-5.

Greenblatt M, Grosser GH, Wechsler H. Differential response of hospitalized patients to somatic therapy. *Am J Psychiatry* 1964; 121: 935-43.

Haller E, Binder RL. Clozapine and seizures. *Am J Psychiatry* 1990; 147: 1069-71.

Hauser WA, Annegers JF, Kurland LT. Prevalence of epilepsy in Rochester, Minnesota: 1940-1980. *Epilepsia* 1991; 32: 429-45.

Hauser WA, Annegers JF, Kurland LT. Incidence of epilepsy and unprovoked seizures in Rochester, Minnesota: 1935-1984. *Epilepsia* 1993; 34: 453-68.

Headache Classification Committee of the International Headache Society. Classification and diagnostic criteria for headache disorders, cranial neuroalgias, and facial pain. Second Edition. *Cephalalgia* 2004; suppl 1: 1-160.

Hemmer SA, Pasternak JF, Zecker SG, Trommer BL. Stimulant therapy and seizure risk in children with ADHD. *PediatrNeurol* 2001; 24: 99-102.

Hempel AM, Frost MD, Ritter FJ, Farnam S. Factors influencing the incidence of ADHD in pediatric epilepsy patients. *Epilepsia* 1995; 36 (suppl 4): 122.

Henriksen B, Juul-Jensen P, Lund M. Mortality of epileptics. In Brackenridge R (ed). *Life assurance medicine*. London: Pitman: 1970: 139-48.

Hesdorffer DC, Ludvigsson P, Hauser WA, Olafsson E, Kjartansson O. Co-occurrence of major depression or suicide attempt and migraine with aura and risk factor for unprovoked seizure. *Epilepsy Research* (in press).

Hesdorffer DC, Hauser WA, Annegers JF, Cascino G. Major depression is a risk factor for seizures in older adults. *Ann Neurol* 2000; 47: 246-9.

Hesdorffer DC, Ludvigsson P, Olafsson E, Gudmundsson, G, Kjartansson O, Hauser WA. ADHD as a risk factor for incident unprovoked seizures and epilepsy in children. *Arch Gen Psychiatry* 2004; 61: 731-6.

Hesdorffer DC, Hauser WA, Ludvigsson P, Olafsson E, Kjartansson O. Depression and attempted suicide as risk factors for incident unprovoked seizures and epilepsy. *Ann Neurology* 2006; 59: 35-41.

Holdsworth L, Whitmore K. A study of children with epilepsy attending ordinary schools. I: their seizure patterns, progress, and behaviour in school. *Dev Med Child Neurol* 1991; 33: 201-15.

Holtmann M, Becker K, Kentner-Figura B, Schmidt MH. Increased frequency of rolandic spikes in ADHD children. *Epilepsia* 2003; 44: 1241-4.

Hughes JR, DeLeo AJ, Melyn MA. The electroencephalogram in attention deficit-hyperactivity disorder: Emphasis on epileptiform discharges. *Epilepsy Behav* 2000; 1: 271-7.

Jabbari B, Bryan GE, Marsh EE, Gunderson CH. Incidence of seizures with tricyclic and tetracyclic antidepressants. *ArchNeurol* 1985; 42: 480-1.

Jacobs BL, Azmitia EC. Structure and function of the brain serotonin system. *Physiol Rev* 1992; 72 (1): 165-229.

Jacoby A, Baker GA, Stgeen N, Potts P, Chadwick DW. The clinical course of epilepsy and its psychosocial findings from a U.K. community study. *Epilepsia* 1996; 37: 148-61.

Jakus R, Graf M, Juhasz G, Gerber K, Levay G, Halasz P, Bagdy G. 5-HT2C receptors inhibit and 5-HT1A receptors activate the generation of spike-wave discharges in a genetic rat model of absence epilepsy. *Exp Neurol* 2003; 184 (2): 964-72.

Jobe PC, Browning RA. The serotonergic and noradrenergic effects of antidepressant drugs are anticonvulsant, not proconvulsant. *Epilepsy Behav* 2005; 7: 602-19.

Jones JE, Hermann BP, Bary JJ, Gilliam FG, Kanner AM, and Meador KJ. Rates and risk factors for suicide, suicidal ideation, and suicide attempts in chronic epilepsy. *Epilepsy Behav* 2003: 4: S31-S38.

Jones JE, Dow C, Sheth R, Koehn M, Watson R, Caplan R, Seidenberg M, Hermann BP. Psychiatric Comorbidity Is Overrepresented in Children Exhibiting Academic Problems Prior to Epilepsy Onset. *Epilepsia* 2006; 47 (s3).

Kaplan HI, Sadock BJ. *Synopsis of Psychiatry: Behavioral Sciences Clinical Psychiatry, sixth edition*. Baltimore, MD: Williams & Wilkins, 1991.

Kendler KS, Roy MA. Validity of a diagnosis of lifetime major depression obtained by personal interview versus family history. *Am JPsychiatry* 1995; 152 (11): 1608-14.

Kennedy N, Everitt B, Boy dell J, Van Os J, Jones PB, Murray RM. Incidence and distribution of first-episode mania by age: results from a 35-year study. *Psychological Med* 2005; 35: 855-863.

Kessler RC, Zhao S, Katz SJ, Kouzis AC, Frank RG, Edlund M, Leaf P. Past-year use of outpatient services for psychiatric problems in the National Comorbidity Survey. *Am J Psychiatry* 1999; 156 (1): 115-23.

Kessler RC, Berglund P, Demler O, Jin R, Merikangas KR, Walters EE. Lifetime prevalence and age-at-onset distributions of DSM-IV disorders in the National Comorbidity Survey replication. *Arch Gen Psychiatry* 2005a; 62: 593-602.

Kessler RC, Berglund P, Borges G, Nock M, Wang PS. Trends in suicide ideation, plans, gestures, and attempts in the United States, 1990-1992 to 2001-2003. *JAMA* 2005b; 293: 2487-95.

Kessler RC, Brandenburg N, Lane M, Roy-Byrne P, Stang PD, Stein DJ, Wittchen H-U. Rethinking the duration requirement for generalized anxiety disorder: evidence from the National Comorbidity Survey Replication. *Psychological Med* 2005c; 3 (5): 1073-82.

Kooij JJS, Buitelaar JK, van den Oord EJ, Furer JW, Rijnders CATh, Hodiamont PPG. Internal and external validity of Attention-Deficit Hyperactivity Disorder in a population-based sample of adults. *Psychological Med* 2005; 3 (5): 817-27.

Lavados J, Germain I, Morales A, Campero M, Lavados P. A descriptive study of epilepsy in the District of El Salvador, Chile 1984-1988. *Acta Neurol Scand* 1992; 91: 718-29.

Lehtinen V, Sohlman B, Nummelin T, Salomaa M, Ayuso-Mateos J-L, Dowrick C. The estimated incidence of depressive disorder and its determinants in the Finnish ODIN sample. Soc *Psychiatry Psychiatr Epidemiol* 2005; 40: 778-84.

Leniger T, von den Driesch S, Isbruch K, Diener HC, Hufnagel A. Clinical characteristics of patients with comorbidity of migraine and epilepsy. *Headache* 2003; 43: 672-7.

Li S, Hauser LA, Gao B. Suicide in Travis County, Texas, from 1994 through 1998. *Texas Medicine* 2001; 97: 64-8.

Lieb R, Becker E, Altamura C. The epidemiology of generalized anxiety disorder in Europe. *Eur Neuropsychopharmacology* 2005; 15: 445-52.

Lilienfeld SO, Waldman ID, Israel AC. A critical examination of the use of the term and concept of comorbidity in psychopathology research. *Clin Psychol Sci Prac* 1994; 1: 71-83.

Lindsay J, Ounsted C, Richards P. Long-term outcome in children with temporal lobe epilepsy. *DevMed ChildNeurol* 1984; 26: 25-32.

Logothetis J. Spontaneous epileptic seizures and electroencephalographic changes in the course of phenothiazine therapy. *Neurology* 1967; 17: 869-77.

Luchins DI, Oliver AP, Wyatt RJ. Seizures with antidepressants: an *in vitro* technique to assess relative risk. *Epilepsia* 1994; 25: 25-32.

Lu KT, Gean PW. Endogenous serotonin inhibits epileptiform activity in rat hippocampal CA1 neurons via 5-hydroxytryptamine1 A receptor activation. *Neuroscience* 1998; 86 (3): 729-37.

Ludvigsson P, Hesdorffer D, Olafsson E, Kjartansson O, Hauser WA. Migraine with aura is a risk factor for unprovoked seizures in children. *Ann Neurol* 2006; 59 (1): 210-3.

Mann JJ. Neurobiology of suicidal behavior. *Nature Reviews Neuroscience* 2003; 4: 819-28.

McDermott S, Mani S, Krishnaswami S. A population-based analysis of specific behavior problems associated with childhood seizure disorders. *J Epilepsy* 1995; 8: 110-18.

McIntosh JL, Jewell BL. Sex difference trends in completed suicide. *Suicide Lefe Treat Behav* 1986; 16: 16-27.

Merali Z. Du L, Hrdina P, Palkovits M, Faludi G, Poulter MO, Anisman H. Dysregulation in the suicide brain: mRNA expression of corticotropin-releasing hormone receptors and GABA(A) receptor subunits in frontal cortical brain region. *J Neuroscience* 2004; 24: 1478-85.

Merikangas KR, Risch NJ, Merikangas JR, Weissman MM, Kidd KK. Migraine and depression: association and familial transmission. *J Psychiatr Res* 1988; 22 (2): 119-29.

Messing RO, Closson RG, Simon RP. Drug-induced convulsions: a 10-year experience. *Neurology* 1984; 34: 582-6.

Moreno FA, Heninger GR, McGahuey CA, Delgado PL. Tryptophan depletion and risk of depression relapse: a prospective study of tryptophan depletion as a potential predictor of depressive episodes. *Biol Psychiatry* 2000; 48 (4): 327-9.

Murphy JM, Laird NM, Monson RR, Sobol AM, Leighton AH. A 40-year perspective on the prevalence of depression: the Stirling County Study. *Arch Gen Psychiatry* 2000a; 57: 209-15.

Murphy JM, Laird NM, Monson RR, Sobol AM, Leighton AH. Incidence of depression in the Stirling County Study: historical and comparative perspectives. *Psychol Med* 2000b; 30: 505-14.

Murray RE, Abou-Khalil B, Griner L. Evidence for familial association of psychiatric disorders and epilepsy. *Biol Psychiatry* 1994; 36 (6): 428-9.

Newman SC, Bland RC. Incidence of mental disorders in Edmonton: estimates of rates and methodological issues. *J Psychiatr Res* 1998; 32: 273-82.

Ng SKC, Brust JCM, Hauser WA, Susser M. Illicit drug use and the risk of new-onset seizures. *Am J Epidemiol* 1990; 132: 47-57.

Nierenberg AA, Pava JA, Clancy KP, Rosenbaum JF, Fava M. Are neurovegetative symptoms stable in relapsing or recurrent atypical depressive episodes? *Biol Psychiatry* 1996; 40: 691-6.

Nilsson L, Tomson T, Farahmand BY, Diwan V, Persson PG. Cause-specific mortality in epilepsy: A cohort study of more than 9;000 patients once hospitalized for epilepsy. *Epilepsia* 1997; 38: 1062-8.

Nilsson FM, Kessing LV, Bolwig TG. On the increased risk of developing late-onset epilepsy for patients with major affective disorder. *J Affective Dis* 2003; 76: 39-48.

O'Donoghue MF, Goodridge DM, Redhead K, Sander JW, Duncan JS. Assessing the psychosocial consequences of epilepsy: a community-based study. *Br J Gen Practice* 1999; 49: 211-4.

Oguz A, Kurul S, Dirik E. Relationship of epilepsy-related factors to anxiety and depression scores in epileptic children. *J Child Neurol* 2002; 17: 37-40.

Ohayon MM, Priest RG, Guilleminault C, et al. The prevalence of depressive disorders in the United Kingdom. *BiolPsychiatry* 1999; 45: 300-7.

Olafsson E, Ludvigsson P, Gudmundsson G, Hesdorffer DC, Kjartansson O, Hauser WA. Incidence of unprovoked seizures and epilepsy: Limited usefulness of the epilepsy syndrome classification in a population-based study. *Lancet Neurology* 2005; 4: 627-34.

Olfson M, Das AK, Gameroff MJ, Pilowsky D, Feder A, Gross R, Lantigua R, Shea S, Weissman MM. Bipolar depression in a low-income primary care clinic. *Am J Psychiatry* 2005; 162: 2146-51.

Oquendo MA, Lizardi D, Greenwald S, Weissman MM, Mann JJ. Rates of lifetime suicide attempt and rates of lifetime major depression in different ethnic groups in the United States. *Acta Psychiatr Scand* 2004; 110: 446-51.

Ott D, Caplan R, Guthrie D, Siddarth P, Komo S, Shields WD, Sankar R, Kornblum H, Chayasirisobhon S. Measures of psychopathology in children with complex partial seizures and primary generalized epilepsy with absence. *J Am Acad Child Adolesc Psychiatry* 2001; 40: 907-14.

Ottman R, Lipton RB. Comorbidity of migraine and epilepsy. *Neurology* 1994; 44: 2105.

Ottman R, Lipton RB. Is the comorbidity of epilepsy and migraine due to a shared genetic susceptibility? *Neurology* 1996; 47: 918-24.

Owens MJ, Nemeroff CB. Role of serotonin in the pathophysiology of depression: focus on the serotonin transporter. *Clin Chem* 1994; 40 (2): 288-95.

Patel NV, Bigal ME, Kolodner KB, Leotta C, Lafata JE, Lipton RB. Prevalence and impact of migraine and probable migraine in a health plan. *Neurology* 2004; 63: 1432-8.

Pauls DL, Shaywitz SE, Kramer PL, Shaywitz BA, Cohen DJ. Demonstration of vertical transmission of attenetion deficit disorder. *Ann Neurol* 1983; 14: 363.

Pich EM, Lorang M, Yegeneh M, Rodriguez de Fonseca F, Raber J, Koob GF, Weiss F. Increase of extracellular corticotrophin-releasing factor-like immunoreactibity levels in the amygdale of awake rats during restraint stress and ethanol withdrawal as measured by microdialyssi. *J Neuroschi* 1995; 15: 5439-47.

Pincus HA, Tanielian TL, Marcus SC, Olfson M, Zarin DA, Thompson J, Zito JM. Prescribing trends in psychotropic medications: Primary care, psychiatry, and other medical specialties. *JAMA* 1998; 279: 526-31.

Pini S, de Queiroz V, Pagnin D, Pezawas L, Angst J, Cassano GB, Wittchen H-U. Prevalence and burden of bipolar disorders in European countries. *Eur Neuropsychopharmacology* 2005; 15: 425-34.

Pisani F, Oteri G, Costa C, Di Raimondo G, Di Perri R. Effects of psychotropic drugs on seizure threshold. *Drug Safety* 2002; 25: 91-110.

Placencia M, Sander JW, Roman M, Madera A, Crespo F, Cascante S, Shorvon SD. The characteristics of epilepsy in a largely untreated population in rural Ecuador. *J Neurol Neurosurg Psychiatry* 1994; 57: 320-50.

Prudhomme C. Epilepsy and suicide. *J Nerv Ment Dis* 1941; 94: 722-31.

Racine R. Kindling: the first decade. *Neurosurgery* 1978; 3: 234-52.

Rafnsson V, Olafsson E, Hauser WA. Cause-specific mortality in adults with unprovoked seizures: A population-based incidence cohort study. *Neuroepidemiology* 2001: 20: 232-6.

Ramasubbu R, Tobias R, Buchan AM, Bech-Hansen NT. Serotonin transporter gene promoter region polymorphism associated with poststroke major depression. *J Neuropsychiatry Clin Neurosci* 2006; 18 (1): 96-9.

Riad M, Garcia S, Watkins KC, Jodoin N, Doucet E, Langlois X, El Mestikawy S, Hamon M, Descarries L. Somatodendritic localization of 5-HT1A and preterminal axonal localization of 5-HT1B serotonin receptors in adult rat brain. *JComp Neurol* 2000; 417 (2): 181-94.

Rorsman B, Grasbeck A, Hagnell O, Lanke J, Ohman R, Ojesjo L, Otterbeck L. A prospective study of first-incidence depression. TheLundby study, 1957-72. *Br J Psychiatry* 1990; 156: 336-42.

Russell MB, Olesen J. Increased familial risk and evidence of genetic factor in migraine. *BMJ* 1995; 311: 541-4.

Russel MB, Rasmussen BK, Fenger K, Olesen J. Migraine without aura and migraine with aura are distinct clinical entities: a study of four hundred and eighty-four male and female migraineurs from the general population. *Cephalagia* 1996; 16: 239-45.

Rutter M. Comorbidity: Meanings and Mechanisms. *Clin Psychol Sci Prac* 1994; 1: 100-3.

Sackeim HA, Decina P, Prohovnik I, Malitz S, Resor SR. Anticonvulsant and antidepressant properties of electroconvulsive therapy: a proposed mechanism of action. *Biol Psychiatry* 1983; 18: 1301-10.

Sanacora G, Gueorguieva R, Epperson CN, Wu Y-T, Appel M, Rothman DL, Krystal JH, Mason GF. Subtype-specific alterations of gamma-aminobutyric acid and glutamate in patients with major depression. *Arch Gen Psychiatry* 2004; 61 (7): 705-13.

Sareen J, Houlahan T, Cox BJ, Asmundson GJG. Anxiety disorders associated with suicidal ideation and suicide attempts in the National Comorbidity Survey. *J Nerv Ment Dis* 2005; 193: 450-4.

Simister RJ, McLean MA, Barker GJ, Duncan JS. Proton MRS reveals frontal lobe metabolite abnormalities in idiopathic generalized epilepsy. *Neurology* 2003; 61 (7): 897-902.

Sotelo C, Cholley B, El Mestikawy S, Gozlan H, Hamon M. Direct Immunohistochemical Evidence of the Existence of 5-HT1A Autoreceptors on Serotoninergic Neurons in the Midbrain Raphe Nuclei. *Eur J Neurosci* 1990; 2 (12): 1144-54.

Steljes TPV, Fullerton-Gleason L, Kuhls D, Shires GT, Fildes J. Epidemiology of suicide and the impact on Western Trauma Centers. *J Trauma* 2005; 58: 772-7.

Statnick MA, Maring-Smith ML, Clough RW, Wang C, Dailey JW, Jobe PC, Browning RA. Effect of 5,7-dihydroxytryptamine on audiogenic seizures in genetically epilepsy-prone rats. *Life Sci* 1996; 59 (21): 1763-71.

Stewart WF, Staffa J, Lipton RB, Ottman R. Familial risk of migraine: A population-based study. *Ann Neurology* 1997; 41: 166-72.

Suominen K, Isometsa E, Suokas J, Haukka J, Achte K, Lönnqvist J. Completed suicide after suicide attempt: A 37-year follow-up study. *Am J Psychiatry* 2004; 161: 563-4.

Ulrich V, Gervil M, Kyvik KO, Olesen J, Russell MB. The inheritance of migraine with aura estimated by means of structural equation modeling. *J Med Genet* 1999; 36: 225-7.

Velioglu SK, Boz C, Ozmenoglu M. The impact of migraine on epilepsy: a prospective prognosis study. *Cephalalgia* 2005; 25 (7): 528-35.

Wang W, Dow KE, Fraser DD. Elevated corticotrophin releasing hormone/corticotrophin releasing hormone-R1 expression in postmortem brain obtained from children with generalized epilepsy. *Ann Neurol* 2001; 50: 404-9.

Watanabe K, Minabe Y, Ashby CR, Jr., Katsumori H. Effect of acute administration of various 5-HT receptor agonists on focal hippocampal seizures in freely moving rats. *Eur J Pharmacol* 1998; 350: 2.

Weissman MM, Bland RC, Canino GJ, Greenwald S, Hwu H-G, Joyce PR, Daram EG, Lee C-K, Lellouch J, Lepine JP, newman SC, Rubio-Stipec M, Wells JE, Wickramaratne PJ, Wittchen H-U, Yeh EK. Prevalence of suicide ideation and suicide attempt in nine countried. *Psychological Med* 1999; 29: 9-17.

Williams J, Griebel ML, Dykman RA. Neuropsychological patterns in pediatric epilepsy. *Seizure* 1998; 7: 223-8.

Williams J, Schultz EG, Griebel ML. Seizure occurrence in children diagnosed with ADHD. *Clin Pediatrics* 2001; 40: 221-4.

Williams J Steel C, Sharp GB, DelosReyes E, Phillips T, Bates S, Lange B, Griebel ML Anxiety in children with epilepsy. *Epilepsy Behav* 2003; 4: 729-32.

Wittchen HU, Knauper B, Kessler RC. Lifetime risk of depression. *Br J Psychiatry Suppl* 1994 Dec; 16-22.

Yehuda R, Teicher MH, Trestman RL, Levengood RA, Siever LJ. Cortisol regulation in posttraumatic stress disorder and major depression: A chronobiological analysis. *Biol Psychiatry* 1996; 40: 79-88.

Zaccara O, Muscas C, Messori A. Clinical feature, pathogenesis and management of drug-induced seizures. *Drug Safety* 1990; 5: 109-51.

Commentary by Andres M. Kanner

Professor of Neurological Sciences and Psychiatry, Rush Medical College
Director, Laboratory of EEG and Video-EEG-Telemetry, Rush University Medical Center, Chicago, Illinois, USA

The data presented by Dr. Hersdorffer is expected to revolutionize the way we think of the relationship between psychiatric and epileptic disorders, as they demonstrate that not only are patients with epilepsy more likely to suffer from depression, anxiety and attention deficit disorders but patients with depression and attention deficit disorders have a significant greater risk to develop epilepsy (Forsgren, 1990; Hesdorffer, 2000; 2004; 2006). These data do not suggest that the former are a cause of the latter or vice-versa but suggest the presence of common pathogenic mechanisms shared by these conditions. Dr. Hersdorffer made brief mention of some of the common pathogenic mechanisms operant in depression and epilepsy. In this commentary I will expand on this topic.

Common neurotransmitter abnormalities in depression and seizure disorders

The neurotransmitters norepinephrine (NE), serotonin (5-hydroxytryptamine, 5HT), dopamine (DA) gamma-amino-butyric acid (GABA), glutamate and neuropeptides operant in the hypothalamic-pituitary-axis, particularly corticotropin releasing hormone (CRH) have been found to play important pathogenic mechanisms in the development of depression, anxiety and epileptic disorders.

Serotonergic and noradrenergic abnormalities

The pathogenic roles of serotonergic and noradrenergic mechanisms have been recognized for a long time and are the bases of the pharmacologic treatment of both psychiatric disorders. In the case of epilepsy, decreased 5HT and NE activity has been shown to facilitate the kindling of seizures, to exacerbate seizure severity and intensify seizure predisposition in some animal models of epilepsy, such as the genetically epilepsy prone rats (GEPR) (Jobe, 1999) with its two strains, GEPR-3 and GEPR-9. These animals have a genetically determined predisposition to sound-induced generalized tonic/clonic seizures (GTCS) (Jobe, 1994, 1999a, b; Dailey, 1989; Coffey, 1996; Yan, 1993). Both strains of rats have innate pre and postsynaptic noradrenergic and serotonergic transmission deficits, the former resulting from deficient arborization of neurons arising from the locus coeruleus coupled with excessive presynaptic suppression of stimulated NE release in the terminal fields and lack of postsynaptic compensatory up-regulation (Jobe, 1994, 1999a, b; Dailey, 1989; Coffey, 1996; Yan, 1993). Abnormal serotonergic arborization has also been identified in the GEPR's brain coupled with deficient postsynaptic serotonin$_{1A}$-receptor density in the hippocampus (Dailey, 1992). Of note, GEPRs display similar endocrine abnormalities to those identified in patients with major depressive disorder, such as increased cortisol serum levels, deficient secretion of growth hormone and hypothyroidism (Jobe).

A dose-dependent seizure-frequency reduction has been demonstrated in the GEPR that resulted from increments of either NE and/or 5HT transmission with the selective serotonin-re-uptake inhibitor (SSRIs) sertraline (Yan, 1993; 1995). In addition, the 5-HT precursor 5-HTP has been shown to have anticonvulsant effects when combined with a monoaminooxidase inhibitor (MAOI) (Meldrum, 1982), while SSRIs and MAOIs have been found to exert anticonvulsant effects in genetically prone epilepsy mice (Yan, 1993; 1995; Daily, 1992;

Jobe), baboons, non genetically-prone cats, rabbits and rhesus monkeys (Meldrum, 1982; Polc, 1979; Piette, 1963; Yanagita, 1980). Conversely, drugs that interfere with the release or synthesis of NE or 5HT have been found to exacerbate seizures in the GEPRs (Yan, 1993; 1995; Daily, 1992; Jobe, 1994); these include NE storage vesicle inactivators, reserpine or tetrabenazine, the NE false transmitter a-methyl-m-tryosine, the NE synthesis inhibitor a-Methyl-(D-tyrosine and the 5-HT synthesis inhibitor (D-chlorophenylalanine, all of which have also been found to facilitate seizure occurrence in humans (Naidoo, 1955; Noce, 1955; Tasher, 1955).

Lopez Meraz et al., reported an anticonvulsant effect of serotonergic activity in epilepsy models with Wistar rats (Lopez-Merez, 2005). They studied the impact of two $5HT_{1A}$ receptor agonists, 8-OH-DPAT and Indorenate, in three animal models of epileptic seizures (clonic-tonic induced by pentylenetetrazol (PTZ), status epilepticus of limbic seizures induced by kainic acid (KA) and tonic-clonic seizures induced by amygdala kindling) and found that 8-OH-DPAT lowered the incidence of seizures and the mortality induced by PTZ, increased the latency and reduced the frequency of wet-dog shake and generalized seizures induced by KA and at high doses diminished the occurrence and delayed the establishment of status epilepticus. Indorenate increased the latency to the PTZ-induced seizures and decreased the percentage of rats that showed tonic extension and death, augmented the latency to wet-dog shake and generalized seizures and diminished the number of generalized seizures.

Furthermore, AEDs with established psychotropic effects (CBZ, VPA and LTG) have been found to cause an increase in 5HT in animal models (Yan, 1992; Dailey, 1997a, b; 1998; Southman, 1998; Whitton, 1991). For example, the anticonvulsant protection of CBZ can be blocked with 5HT depleting drugs in GEPRs (Yan, 1992). Likewise, in a recent study, Clinkers et al., investigated the impact of oxcarbazepine (OXC) infusion on the extracellular hippocampal concentration of 5HT and DA in the focal pilocarpine model for limbic seizures (Clinckers, 2005a). When OXC was administered together with verapamil or probenecid (so as to ensure its passage through the blood-brain barrier), complete seizure remission was obtained associated with an increase in 5HT and DA extracellular concentrations (Clinckers, 2005b).

In addition, it has been suggested that the anticonvulsant effect of the vagal nerve stimulator (VNS) in the rat could be mediated by noradrenergic and serotonergic mechanisms, as destruction of noradrenergic and serotonergic neurons in the rat prevents or reduces significantly the anticonvulsant effect of VNS against electroshock or pentylenetetrazol induced seizures (Naritokku, 1995; Browning, 1997). Furthermore, it is believed that the effect of VNS on the locus coeruleus and raphe may be responsible for its antidepressant effects identified in humans (Nahas, 2005).

The impact of pharmacologic augmentation or reduction of 5HT and NE transmission on seizures in patients with epilepsy (PWE) has been rather sparse and mostly based on uncontrolled data. As already stated above, depletion of monoamines with reserpine has been associated with an increase in frequency and severity of seizures in PWE (Naidoo, 1956; Noce, 1955), while the use of reserpine was found to lower the electroshock seizure threshold and the severity of the resulting seizures in patients with schizophrenia (Tasher, 1955). The tricyclic antidepressant imipramine, with reuptake inhibitory effects of NE and 5HT was reported to suppress absence and myoclonic seizures in double-blind placebo-controlled studies (Fromm, 1971; 1972; 1978). Open trials with the SSRIs fluoxetine and citalopram yielded an improvement in seizure frequency, but no controlled studies with this class of antidepressants have been performed as of yet (Favale, 1995; Specchio, 2004). In a recent study, Alper et al. compared the incidence of seizures between patients with depression randomized to placebo or an antidepressant of the SSRI family, the serotonin-norepinephrine reuptake inhibitor (SNRI) venlafaxine or the α2 antagonist mirtazapine in regulatory studies submitted to the Food and Drug Administration (Alper, 2007). While the incidence of epileptic seizures in depressed patients randomized to placebo and an antidepressant was higher than that expected in the general population, patients treated with an antidepressant agent had significantly less seizures than those randomized to placebo. This study confirms the higher risk of depressed patients to experience epileptic seizures but suggest a protective effect of the antidepressants.

Dysfunction of the hypothalamic-pituitary-adrenal-axis in depressive disorders and epilepsy

The hypothalamic-pituitary-axis (HPA) plays a fundamental pathogenic role in mood disorders and epilepsy (Romero, 1996; Charney, 2004). Neurons in the paraventricular nucleus of the hypothalamus secrete CRH which stimulates the secretion of ACTH from the pituitary gland. ACTH, in turn, releases glucocorticoids from the adrenal gland, which have an impact on various brain regions and once in the circulation they exert an inhibitory effect on the HPA axis (Reul, 2002). Under normal conditions, hippocampus and amygdala play a role in the inhibition of the HPA axis as well (Herman, 1997). High levels of CRH and glucocorticoids occur in acute and chronic stress, in anxiety disorders, particularly post-traumatic stress disorder and depressive disorders (Van Praag, 2004). As shown below, both hormones at high concentrations have been associated with damage to neuronal cells in the hippocampal formation.

By the same token, an activation of the HPA axis demonstrated by an increase in the secretion of CRH, ACTH and cortisol has been found in humans postictally following generalized tonic-clonic and complex partial seizures as well as interictally. Wang et al. found significantly higher brain concentrations of CRH in postmortem brains from children with epilepsy compared to controls (Wang, 2001). A direct pathogenic role of CRH was suggested by Baram et al. in studies of infants with infantile spasms which were found to have low CSF ACTH and cortisol, which reflect a high brain CRH (Baram, 1999).

Glutamate: The interplay between the impact of high glucocorticoid levels and glutamate secretion in the hippocampus is of significant relevance in our attempts to understand the bidirectional relationship between depression and epilepsy. The role excitatory neurotransmitters and the glutamate receptor, N-methyl-D-aspartate (NMDA) site has been well established in epilepsy. Indeed, NMDA antagonists have been shown to have antiepileptogenic properties in the "kindling" animal model and to display as well antiepileptic properties. Recent data suggest their potential pathogenic role in depression (Del Rio, 2005). First, disturbances in glutamate metabolism, NMDA, and mGluR1,5 receptors have been implicated in depression and suicidality. Secondly, the NMDA receptor antagonists, group I metabotropic glutamate receptor (mGluR1 and mGluR5) antagonists, as well as positive modulators of alpha-amino-3-hydroxy-5-methyl-4-isoxazolepropionic acid (AMPA) receptors have been found to display antidepressant-like activity in a variety of preclinical models. Thirdly, a single intravenous dose of an NMDA receptor antagonist has been found to be sufficient to produce sustained relief from depressive symptoms.

The use of positron emission tomography (PET) and single photon emission tomography (SPECT) studies have yielded significant data suggestive of abnormal 5HT activity in primary depressive disorders and in epilepsy, with particular involvement of $5HT_{1A}$ receptors. Deficits in 5HT transmission in human depression is thought to be partially related to a paucity of serotonergic innervation of its terminal areas suggested by a scarcity of 5HT levels in brain tissue, plasma and platelets and with a deficit in serotonin transporter binding sites in postmortem human brain (Asberg, 1976; Brown, 1982; 1990; Roy, 1989; Langer, 1988; Nemeroff, 1988; Malison, 1998; Ogilvie, 1996; 1997; Cheetham, 1989, 1990; Stanley, 1982; Perry, 1983; Leake, 1991; Briley, 1980; Langer, 1981; Stockmeier, 1998). With respect to abnormal serotonergic activity in functional neuroimaging studies of patients with primary major depression, Sargent et al. demonstrated reduced $5HT_{1A}$ receptors binding potential of values in frontal, temporal, and limbic cortex with PET studies using [11C]WAY-100635 in both unmedicated and medicated depressed patients compared with healthy volunteers (Sragent, 2000). Of note, binding potential values in medicated patients were similar to those in unmedicated patients. Drevets et al. using the same radioligand reported a decreased binding potential of $5HT_{1A}$ receptors in mesial-temporal cortex and in the raphe in 12 patients with familial recurrent major depressive episodes, compared to controls (Drevets, 1999). A deficit in the density or affinity of postsynaptic $5HT_{1A}$ receptors has been identified in the hippocampus and amygdala of untreated depressed patients who committed suicide (Oguendo, 2003). In addition, impaired serotonergic transmission has been associated to defects in the dorsal raphe nuclei of suicide victims with major depressive disorder consisting of an excessive density of serotonergic somatodendritic impulse suppressing $5HT_{1A}$ autoreceptors (Leake, 1991).

Similar abnormalities have been reported in patients with epilepsy. In PET studies of patients with TLE using the $5HT_{1A}$ receptor antagonist ([18F] trans-4-fluro-N-2-[4-(2-methoxyphenyl)piperazin-1-yl]ethyl-N-(2-pyridyl) cyclohexanecarboxamide), reduced $5HT_{1A}$ binding were found in mesial temporal structures ipsilateral to the seizure focus in patients with and without hippocampal atrophy. Reduced serotonergic activity was independent of the presence or absence of hippocampal atrophy on MRI and reduced volume of distribution and binding remained significant after partial volume correction (Toczek, 2003). In addition a 20% binding reduction was found in the raphe and a 34% lower binding in the ipsilateral thalamic region to the seizure focus. In a separate PET study aimed at quantifying $5HT_{1A}$ receptor binding in 14 patients with TLE, a decreased binding was identified in the epileptogenic hippocampus, amygdala, anterior cingulate and lateral temporal neocortex ipsilateral to the seizure focus, as well as in the contralateral hippocampi, but to a lesser degree and in the raphe nuclei (Savic, 2004). A study using the $5HT_{1A}$ tracer, 4,2-(methoxyphenyl)-1-[2-(N-2-pyridinyl)-p-fluorobenzamido]ethylpiperazine ([^{18}F]MPPF), revealed that the decrease in binding of $5HT_{1A}$ was significantly greater in the areas of seizure-onset and propagation identified with intracranial electrode recordings. As in the other studies, reduction in $5HT_{1A}$ binding was present even when quantitative and qualitative MRI were normal (Merlet, 2004).

Dopamine: Tremblay et al., have recently demonstrated abnormal dopaminergic function in the brain of patients with primary major depressive disorders (Tremblay, 2005). Using functional MRI blood oxygen level-dependent activation during a controlled task and measurement of dextro-amphetamine subjective effects, patients with major depression had a two-fold increase in the response to the rewarding effects of dextro-amphetamine, compared to a group of 12 healthy controls. Abnormal brain activation was identified in the ventrolateral prefrontal cortex and orbitofrontal cortex as well as the caudate and putamen in the patient group.

Likewise, abnormal dopamine activity in the brain of patients with refractory epilepsy has been recently suggested in a PET study using 18F-fluoro-DOPA (Bouilleret, 2005). Three groups of patients were included: one consisted of 16 patients with a ring chromosome 20 (r20); a second group included 10 patients with absence-like epilepsy, while the third was integrated by nine patients with intractable TLE. Compared to a group of 10 healthy volunteers, patients from all three epilepsy groups displayed a decrease of 18F-fluro-DOPA uptake, but only patients with TLE was the decreased uptake lateralized to the side of the seizure focus. A bilateral uptake was found in the substantia nigra in all three patients groups.

Common neuroanatomical structures involved in depression and epilepsy

Structural changes in temporal lobes

Temporal lobe epilepsy is the most frequent type of epilepsy in adults and the most frequently associated with mood disorders, in addition to frontal lobe epilepsy. Mesial temporal sclerosis which consists of atrophy of mesial temporal structures is the most frequent type of TLE. Of note, structural changes in mesial temporal structures have been reported in patients with primary mood disorders. Indeed, Sheline *et al.* reported bilateral smaller hippocampal volumes in two separate studies of patients with a history of primary major depressive disorders in remission when compared to hippocampal volumes of age, sex and height-matched normal controls (Sheline, 1996; 1999). They also identified large hippocampal low signal foci ≥ 4.5 mm in diameter) and their number correlated with the total number of days depressed. A significant inverse correlation between the duration of depression and left hippocampal volume was also demonstrated, suggesting that patients with more chronic and active disease were more likely to have hippocampal atrophy. Atrophy has also been identified in entorhinal cortex and amygdala (Sheline, 1996; Bell-McGinty, 2002; Posener, 2003). Furthermore, in a neuropathologic study of amygdala and entorhinal cortex, a significant reduction of glial cells and of glial/neurons ratio were found in left amygdala and to a lesser degree in left entorhinal cortex of patients with major depressive and bipolar disorders compared to those of controls (Sheline, 1998).

By the same token, abnormalities of mesial temporal structures are among the most frequently identified in PWE and comorbid depression. In three studies of patients with TLE, higher scores of depression were associated with the presence of mesial temporal sclerosis (MTS), decreased temporal lobe and frontal lobe perfusion on (99m) Tc-HMPAO SPECT scans and a greater abnormalities identified with magnetic resonance spectroscopy (Gilliam, 2000; Quiske, 2000; Schmitz, 1997).

Hippocampal atrophy in primary major depressive disorders has been attributed to two potential pathogenic mechanisms: 1. An alteration in neurotrophic factors resulting from the mood disorder (Smith, 1995; Nibuya, 1995; Chen, 2001) and 2. high glucocorticoid exposure (Holsboer, 2001; 2003; Reul, 2002; Sapolsky, 2000).

Acute and chronic stress decreases levels of brain-derived neurotrophic factor (BDNF) in the dentate gyrus, pyramidal cell layer of hippocampus, amygdala and neocortex which may contribute to structural hippocampal changes (Smith, 1995). These changes are mediated by glucocorticoids and can be overturned with antidepressant therapy, as chronic administration of antidepressant drugs increased BDNF expression and also prevent a stress-induced decrease in BDNF levels (Nibuya, 1995; Chen, 2001). There is also evidence that antidepressant drugs can increase hippocampal BDNF levels in humans (Holsboer, 2001). These data indicate that antidepressant-induced upregulation of BDNF can hypothetically repair damage to hippocampal neurons and protect vulnerable neurons from additional damage.

The high glucocorticoid exposure mediating hippocampal atrophy is based on the excessive activation of the hypothalamic-pituitary-adrenal axis identified in almost half of individuals with depression resulting in impaired dexamethasone suppression of ACTH and cortisol. These changes are reversible to treatment with antidepressants (Holsboer, 2003). In experimental studies with rats and monkeys, prolonged increased concentrations of glucocorticoids have been found to damage hippocampal neurons, particularly CA3 pyramidal neurons, possibly by reduction of dendritic branching and loss of dendritic spines that are included in glutamatergic synaptic inputs (Sapolsky, 2000). Hypercortisolemia has also been found to interfere with the development of new granule cell neurons in the adult hippocampal dentate gyrus. Deleterious effects of chronic glucocorticoid exposure may lead initially to a transient and reversible atrophy of the CA3 dendritic tree, to an increased vulnerability to a variety of insults and finally result in cell death under extreme and prolonged conditions (Sapolsky, 2000).

Structural changes in frontal lobes

As stated above, frontal lobe epilepsy is among the seizure disorders with a relatively high comorbid mood disorders. In primary mood disorders, structural changes have been identified in the orbito-frontal and prefrontal cortex, cingulate gyrus as well as in their white matter, including smaller volume of orbito-frontal cortex in young adults and geriatric patients with major depressive disorder (Lai, 2000; Taylor, 2003a, b; Kumar, 1998). Involvement of frontal lobes in primary depression has also been demonstrated with functional neuroimaging (PET, SPECT) and neuropsychological studies (Liotti, 2002; Bromfield, 1990; Jokeit, 1997; Seidenberg, 1996; Hermann, 1987; Hempel, 1996). For example, executive abnormalities are consistently found among studies, and are more apparent in more severe depressive disorders. These neuropsychological disturbances correlated with reduced blood flow in mesial prefrontal cortex (Liotti, 2002). Furthermore, in tests demanding executive function, cingulate cortex and striatum could not be activated in patients with major depressive disorders. Functional disturbance of frontal lobe structures has been recognized in TLE and particularly among patients with TLE and comorbid depression, as they have been found to have bilateral reduction in infero-frontal metabolism (Bromfield, 1990; Jokeit, 1997). Likewise, neuropsychological testing with the Wisconsin Card Sorting Test (WCST), which is highly sensitive to executive dysfunction, has revealed poor performance in patients with TLE and comorbid depression (Seidenberg, 1996; Hermann, 1987; Hempel, 1996).

Neuropathological studies have also documented structural cortical changes in frontal lobes of depressed patients. Rajkowska *et al.* found decrease in cortical thickness, neuronal sizes, and neuronal densities in layers II, III and IV of the rostral orbito-frontal region in the brains of depressed patients (Rajkowska, 1999). In the caudal orbito-frontal cortex there were significant reductions in glial densities in cortical layers V and VI that were also associated with decreases in neuronal sizes. Finally in the dorsolateral prefrontal cortex there was a decrease in neuronal and glial density and size in all cortical layers.

Clinical implications

Clearly, the data presented above supports the suggestion that pathogenic mechanisms that are common to both depression and epilepsy may explain their bi-directional relationship. Of greater significance to the clinician is the question of the potential impact that such bi-directional relationship may have on the response to therapy when both conditions occur together. In other words, do the structural and functional neurologic abnormalities resulting from a lifetime depressive disorder change the response to pharmacologic and surgical treatment of epileptic seizures? Some data appear to suggest such possibility. For example, in a study of 890 patients with new onset epilepsy, Mohanraj and Brodie found that individuals with a history of psychiatric disorders were more than three times *less likely* to be seizure-free with antiepileptic drugs (median follow-up period was 79 months) than patients without a history of psychiatric disorders (Mohanraj, submitted). Similarly, among 121 patients who underwent a temporal lobectomy, Anhoury *et al.* reported a worse postsurgical seizure outcome for patients with a psychiatric history compared with those without a psychiatric history (Anhoury, 2000).

Given that depression (along with anxiety) is one of the most frequent psychiatric comorbidities in epilepsy, can depression predict a worse postsurgical outcome for patients who undergo a temporal lobectomy? In a study of 100 patients who had a temporal lobectomy and were followed for a mean period of 8.0 ± 3.3 years, the role of a lifetime history of depression as a predictor of postsurgical seizure outcome was investigated at the Rush Epilepsy Center (Kanner, 2006). Using a multivariate logistic regression model, we evaluated the covariates of a lifetime history of depression and psychiatric history in general, cause of temporal lobe epilepsy (*i.e.*, mesial temporal sclerosis, lesional, or idiopathic), duration of seizure disorder, occurrence of generalized tonic-clonic seizures and extent of resection of mesial temporal structures. We found that a lifetime history of depression and extent of resection of mesial temporal structures were two independent predictors of persistent auras in the absence of disabling seizures, while the cause of the temporal lobe epilepsy and a lifetime history of depression were both significant predictors of failure to achieve freedom from disabling seizures. The data in these three studies raise the question of whether a history of depression may be a marker of a more severe form of epilepsy.

These data raise the question of whether the existence of comorbid psychiatric disorders, and specifically mood disorders should be included among the variables to consider as potential predictors of response to therapy after a first epileptic seizure?

References

Alper K, Schwartz KA, Kolts RL, Khan A. Seizure Incidence in Psychopharmacological Clinical Trials: An Analysis of Food and Drug Administration (FDA) Summary Basis of Approval Reports. *Biol Psychiatry* 2007, in press.

Anhoury S, Brown RJ, Krishnamoorthy ES and Trimble MR. Psychiatric outcome after temporal lobectomy: a predictive study. *Epilepsia* 2000; 41: 1608-15.

Asberg M, Traskman L, Thoren P. 5-HIAA in the cerebrospinal fluid. A biochemical suicide predictor? *Arch Gen Psychiatry* 1976; 33: 1193-7.

Baram TZ, Mitchell WG, Brunson K, Haden E. Infantile spasms: hypothesis-driven therapy and pilot human infant experiments using corticotropin-releasing hormone receptor antagonists. *Dev Neurosci* 1999; 21 (3-5): 281-9.

Bell-McGinty S, Butters MA, Meltzer CC, Greer PJ, Reynolds CF 3rd, Becker JT. Brain Morphometric Abnormalities in Geriatric Depression: Long Term Neurobiological Effects of Illness Duration. *American Journal of Psychiatry* 2002; 159 (8): 1424-7.

Bouilleret V, Semah F, Biraben A, Taussig D, Chassoux F, Syrota A, Ribeiro MJ. Involvement of the basal ganglia in refractory epilepsy: an 18-F-fluoro-L-DOPA PET study using 2 methods of analysis. *J Nucl Med* 2005; 46: 540-7.

Briley MS, Langer SZ, Raisman R, Sechter D, Zarifian E. Tritiated imipramine binding sites are decreased in platelets of untreated depressed patients. *Science* 1980; 209: 303-5.

Bromfield E, Altshuler L, Leiderman D. Cerebral metabolism and depression in patients with complex partial seizures. *Epilepsia* 1990; 31: 625.

Brown GL, Ebert MH, Goyer PF *et al.* Aggression, suicide, and serotonin: relationships to CSF amine metabolites. *Am J Psychiatry* 1982; 139: 741-6.

Brown GL, Linnoila MI. CSF serotonin metabolite (5-HIAA) studies in depression, impulsivity, and violence. *J Clin Psychiatry* 1990; 51 (suppl): 31-41.

Browning, Ra, Clark KB, Naritoku, DK, Smith DC and Jensen RA. Loss of anticonvulsant effect of vagus nerve stimulation in the pentylenetetrazol seizure model following treatment with 6-hydroxydopamine or 5,7-dihydroxy-tryptamine. *Soc Neurosci* 1997; 23: 2424.

Charney DS and Bremner JD. The neurobiology of anxiety disorders. In: *Neurobiology of Mental Illness*, Second Edition. DS Charney, EJ Nestler, eds. New York, Oxford University Press, 2004: 605-27.

Cheetham SC, Crompton MR, Czudek C, Horton RW, Katona CL, Reynolds GP. Serotonin concentrations and turnover in brains of depressed suicides. *Brain Res* 1989; 502: 332-40.

Cheetham SC, Crompton MR, Katona CL, Horton RW. Brain 5-HT1 binding sites in depressed suicides. *Psychopharmacology* 1990; 102: 544-8.

Chen B, Dowlatshahi D, MacQueen GM, Wang JF, Young LT. Increased hippocampal BDNF immunoreactivity in subjects treated with antidepressant medication. *Biol Psychiatry* 2001; 50: 260-5.

Clinckers R, Smolders I, Meurs A, Ebinger G, Michotte Y. Hippocampal dopamine and serotonin elevations as pharmacodynamic markers for the anticonvulsant efficacy of oxcarbazepine and 10,11-dihydro-10-hydroxicarbamazepine. *Neurosci Lett* 2005a; 16: 390: 48-53.

Clinckers R, Smolders I, Meurs A, Ebinger G, Michotte Y. Quantitative in-vivo microdialysis study on the influence of multidrug transporters on the blood-brain barrier passage of oxcarbazepine: concomitant use of hippocampal monoamines as pharmacodynamic markers for the anticonvulsant activity. *J Pharmacol Exp Ther* 2005b; 314: 725-31.

Coffey LL, Reith MEA, Chen NH, Jobe PC, Mishra PK. Amygdala Kindling of Forebrain Seizures and the Occurrence of Brainstem Seizures in Genetically Epilepsy-Prone Rats. *Epilepsia* 1996; 37: 188-97.

Dailey JW, Mishra PK, Ko KH, Penny JE, Jobe PC. Serotonergic abnormalities in the central nervous system of seizure-naive genetically epilepsy-prone rats. *Life Sci* 1992; 50: 319-26.

Dailey JW, Reigel CE, Mishra PK, Jobe PC. Neurobiology of seizure predisposition in the genetically epilepsy-prone rat. *Epilepsy Res* 1989; 3: 3-17.

Dailey JW, Reith ME, Steidley KR, Milbrandt JC, Jobe PC. Carbamazepine-induced release of serotonin from rat hippocampus in vitro. *Epilepsia* 1998; 39 (10): 1054-63.

Dailey JW, Reith MEA, Yan QS, Li MY, Jobe PC. Anticonvulsant doses of carbamazepine increase hippocampal extracellular serotonin in genetically epilepsy-prone rats: dose response relationships. *Neurosci Lett* 1997a; 227 (1): 13-6.

Dailey JW, Reith ME, Yan QS, Li MY, Jobe PC. Carbamazepine increases extracellular serotonin concentration: lack of antagonism by tetrodotoxin or zero Ca2+. *Eur J Pharmacol* 1997b; 328 (2-3): 153-62.

Del Rio J, Frechilla D. Glutamate and depression. In *Dopamine and Glutamate in Psychiatric Disorders*. WJ Schmidt, MEA Reith, eds, Humana Press, Totowa, NJ, 2005: 205-36.

Drevets WC, Frank E, Price JC, Kupfer DJ, Holt D, Greer PJN, Huang Y, Gautier C, Mathis C. PET imaging of serotonin 1A receptor binding in depression. *Biol Psychiatry* 1999; 46: 1375-87.

Favale E, Rubino V, Mainardi P, Lunardi G, and Albano C. The anticonvulsant effect of fluoxetine in humans. *Neurology* 1995; 45: 1926.

Forsgren L, Nystrom L. An incident case referent study of epileptic seizures in adults. *Epilepsy Research* 1990; 6: 66-81.

Fromm GH, Amores CY and Thies W. Imipramine in epilepsy, *Arch Neurol* 1972; 27: 198.

Fromm GH, Rosen JA and Amores CY. Clinical and experimental investigation of the effect of imipramine on epilepsy. *Epilepsia* 1971; 12: 282.

Fromm GH, Wessel HB, Glass JD, Alvin JD, VanHorn G. Imipramine in absence and myoclonic-astatic seizures. *Neurology* 1978; 28: 953.

Gilliam F, Maton B, Martin RC et al., Extent of 1H spectroscopy abnormalities independently predicts mood status and quality of life in temporal lobe epilepsy. *Epilepsia* 2000; 41 (suppl): 54.

Hempel A, Risse GL, Mercer K, Gates J. Neuropsychological evidence of frontal lobe dysfunction in patients with temporal lobe epilepsy. *Epilepsia* 1996; 37 (suppl 5): 119.

Hermann BP, Wyler AR, Richey ET. Epilepsy, frontal lobes and personality. *Biol Psychiatry* 1987; 22: 1055-7.

Hermann BP, Wyler AR, Richey ET. Wisconsin card sorting test performance in patients with complex partial seizures of temporal-lobeorigin. *J Clin Exp Neuropsychol* 1988; 10: 467-76.

Herman JP and Cullinan WE. Neurocircuitry of stress: central control of the hypothalamo-pituitary-adrenocortical axis. *Trends Neurosci* 1997; 20: 78-84.

Hesdorffer DC, Hauser WA, Annegers JF et al. Major depression is a risk factor for seizures in older adults. *Annals of Neurology* 2000; 47: 246-9.

Hesdorffer DC, Ludvigsson P, Olafsson E, Gudmundsson, G, Kjartansson O, Hauser WA. ADHD as a risk factor for incident unprovoked seizures and epilepsy in children. *Archives of General Psychiatry* 2004; 61: 731-6.

Hesdorffer DC, Hauser WA, Olafsson E, Ludvigsson P, Kjartansson O. Depression and suicidal attempt as risk factor for incidental unprovoked seizures. *Ann Neurol* 2006.

Holsboer F. Stress, hypercortisolism and corticosteroid receptors in depression: implications for therapy. *J Affect Disord* 2001; 62: 77-91.

Holsboer F. Corticotropin-releasing hormone modulators and depression. *Curr Opin Investig Drugs* 2003; 4: 46-50.

Jobe PC. Affective Disorder and Epilepsy Comorbidity in the Genetically Epilepsy Prone-Rat (GEPR). In: Gilliam F, Kanner AM, Sheline YI. *Depression and Brain Dysfunction*. London: Taylor & Francis: 121-57.

Jobe PC, Dailey JW, Wernicke JF. A noradrenergic and serotonergic hypothesis of the linkage between epilepsy and affective disorders. *Crit Rev Neurobiol* 1999a; 13: 317-356.

Jobe PC, Mishra PK, Browning RA et al. Noradrenergic abnormalities in the genetically epilepsy-prone rat. *Brain Res Bull* 1994; 35: 493-504.

Jobe PC, Mishra PK, Dailey JW, Ko KH, Reith MEA. Genetic predisposition to partial (focal) seizures and to generalized tonic/clonic seizures: Interactions between seizure circuitry of the forebrain and brainstem. In: Berkovic SF, Genton P, Hirsch E, Picard F, eds. *Genetics of Focal Epilepsies*. Paris: John Libbey, 1999b: 251.

Jokeit H, Seitz RJ, Markowitsch HJ, Neumann N, Witte OW, Ebner A. Prefrontal asymmetric interictal glucosa hypometabolism and cognitive impairment in patients with temporal lobe epilepsy. *Brain* 1997; 12: 2283-94.

Kanner AM, Byrne R, Smith MC, Balabanov AJ, Frey M. *Does a life-time history of Depression predicts a worse postsurgical seizure outcome following a temporal lobectomy?* Presented at the annual meeting of the American Neurological Association, Chicago, IL, 2006.

Kumar A, Zhisong J, Warren B, Jayaram U, Gottlieb G. Late-Onset Minor and Major Depression: Early Evidence for Common Neuroanatomical Substrates Detected by Using MRI. *Proc Natl Acad Sci USA* 1998; 95 (13): 7654-8.

Lai T, Payne ME, Byrum CE, Steffens DC, Krishnan Kr. Reduction of Orbital Frontal Cortex Volume in Geriatric Depression. *Biol Psychiatry* 2000; 48 (10): 971-5.

Langer SZ, Galzin AM. Studies on the serotonin transporter in platelets. *Experientia* 1988; 44: 127-30.

Langer SZ, Zarifian E, Briley M, Raisman R, Sechter D. High-affinity binding of 3H-imipramine in brain and platelets and its relevance to the biochemistry of affective disorders. *Life Sci* 1981; 29: 211-20.

Leake A, Fairbairn AF, McKeith IG, Ferrier IN. Studies on the serotonin uptake binding site in major depressive disorder and control post-mortem brain: neurochemical and clinical correlates. *Psychiatry Research* 1991; 39: 155-65.

Liotti M, Mayberg H, McGinnis S, Brennan SL, Jerabek P. Unmasking disease specific cerebral blood flow abnormalities: mood challenge in patients with remitted unipolar depression. *Am J Psychiatry* 2002; 159: 1830-40.

Lopez-Meraz ML, Gonzalez-Trujano ME, Neri-Bazan L, Hong E, Rocha LL. 5-HT1A receptor agonists modify seizures in three experimental models in rats. *Neuropharmacology* 2005; 49: 367-75.

Malison RT, Price LH, Berman R et al. Reduced brain serotonin transporter availability in major depression as measured by [123I]-2 beta-carbomethoxy-3 beta-(4-iodophenyl)tropane and single photon emission computed tomography. *Biol Psychiatry* 1998; 44: 1090-8.

Meldrum BS, Anlezark GM, Adam HK, and Greenwod DT. Anticonvulsant and proconvulsant properties of viloxazine hydrohloride: pharmacological and pharmacokinetic studies in rodents and epileptic baboon. *Psychopharmacology* 1982; 76: 212.

Merlet I, Ostrowsky K, Costes N, Ryvlin P, Isnard J, Faillenot I, Lavenne F, Dufournel D, Le Bars D, Mauguiere F. 5-HT1A receptor binding and intracerebral activity in temporal lobe epilepsy: an [18F]MPPF-PET study. *Brain* 2004; 127: 900-13.

Mohanraj R and Brodie MJ. Predicting outcomes in newly diagnosed epilepsy. *Epilepsia* 2003; 44 (suppl 9): 15 (Abstract).

Nahas Z, Marangell LB, Husain MM, Rush AJ, Sackeim HA, Lisanby SH, Martinez JM, George MS. Two-year outcome of vagus nerve stimulation (VNS) for treatment of major depressive episodes. *J Clin Psychiatry*. 2005; 66 (9): 1097-104.

Naidoo D. The effects of reserpine (serpasil) on the chronic disturbed schizophrenic: a comparative study of rauwolfia alkaloids and electroconvulsive therapy. *J Nerv Ment Dis* 1956: 123.

Naritokku DK, Terry WJ, and Helfert RH. Regional induction of fos immunoreactivity in the brain by anticonvulsant stimulation of the vagus nerve. *Epilepsy Res* 1995; 22: 53.

Nemeroff CB, Knight DL, Krishnan RR et al. Marked reduction in the number of platelet-tritiated imipramine binding sites in geriatric depression. *Arch Gen Psychiatry* 1988; 45: 919-23.

Nibuya M, Morinobu S, Duman RS. Regulation of BDNF and trkB mRNA in rat brain by chronic electroconvulsive seizure and antidepressant drug treatments. *J Neurosci* 1995; 15: 7539-47.

Noce RH, Williams DB and Rapaport W. Reserpine (serpasil) in management of the mentally ill. *JAMA* 1955; 158: 11.

Ogilvie AD, Battersby S, Bubb VJ et al. Polymorphism in serotonin transporter gene associated with susceptibility to major depression. *Lancet* 1996; 347: 731-3.

Ogilvie AD, Harmar AJ. Association between the serotonin transporter gene and affective disorder: the evidence so far. *Mol Med* 1997; 3: 90-3.

Oguendo MA, Placidi GP, Malone KM et al. Positron emission tomography of regional brain metabolic responses to a serotonergic challenge and lethality of suicide attempts in major depression. *Arch Gen Psychiatry* 2003; 60: 14-22.

Perry EK, Marshall EF, Blessed G, Tomlinson BE, Perry RH. Decreased imipramine binding in the brains of patients with depressive illness. *Br J Psychiatry* 1983; 142: 188-92.

Piette Y, Delaunois AL, De Shaepdryver AF and Heymans C. Imipramine and electroshock threshold. *Arch Int Pharmacodyn Ther* 1963; 144: 293.

Polc P, Schneeberger J, and Haefely, W. Effects of several centrally active drugs on the sleep wakefulness cycle of cats. *Neuropharmacology* 1979; 18: 259.

Posener JA, Wang L, Price JL, Gado HM, Province MA, Miller MI, Babb CM, Csernansky JG. High-Dimensional Mapping of the Hippocampus in Depression. *American Journal of Psychiatry* 2003; 160: 83-9.

Quiske A, Helmstaedter C, Lux S et al., Depression in patients with temporal lobe epilepsy is related to mesial temporal sclerosis. *Epilepsy Res* 2000; 39 (2): 121-5.

Rajkowska G, Miguel-Hidalgo JJ, Wei J, Dilley G, Pittman SD, Meltzer HY, Overholser JC, Roth BL, Stockmeier CA. Morphometric Evidence for Neuronal and Glial Prefrontal Cell Pathology in Major Depression. *Biol Psychiatry* 1999; 45 (9): 1085-98.

Reul JM, Holsboer F. Corticotropin-releasing factor receptors 1 and 2 in anxiety and depression. *Curr Opin Pharmacol* 2002; 2: 23-33.

Reul JM, Holsboer F. Corticotropin-releasing factor receptors 1 and 2 in anxiety and depression. *Curr Opin Pharmacol* 2002; 2: 23-33.

Romero LM and Sapolsky RM. Patterns of ACTH secretagog secretion in response to psychological stimuli. *J Neuroendocriol* 1996; 8: 243-58.

Roy A, De Jong J, Linnoila M. Cerebrospinal fluid monoamine metabolites and suicidal behavior in depressed patients. A 5-year follow-up study. *Arch Gen Psychiatry* 1989; 46: 609-12.

Sapolsky RM. Glucocorticoids and hippocampal atrophy in neuropsychiatric disorders. *Arch Gen Psychiatry* 2000; 57: 925-35.

Sargent PA, Kjaer KH, Bench CJ, Rabiner EA, Messa C, Meyer J, Gunn RN, Grasby PM, Cowen PJ. Brain serotonin1A receptor binding measured by positron emission tomography with [11C]WAY-100635: effects of depression and antidepressant treatment. *Arch Gen Psychiatry* 2000; 57: 174-80.

Savic I, Lindstrom P, Gulyas B, Halldin C, Andree B, Farde L. Limbic reductions of 5-HT1A receptor binding in human temporal lobe epilepsy. *Neurology* 2004; 62: 1343-51.

Schmitz EB, Moriarty J, Costa JC et al. Psychiatric profiles and patterns of cerebral blood flow in focal epilepsy: interactions between depression, obsessionality, and perfusion related to the laterality of the epilepsy. *J Neurol Neurosurg Psychiatry* 1997; 62 (5): 458-63.

Seidenberg M, Hermann BP, Noe A. Depression in temporal lobe epilepsy: a possible role for associated frontal lobe dysfunction?. In: *Psychological disturbances in epilepsy*, Sackellares JC, Berent S, ed. Newton, MA: Butterworth-Heinemann, 1996: 143-57.

Sheline YI. Brain structural changes associated with depression. In: Gilliam F, Kanner AM, Sheline YI. *Depression and Brain Dysfunction*. London: Taylor & Francis: 85-104.

Sheline YI, Gado MH, Price JL. Amygdala Core Nuclei Volumes are Decreased in Recurrent Major Depression. *Neuroreport* 22, 1998; 9 (9): 2023-8.

Sheline YI, Sanghavi M, Mintun MA et al., Depression duration but not age predicts hippocampal volume loss in medically healthy women with recurrent major depression. *J Neurosci* 1999; 19 (12): 5034-43.

Sheline YI, Wang PW, Gado MH et al., Hippocampal atrophy in recurrent major depression. *Proc Natl Acad Sci USA* 1996; 93 (9): 3908-13.

Smith MA, Makino S, Kvetnansky R, Post RM. Effects of stress on neurotrophic factor expression in the rat brain. *Ann N Y Acad Sci* 1995; 771: 234-9.

Southam E, Kirkby D, Higgins GA, Hagan RM. Lamotrigine inhibits monoamine uptake *in vitro* and modulates 5-hydroxytryptamine uptake in rats. *Eur J Pharmacol* 1998; 358 (1): 19-24.

Specchio LM, Iudice A, Specchio N, La Neve A, Spinelli A, Galli R, Rocchi R, Ulivelli M, de Tommaso M, Pizzanelli C, Murri L. Citalopram as treatment of depression in patients with epilepsy. *Clin Neuropharmacol* 2004; 27 (3): 133-6.

Stanley M, Virgilio J, Gershon S. Tritiated imipramine binding sites are decreased in the frontal cortex of suicides. *Science* 1982; 216: 1337-9.

Stockmeier CA, Shapiro LA, Dilley GE, Kolli TN, Friedman L, Rajkowska G. Increase in serotonin-1A autoreceptors in the midbrain of suicide victims with major depression-postmortem evidence for decreased serotonin activity. *J Neurosci* 1998; 18: 7394-401.

Tasher, DC and Chermak, MW. The use of reserpine in shock-reversible patients and shock-resistent patients. *Ann NY Acad Sci* 1955; 61: 108.

Taylor WD, MacFall Jr, Steffens DC, Payne ME, Provenzale JM, Krishnan KR. Localization of Age-Associated White Matter Hyperintensities in Late-Life Depression. *Prog Neuropsychopharmacol Biol Psychiatry* 2003b; 27 (3): 539-44.

Taylor WD, Steffens DC, McQuoid DR, Payne ME, Lee SH, Lai TJ, Krishnan Kr. Smaller Orbital frontal Cortex Volumes Associated with Functional Disability in Depressed Elders. *Biol Psychiatry* 2003a; 53 (2): 144-9.

Toczek MT, Carson RE, Lang L, Ma Y, Spanaki MV, Der MG, Fazilat S, Fazilat S, Kopylev L, Herscovitch P, Eckelman WC, Theodore WH. PET imaging of 5-HT1A receptor binding in patients with temporal lobe epilepsy. *Neurology* 2003; 60: 749-56.

Tremblay LK, Naranjo CA, Graham SJ, Herrmann N, Mayberg H, Hevenor S, Busto UE. Functional neuroanatomical substrates of altered reward processing in major depressive disorder revealed by a dopamine probe. *Arch Gen Psychiatry* 2005; 62: 1228-36.

Van Praag HM, de Kloet R, van Os J. Stress the brain and depression. In: *Stress the brain and Depression*, Cambridge University Press, 2004: 225-59.

Wang W, Dow KE, Fraser DD. Elevated corticotropin releasing hormone/corticotropin releasing hormone-R1 expression in postmortem brain obtained from children with generalized epilepsy. *Ann Neurol* 2001; 50 (3): 404-9.

Whitton PS, Fowler LJ. The effect of valproic acid on 5-hydroxytryptamine and 5-hydroxyindoleacetic acid concentration in hippocampal dialysates *in vivo*. *Eur J Pharmacol* 1991; 200: 167-9.

Yanagita T, Wakasa Y and Kiyohara H. Drug- dependance potential of viloxazine hydrochloride tested in rhesus monkeys. *Pharmacol BiochemBehav* 1980; 12: 155.

Yan QS, Jobe PC, Dailey JW. Thalamic deficiency in norepinephrine release detected via intracerebral microdialysis: a synaptic determinant of seizure predisposition in the genetically epilepsy-prone rat. *Epilepsy Res* 1993; 14: 229-36.

Yan QS, Jobe PC, Dailey JW. Further evidence of anticonvulsant role for 5-hydroxytryptamine in genetically epilepsy prone rats. *Br J Pharmacol* 1995; 115: 1314-8.

Yan QS, Jobe PC, Dailey JW. Evidence that a serotonergic mechanism is involved in the anticonvulsant effect of fluoxetine in genetically epilepsy-prone rats. *Eur J Pharmacol* 1993; 252 (1): 105-12.

Yan QS, Mishra PK, Burger RL, Bettendorf AF, Jobe PC, Dailey JW. Evidence that carbamazepine and antiepilepsirine may produce a component of their anticonvulsant effects by activating serotonergic neurons in genetically epilepsy-prone rats. *J Pharmacol Exp Ther* 1992; 261: 652-9.

Epileptic seizures in the context of the dysimmune syndromes

Sean T. Hwang, Frank G. Gilliam

The Neurological Institute, Columbia University, New York, USA

Anecdotal evidence in the literature suggests an association of seizures and epilepsy with a various number of autoimmune disorders. Seizures have been recognized to occur in a relatively higher rate than expected in type 1 diabetes, autoimmune thyroiditis, systemic lupus erythematous, celiac disease, sarcoidosis, Sjogren syndrome, and Bechet disease among others. Whether seizures and epilepsy occur as a direct effect of the autoimmune process, as a complication of the underlying disease, or due to a common genetic propensity, has yet to be discerned. Additionally, a number of epilepsy syndromes have come under scrutiny, due to possible associations with underlying dysimmune processes, such as Rasmussen encephalitis, Landau Kleffner syndrome, West syndrome, and Lennox-Gastaut syndrome.

Serologic markers now exist for several of the autoimmune disorders. Autoantibodies associated with several of the disorders, may be helpful in their diagnosis, and may additionally offer insight into their pathogenesis and treatment. In the case of one or more organ specific autoantibodies associated with an immune processes, it may be hypothesized that the antibodies manage to interfere with the normal function of the brain, creating an environment conducive to seizures, either directly or indirectly. Alternatively, the finding of certain antibodies in the context of systemic disease could ultimately be determined to be incidental, and amount to nothing more than nonspecific markers of the process of associated inflammation.

Ideally, in order to better offer evidence for a disorder, such as a specific epilepsy, being autoimmune mediated, there are a number of conditions that must be met. A target of the immune system should be identifiable. Next, an immune response should be discerned, either by the identification of corresponding antibodies or cell-mediated immunity. A plausible mechanism for the manifestations of the disease should exist, and an analogous autoimmune response should be elicited from experimental animal models (Aarli, 2000; Palace and Lang, 2000). Lastly, a beneficial response to modification of the immune process can be potentially helpful when observed.

Much of the current data is associative rather than offering conclusive causative evidence for the development of epilepsy in the various syndromes. However, these associations may offer further insight into the pathogenic contributions of the immune system in epilepsy, the genetic predispositions towards epilepsy and concurrent illness, and distinct potential modalities of treatment (Table I).

Table I. An overview of antibodies associated with epilepsy

Epilepsy associated autoantibody	Antigen function	Associated clinical syndromes
Glutamic acid decarboxylase antibody (GAD Ab)	Enzymatic conversion of L-glutamic acid to GABA	SPS, T1D, cerebellar ataxia, palatal myoclonus, thyroid disorders, encephalitis
Thyroid peroxidase antibody (TPO Ab)	Enzymatic iodinatation of thyroglobulin	Hashimoto's thyroiditis, Graves' disease, Hashimoto's encephalopathy
Anti-thyroglobulin antibody (TG Ab)	Thyroid hormone precursor	Hashimoto's thyroiditis, Hashimoto's encephalopathy
TSH receptor antibody (TR Ab)	Endocrine receptor	Graves disease
Anti-phospholipid antibodies (aPL Abs)	Proteins bound to cell membrane phospholipid	SLE, APS, medications, Bechet disease
Glutamate receptor subunit 3 antibody (GluR3 Ab)	Ligand gated ion channel receptor component	Rasmussen encephalitis, EPC
Glutamate receptor subunit epsilon 2 (GluRε2 Ab)	Glutamate receptor component	Rasmussen encephalitis, EPC
Antibody to the mammalian analogue to the UNC-18 gene (MUNC-18 Ab)	Involved with exocytic secretion of neurotransmitter	Rasmussen encephalitis
Alpha 7 acetylcholine receptor antibody (A7-nACH Ab)	Nicotinic receptor	Rasmussen encephalitis
Antigliadin antibody (AG Ab)	Gluten component	Celiac disease, cerebral calcifications
Tissue transglutaminase antibody (tTG Ab)	Enzyme modifying gliadin	Celiac disease
Voltage gated potassium channel antibody (VGKC Ab)	Ion channel protein	Isaac syndrome, limbic encephalitis
Anti-GM1 ganglioside antibody (GM-1 Ab)	Synaptic membrane component	SLE, Waldenstrom macroglobulinemia
Anti-mitochondrial antibody	Mitochondrial protein	Primary biliary sclerosis, infections, medications, graft vs host disease, myocardial infarction
Anti-endothelial antibody	Specialized epithelium	Landau-Kleffner syndrome, autism
Myelin basic protein antibody (MBP Ab)	Myelin component	Landau-Kleffner syndrome, autism

GABA, γ-aminobutyric acid; SPS, stiff-person syndrome; T1D, type 1 diabetes; SLE, systemic lupus erythematous; APS, antiphospholipid syndrome; EPC, epilepsy partialis continua

Type 1 diabetes and epilepsy

Type 1 diabetes (T1D), previously called insulin-dependent diabetes mellitus (IDDM) or juvenile-onset diabetes, results from T-cell immune mediated destruction of pancreatic beta cells responsible for the production of insulin and the regulation of blood glucose (Tisch and McDevitt, 1996). The onset of this form of diabetes is typically observed in the young, although it may occur at any age, and accounts for 5 to 10% of all diagnosed cases of diabetes. The NIH estimates the prevalence of T1D in children and adolescents in the U.S. to be between 0.17 to 0.25% (National Institute of Diabetes and Digestive and Kidney Diseases, 2005), although incidence varies by racial and ethnic groups worldwide. Approximately 90% of cases are sporadic, although first-degree relatives of patients with T1D are at increased risk compared to the general population.

Markers of the destructive immune process resulting in the disease include several autoantibodies including those directed towards islet cells, insulin, tyrosine phosphatase IA-2, glutamic acid decarboxylase (GAD Abs) (Baekkeskov et al., 1990; Wasserfall and Atkinson, 2006). These autoantibodies are detected in 80 to 90% of individuals with T1D, and may be present several years prior to the development of the clinical manifestations of the disease (De Aizpurua et al., 1992; Hagopian et al., 1993). Various MHC-class II associations have also been described (She, 1996). In a minority of patients no evidence of autoimmunity is present, and in such circumstances the disease is considered idiopathic (Expert Committee on the Diagnosis and Classification of Diabetes Mellitus, 2003). Patients with autoimmune T1D also have a higher incidence of other autoimmune disorders such as Graves disease, Hashimoto thyroiditis, celiac disease, Addison disease, vitiligo, and pernicious anemia (Barker, 2006).

Seizures as a consequence of hypoglycemia are well known to occur (The Diabetes Control and Complications Trial Research Group, 1997). Type 1 diabetics in hyperglycemic ketoacidosis experience seizures less frequently in contrast to patients in non-ketotic hyperglycemia or hyperosmolar coma, as typically seen in type 2 diabetics, who more commonly have seizures as a complication. Theoretically, this may be due to the protective effect of ketoacidosis increasing the availability γ-aminobutyric acid (GABA) (Singh and Strobos, 1980).

Several EEG abnormalities have been described in individuals with T1D. In comparison to healthy controls, adolescents with T1D have a greater degree of slow wave activity and a lower peak alpha frequency in the frontal regions, as well as decreased fast frequency activity in the posterior temporal regions (Hyllienmark et al., 2005). Adults with T1D generally have decreased alpha and beta activity in the posterior temporal regions, and a lower peak frequency bilaterally in the temporo-central regions (Brismar et al., 2002).

Earlier neurophysiologic studies of children with T1D, noted paroxysmal non-rhythmic generalized slow-wave abnormalities were observed in patients with a specific history of recurrent hypoglycemia (Eeg-Olofsson, 1977). Children with labile glycemic control have been found to be more likely to have abnormalities on EEG including including generalized discharges and focal sharp waves (Halonen et al., 1983). Quantitative EEG methods, have demonstrated that a history of severe hypoglycemia is correlated with an increase in fronto-central theta activity and a decrease in alpha power in children (Bjorgaas et al., 1996), a global increase in theta activity in adolescents (Hyllienmark et al., 2005), and decreased global beta activity in adults (Howorka et al., 2000). Poor metabolic control, as measured by acute and chronic hemoglobin A1C levels, has been shown in adolescents to be associated with increased delta activity and a decrease in peak alpha frequency (Hyllienmark et al., 2005).

While some of the EEG abnormalities that have been observed in persons with T1D have been attributed to a consequence of hypoglycemic episodes, others are not. Eeg-Olofson observed an 11% prevalence of paroxysmal epileptiform abnormalities on EEG in comparison to that of 2.7% in normal control subjects, representing a four-fold increase (Eeg-Olofsson, 1977).

A recent publication from the U.K. examined the relationship between T1D and idiopathic generalized epilepsy (IGE) (McCorryc et al., 2006). The investigators observed a two to nine fold increase in the prevalence of insulin dependent diabetes in a cohort of 518 patients ages 15-30 years-old with a diagnosis of idiopathic generalized epilepsy, compared to the a background population of 150,000 patients from a regional area. Seven patients in the IGE cohort were found to have insulin dependent diabetes, in comparison to the expected rate of 0.3% observed in the general population. The diagnosis of T1D preceded that of epilepsy in all of the cases where such information was available. In the patients with a concomitant diagnosis of idiopathic generalized epilepsy and T1D, an EEG pattern of generalized spike and wave abnormalities was observed. Absence epilepsy was notably absent. The authors appropriately advised approaching the data with caution given the cohort size and its derivation from the database of a tertiary epilepsy center, possibly subject to referral bias. Nevertheless, this was the first published study to suggest an association between IGE and T1D.

Of the several immunological markers of T1D, special attention has been directed to the association of glutamic acid decarboxylase antibodies (GAD Abs) with several neurological diseases. GAD Abs have been observed in up to 70 to 80% of patients with T1D (Baekkeskov et al., 1982). In addition to epilepsy, GAD Abs have also been implicated in the pathogenic processes associated with stiff-person syndrome (SPS) (Solimena et al., 1988), chronic cerebellar ataxia (Honnorat et al., 1995; Saiz et al., 1997), branchial muscle myoclonus (Nemni et al., 1994), and juvenile neuronal ceroid lipofuscinoses or Batten disease (Pearce et al., 2004; Ramirez-Montealegre et al., 2005). The association of GAD Abs with these syndromes is not accounted for simply by the presence of coexisting T1D. In SPS, rates of positivity to GAD Abs have been reported as high as 60 to 88%, while the rate of T1D in SPS is between 30 to 40% (Solimena et al., 1990; Barker et al., 1998). Higher GAD Ab titers are also typically observed when associated with neurological syndromes than for those in autoimmune T1D. Although the presence of GAD Abs may suggest a common mechanism among the neurological syndromes, the reason for the variation in clinical phenotype remains unaccounted for at this time.

The enzyme GAD normally functions to convert L-glutamic acid to GABA. The release of GABA from vesicles in beta cells may regulate the inhibition of insulin secretion via GABA receptors, although the exact mechanism has not been fully elucidated (Ellis and Atkinson, 1996; Shi et al., 2000). GAD is also expressed in the CNS and is present in GABA-ergic neuronal cytoplasm and secretory vesicles. GAD is also expressed in the testis, fallopian tube, liver, kidney, and adrenal gland (Erdo and Wolff, 1990).

There exist two isoforms of GAD, encoded by two distinct, independently regulated genes. The 65.4 kDa isoform (GAD65) is produced by a gene located on chromosome 2, while the gene for the 66.6 kDa isoform (GAD67) is located on chromosome 10. Both isoforms have been observed in the CNS, but differ in subcellular localization, in membrane interaction, and possibly mode of cellular GABA release. The relative preponderance of a specific GAD isoform may be influenced by the underlying function of the GAD containing population of neurons (Esclapez et al., 1994; Soghomonian and Martin, 1998). GAD65 is the only isoform produced in pancreatic beta cells, and has also been shown to be the more prevalent isoform in the dentate gyrus and CA1 of the rat hippocampus (Sloviter et al., 1996; Soghomonian and Martin, 1998).

Variation exists in the antigens to which the GAD Abs may recognize. It has been observed that GAD Abs recognize different epitopes specific to T1D, distinct from those detected in the various neurological syndromes (Butler et al., 1993; Kim et al., 1994; Daw et al., 1996; Ramirez-Montealegre et al., 2005). In rat hippocampal neurons, GAD Abs from the sera of epileptic patients and T1D were shown to differ in the ability to recognize cellular structures, resulting in differential peri-nuclear staining in comparison to GAD Abs obtained from the sera of patients with other neurological syndromes (Vianello et al., 2006). Specific populations of GABAergic neurons may differ in epitope specificity, resulting in distinct susceptibility to GAD Abs, and hence, variation in clinical phenotype (Butler et al., 1993). Confounding differences between method of detection, antibody specificity, and antigenic recognition has been suggested as possible explanations as to the discrepancies among the results of some studies (McKnight et al., 2005; Vianello et al., 2005).

The role of reduced GABA mediated inhibition, has been studied extensively as a mechanism of epilepsy (Chang and Lowenstein, 2003). GABA A receptors are predominantly inhibitory, causing chloride ion influx upon activation, and hyperpolarization of the neuron. Theoretically, the reduced availability of GAD secondary to GAD Abs could potentially impair the conversion of glutamate to GABA, resulting in decreased inhibitory synaptic transmission, neuronal hyperexcitability, and a lowered seizure threshold. It has been hypothesized that GAD Abs may act at nerve terminals to interfere with GAD and to reduce the synthesis and exocytosis of GABA (Vianello et al., 2002). In knockout mice deficient in GAD65, seizure susceptibility is dramatically increased (Kash et al., 1997). It has been proposed that GAD Abs may be implicated in patients who develop both T1D and IGE given the higher than expected rates of concurrence (Ruegg, 2006; Vulliemoz and Seeck, 2006). GAD Abs have also been reported to be associated with other forms of epilepsy, including in focal epilepsy syndromes.

Problematic to this hypothesis is the observation that GAD is localized intracytoplasmically, and is not normally exposed to the outside of the neuronal membrane. However, other mechanisms may exist for penetration of Abs into intact cells, or presentation of GAD to the cell surface (Kim et al., 1994; Vianello et al., 2002). It has been hypothesized that GAD Abs may cause their effects by an alternative mechanism such as direct interference with the GABA receptor binding site. Also of note, is though differences in absolute GAD Ab titers may exist between clinical syndromes, a clear dose response relationship has also not been observed in regards to severity of clinical course (Vianello et al., 2005).

In the early case reports of patients with elevated GAD Abs, several included a depiction of seizures occurring in the context of other syndromes including SPS (Martinelli et al., 1978; Solimena et al., 1990), palatal myoclonus (Nemni et al., 1994), cerebellar ataxia and T1D (Saiz et al., 1997). A case of a patient with new onset medically refractory temporo-parietal lobe epilepsy and behavioral changes was later discovered to have an encephalitic process with elevated GAD Ab titers present both in serum and CSF. The authors noted clinical improvement in the patient's clinical condition after empiric steroid immunotherapy (Giometto et al., 1998). A similar course was described an a unique case study, describing epilepsia partialis continua occurring in a recently diagnosed T1D child with elevated GAD65 Abs. Full abatement of seizures also only occurred after the institution of high dose steroids, intravenous immunoglobulins (IVIG), and plasma exchange (PE). Clinical improvement after immunotherapy corresponded with reduction in absolute GAD Ab titers (Olson et al., 2002).

An abnormal immune state owing to medications has been described, however differences in GAD Ab levels correlated to the use of antiepileptic drug use has not been observed in several preliminary studies (Peltola et al., 2000a; Sokol et al., 2004; Aykutlu et al., 2005).

In an early, uncontrolled pilot study of 105 epileptic patients, positive GAD Abs by radioimmunassay were detected in four patients, all with uncontrolled epilepsy. Of those four patients, two had a previous diagnosis of MTS, one patient carried a diagnosis of JME, and one had known cortical dysplasia. None of the subjects in the study were known to have T1D, however, three of the patients with GAD Abs also tested positive for islet cell Abs. Of interest, by history, GABA-ergic treatments had not been more successful in the treatment of these patients. The absolute GAD titers between groups of patients with controlled or uncontrolled epilepsy were no different (Kwan et al., 2000). A separate study of 114 unselected children with various types of epilepsy, including a small minority of 7 patients with medically refractory seizures, failed to detect GAD Abs in any patients (Rantala et al., 1999). Similarly, a later study of 74 unselected children with epilepsy, found no significant difference in the presence of GAD Abs in comparison to control subjects, between type of epilepsy, or between the 22 patients with medically refractory epilepsy versus the 52 patients who were seizure-free. Ultimately, 4 patients with epilepsy and 2 control subjects tested positive for the antibody (Verrotti et al., 2003).

A study focusing entirely on the association between GAD Abs and patients with medically refractory epilepsy, found GAD Abs present in 8/51 patients, exclusively from the partial epilepsy cohort. None of the eight subjects had T1D, or a clinical course distinct from the other groups tested, including 49 patients with generalized epilepsy, 48 healthy patients, 38 patients with other neurological diseases, and 124 patients with T1D (Peltola et al., 2000a). Notably, the two patients with the highest GAD Ab titers, also had evidence for the presence of other autoimmune processes. One had a clinical history of abnormal thyroid function, and the other with elevated anticardiolipin Abs, anti-thyroid peroxidase antibodies Abs, antigliadin Abs, and islet cell Abs also present. A contradictory later study of 39 exclusively therapy resistant epileptic patients, most with MTS, found elevated GAD Abs in only a single patient, again, clinically indistinct from the others (Sokol et al., 2004). Of interest, in an investigation of 30 patients with Rasmussen encephalitis, 3 patients were found to harbor antibodies to GAD. GAD Abs were absent in 49 other patients with intractable epilepsy of other etiology and 23 control subjects who were also tested (Watson et al., 2004).

Research has attempted to address the prevalence of GAD Abs specifically in IGE. In a cross-sectional pilot study, 69 patients with juvenile myoclonic epilepsy (JME) were screened for GAD Abs, 10 of which had a history of therapy-resistant epilepsy, *versus* 25 control subjects. Differences did not reach significance, however, four of the patients with JME (5.8%) had elevated titers of at least 2 SD above the control group mean, in comparison to a single pregnant control subject. None of the patients were observed to have concomitant T1D. Three patients were photosensitive, but did not have any other differences in regards to clinical syndrome compared to other patients in the JME group. There was no statistical difference overall in regards GAD ab titers for patients in the therapy resistant group compared to those with epilepsy under better seizure control (Aykutlu et al., 2005).

Most of the studies investigating the role of GAD Abs in the various forms of epilepsy have carried similar potential limitations in regards to study size and power. To date, only a small total number of cases have been described in the literature with concurrent epilepsy and elevation in GAD Ab titers. It is difficult to draw conclusions at this time in regards to the recommendations for routine screening much less for immunosuppressive treatment, based strictly on anecdotal evidence. Currently, based on existing data, routine screening for GAD Abs in unselected patients with epilepsy is not recommended. Nonetheless, GAD Abs continue to be of specific interest in patients with medically refractory focal and generalized epilepsies in an out of association with other neurological syndromes and autoimmune processes including T1D. The data remains intriguing as to the potential contribution of the immune system to the pathogenesis of epilepsy in certain patient populations.

While GAD Abs may serve as potential evidence such an underlying immune process, further investigation is required. Several questions remain unanswered. As illustrated above, it is not clearly known under what conditions GAD Abs are generated. It has not been established in what epilepsy syndromes GAD Abs are consistently elevated, or during what course of the disease. Work continues to further characterize the GAD antibody, potential epitopes, and the manner in which it may contribute to lower seizure threshold. And though a link between T1D and IGE has been established, the prevalence of T1D related autoantibodies, such as GAD Ab, in those specific patients has not been addressed.

A recent report in the literature described a GAD Ab positive adult with concurrent late onset T1D, late onset partial epilepsy, as well as autoimmune thyroiditis as evidenced by an abnormally elevation of anti-thyroid peroxidase Abs, anti-thyroglobulin Abs, and an elevated TSH (Yoshimoto et al., 2005). Such a case further illustrates the potential convergence of several potentially immunologically mediated syndromes, and a possible common immunological process yet to be delineated *(Table II)*.

■ Autoimmune thyroid disorders and epilepsy

Goitrous chronic lymphocytic thyroiditis was described histologically by Hashimoto in 1912. Also known as Hashimoto thyroiditis, the disorder is characterized by autoimmune destruction of the follicle cells of the thyroid gland. Autoimmune thyroiditis is the most common cause of primary hypothyroidism in the United States, and the disease incidence is 7 times higher among women than among men. It is also more frequently observed with increasing age, in those with a family history of thyroid disorders, and in patients with chromosomal abnormalities such as Down, Turner, and Klienfelter syndrome. Among patients with Hashimoto thyroiditis, there is a higher incidence of other autoimmune disorders such as T1D, Addison's disease, vitiligo, pernicious anemia, myasthenia gravis, and rheumatic diseases (Roberts and Ladenson, 2004). The condition may occur without the presence of a goiter, and potentially, during the course of the disease patients may be euthyroid or even hyperthyroid. Treatment consists of thyroid hormone replacement when indicated (American Association of Clinical Endocrinologists, 2002).

High serum thyroid autoantibodies, particularly thyroid peroxidase antibodies (TPO Abs), previously known as antimicrosomal antibodies, are detected in up to 95% of patients with Hashimoto's thyroiditis. In addition, 60% of patients will also be positive for anti-thyroglobulin antibodies (TG Abs) (Roberts and Ladenson, 2004). Although these antibodies are markers of the underlying autoimmune process and are helpful diagnostically, they have not been established as causative. Antibodies directed against thyroxine (T_4) and thiiodothyronine (T_3) have also been observed.

The syndrome of encephalopathy associated with autoimmune thyroiditis, also known as Hashimoto encephalopathy (HE), has been a clinical entity of significant interest. Debate continues on as to the proper nomenclature for the disease due to the unknown pathogenesis of the disorder despite the association with thyroid antibodies, the lack of literature to support Hashimoto reported the syndrome, and ongoing debate over the use of steroid responsiveness as a diagnostic criterion (Canton et al., 2000; Sawka et al., 2002; McKeon et al., 2004; Castillo et al., 2006). The diagnosis is generally suspected in a patient with relapsing-remitting or subacute progressive neuropsychiatric symptoms, in the setting of elevated anti-thyroid antibodies, and after careful exclusion of other metabolic, infectious, vascular, and neoplastic causes.

The first reported case in the literature is attributable to Brain et al. in 1966 (Brain et al., 1966). While episodes of unexplained loss of consciousness and periodic confusion were described, overt seizures were not. EEG was performed on this patient on several occasions and was notable for generalized slowing of the background, progressing in parallel with deteriorations in the patient's condition, which eventually

Table II. A summary of the clinical studies of antibodies to glutamic acid decarboylase (GAD Abs) in epilepsy

Investigators	Subjects (n)	# of GAD Ab+ Patients	Associated clinical features of GAD Ab+ patients (n)
(Martinelli et al., 1978)	SPS with epilepsy (1)	1	
(Solimena et al., 1988)	SPS with epilepsy (1)	1	T1D, Elevated oligoclonal bands
(Nemni et al., 1994)	Epilepsy and palatal myoclonus (1)	1	Impaired glucose tolerance
(Saiz et al., 1997)	Cerebellar ataxia (1)	1	Diabetes
(Giometto et al., 1998)	Encephalitis and LRE (1)	1	CSF pleocytosis
(Rantala et al., 1999)	Pediatric epilepsy (114) [medically refractory (7)]	None	
(Kwan et al., 2000)	Epilepsy (105) [medically refractory (74)] [MTS (40), CD (22), gliosis (24), JME (19)]	4 refractory only [2 MTS, 1 JME, 1 CD]	+Islet cell Abs in (3)
(Peltola et al., 2000a)	Medically refractory epilepsy (100) [LRE (51), GE (49)] Controls (86) [other neuro dx (38)]	8 in LRE only	Hypothyroidism (1), Pt with TPO Abs, anticardiolipin Abs, AG Abs, islet cell Abs (1)
(Olson et al., 2002)	Epilepsia partialis continua (1)	1	T1D, Transient MRI lesions of cerebellar and cortical grey matter
(Verrotti et al., 2003)	Children with epilepsy (74) [medically refractory (22)] Controls (50)	1 refractory 3 seizure free 2 controls	
(Sokol et al., 2004)	Medically refractory epilepsy (39)	1	HTN
(Watson et al., 2004)	Rasmussen encephalitis (30) Intractable epilepsy (49), Controls (23)	3 RE	Voltage gated calcium channel Abs (1)
(Aykutlu et al., 2005)	JME (96), Controls (25)	4 JME 1 pregnant control	
(Yoshimoto et al., 2005)	T1D and LRE (1)	1	Subclinical hypothyroidism, TPO Abs, TG Abs, elevated TSH
(McKnight et al., 2005)	Epilepsy (139) Controls (150) [other neuro dx (131)]	5 refractory 2 controls with stroke	T1D and hypothyroid (1)
(Majoie et al., 2006)	Females with Epilepsy (106)	None	

SPS, stiff-person syndrome; T1D, type 1 diabetes; LRE, localization related epilepsy; MTS, mesial temporal sclerosis; CD, cortical dysplasia; GE, generalized epilepsy; TPO Abs, thyroid peroxidase antibodies; AG Abs, antigliadin antibodies; TG Abs, thyroglobulin antibodies; RE, Rasmussen encephalitis; JME, juvenile myoclonic epilepsy; pt(s), patients improved after courses of prednisone, thyroxin, and apparently, anticonvulsants. The first case of seizures occurring in a patient with HE was reported in 1974 by Thrush and Boddie (Thrush and Boddie, 1974). Their clinical description of a 38 year-old female with recurrent seizures, myoclonus, depression, and hallucinations responsive to immunosuppressive therapy with steroids and cyclophosphamide was prototypical.

In addition to seizures, the spectrum of symptoms that have been reported in association with HE has included confusion, delirium, subacute cognitive deterioration, psychiatric symptoms, headache, fatigue, myoclonus, ataxia, clonus, tremor, as well as focal motor or sensory deficits (Ferracci and Carnevale, 2006). Symptoms are typically relapsing-remitting or progressive and have been described to occur in isolation, although by strict criterion an encephalopathy should be part of the clinical picture (Chong et al., 2003). The occurrence of symptoms are not directly attributable to thyroid dysfunction or abnormal thyroid hormone levels, and may occur in the setting of euthyroidism.

Neuroimaging, in some cases, may reveal global or focal cerebral atrophy, nonspecific focal subcortical lesions, or more extensive white matter abnormalities. In some, imaging may be normal (Bohnen et al., 1997; Chong et al., 2003; Ferracci and Carnevale, 2006). Diagnosis rests on the detection of thyroid antibodies in the serum of affected patients. CSF investigations have not yielded consistent results, although elevated intrathecal TPO and TG Abs, mild lymphocytic pleocytosis, and frequently elevated protein levels have been reported (Chong et al., 2003; Ferracci et al., 2003; Ferracci and Carnevale, 2006).

A recent review of the literature available in the English language, found a total of 121 cases of neurological dysfunction attributed to autoimmune thyroiditis, with patients ranging from age 8 to 86 years (Ferracci and Carnevale, 2006). An overall female to male predominance was reported at a ratio of 4:1. Seizures complicated HE in 63 of 121 patients (52%). Of those cases, generalized seizures were observed in 78%, partial seizures with or without generalization in 17%. Status epilepticus was described in 13% of those patients who experienced seizures. Additional patients with seizures or status epilepticus in the setting of HE have also been recently described (Ferlazzo et al., 2006; Striano et al., 2006). Using stricter inclusion criteria, an earlier comprehensive review by Chong et al. found 85 patients with HE, occurring in a similar male to female ratio, with 66% of patients having had seizures. 30% of patients were either euthyroid or euthyroid on replacement therapy, 35% were subclinically hypothyroid, 20% were hypothyroid, and 7% were hyperthyroid (Chong et al., 2003).

Studies conducted to examine the EEG abnormalities associated with HE, have revealed relatively nonspecific findings. Generalized slowing, is the most common finding in patients with HE. The degree of slowing corresponds to the clinical severity of the underlying encephalopathy, and may normalize parallel to clinical improvement, or deteriorate with recurrent encephalopathy (Henchey et al., 1995; Schauble et al., 2003). Triphasic waves, fluctuating focal slow wave activity, generalized sharp and slow waves discharges, focal and multifocal sharp waves, periodic lateralized discharges, and a photomyogenic response have also been described (Thrush and Boddie, 1974; Bohnen et al., 1997; Forchetti et al., 1997; Vasconcellos et al., 1999; Nolte et al., 2000; Arain et al., 2001; Schauble et al., 2003; McKeon et al., 2004; Rodriguez et al., 2006). The myoclonic jerks associated with HE are not typically associated with EEG abnormalities (Schauble et al., 2003). The overall utility of the EEG may lie in the exclusion of active seizures and other diagnoses.

The cause of the neuropsychiatric symptoms in HE, and the role of anti-thyroid antibodies in the disease are controversial. The enzyme thyroid peroxidase functions to prepare iodine for attachment to the protein thyroglobulin during the synthesis of thyroid hormone, and does not have any known functional role outside of the thyroid gland (Chong et al., 2003). Elevated anti-thyroid antibodies maybe found in as many as 10% of normal subjects, and may be an incidental finding in some cases (Shaw et al., 1991). Notably, the absolute titers of the TPO or TG abs have not been shown to correlate with disease severity (Chong et al., 2003; Ferracci et al., 2004; Castillo et al., 2006). The antibodies also do not have any known recognized antigens within the brain, making a hypothesis of an abnormal response due to a mechanism of molecular mimicry less likely (Chong et al., 2003). It is possible that the antibodies are potentially epiphenomena and common markers of another independent disease process, which affect the brains of susceptible persons by a different mechanism altogether (Chong et al., 2003). However, abnormal immune-complex deposition resulting in cerebral vasculitis has been put forth as a possible etiology (Shaw et al., 1991; Kothbauer-Margreiter et al., 1996; Forchetti et al., 1997). Limited histological data has infrequently supported speculation of a vasculitic component to the disease. Separate case studies have reported the findings of mild to marked lymphocytic infiltratation around arterioles and veins in two persons, lymphocytic infiltrate of the leptomeningeal veins in the brainstem in one patient, and perivascular lymphocytic cuffing in another (Shibata et al., 1992; Nolte et al., 2000; Chong et al., 2003; Duffey et al., 2003). Normal biopsy findings have also been reported (Schauble et al., 2003; Castillo et al., 2006). Focal and global hypoperfusion on single photon emission computed tomography (SPECT) has also been observed in HE, potentially related to microvascular compromise (Forchetti et al., 1997), although the data on this subject has been conflicting (Ferracci et al., 2004; Ferracci and Carnevale, 2006). Patients with Hashimoto thyroiditis have also been found to have focal and global perfusion abnormalities by SPECT in the absence of overt neurological symptoms or functional thyroid abnormalities (Piga et al., 2004).

Immunomodulatory therapy with steroids is recommended, with the large majority of patients going into subsequent remission (Chong et al., 2003). Clinical response in association with steroids in the setting of supportive criteria, while suggestive, has not been shown to be diagnostic of HE, as a small minority of patients may not show unambiguous improvement (Ferracci and Carnevale, 2006). However, disease regression in the face of steroids may be helpful in exclusion of other non-steroid responsive degenerative neurological processes (Castillo et al., 2006). Anecdotally, other immunosuppressive agents, IVIG, and PE have been attempted successfully for refractory cases (Kothbauer-Margreiter et al., 1996; Boers and Colebatch, 2001). Levothyroxine and antiepileptic medications should be utilized when warranted.

Seizures may occur as a consequence of severe hypothyroidism, regardless of etiology, and may potentially respond to thyroid hormone replacement therapy (Evans, 1960). Myxedema coma is a rare syndrome resulting from chronic untreated hypothyroidism.

Precipitants may include physical stressors such as infection, hypothermia, hypoglycemia, trauma, surgery, and medications such as beta-blockers, amiodarone, diuretics, narcotics, lithium, and potentially enzyme inducing antiepileptic drugs. In addition to the stigmata of chronic hypothyroidism, the signs and symptoms of myxedema occur along a spectrum, and rarely actually include coma. Patients may present with altered mentation and cognition, headache, cranial nerve palsies, myopathic and neuropathic changes, ataxia, edema, and reflex abnormalities. Hypothermia, hyponatremia, and compromised cardiac output frequently occur as serious complications of myxedema (Wall, 2000; Fliers and Wiersinga, 2003; Jansen et al., 2006).

Seizures occurring in the setting of a comatose myxedematous patient represent a poor prognostic sign, with high mortality rates previously reported to be as high as 30 to 60% (Levin and Daughaday, 1955; Jellinek, 1962; Nielsen and Ranlov, 1964; Yamamoto et al., 1999). Status epilepticus in this setting has also been described (Jansen et al., 2006). The mechanism of seizure provocation is not clear, but may be related to cerebral edema and myxedema associated electrolyte imbalances.

In addition to warming the patient, cardiac support, and correction of other metabolic abnormalities, treatment is primarily with intravenous replacement T4 and potentially oral T3, replaced cautiously due to the risk of inducing cardiac instability. At least theoretically, some antiepileptic medications have the potential to further exacerbate hypothyroidism. Phenobarbital, primidone, phenytoin, carbamazepine, and oxcarbamazepine increase the hepatic clearance of levothyroxine by induction of cytochrome P450 enzymes, and could potentially lead to a subacute increased levothyroxine requirement, or precipitate hypothyroidism in patients with diminished reserve. While data is lacking in regards to the newer agents, such as topiramate and felbamate, it is unlikely that antiepileptic drugs with low or no enzyme induction such as levetiracetam, gabapentin, pregabalin, or lamotrigine have a clinically significant effect on thyroid function (Steinhoff, 2006).

Interestingly, thyroid hormones, in themselves, have been purported to lower the seizure threshold in animals (Timiras and Woodbury, 1956; Seyfried et al., 1981), and to cause a high amplitude paroxysmal photic response in the EEG of normal subjects (Wilson et al., 1964). Focal and generalized seizures have rarely been reported in the setting of thyroxine toxicity (Sundaram et al., 1985; Aydin et al., 2004), as well as in thyrotoxicosis due to other causes including Graves disease (Chapman and Maloof, 1956; Skanse and Nyman, 1956; Korczyn and Bechar, 1976; Jabbari and Huott, 1980; Smith and Looney, 1983; Aiello et al., 1989; Primavera et al., 1990; Radetti et al., 1993). Thyrotoxicosis in Graves disease was also reported to exacerbate seizures in several JME patients (Su et al., 1993; Obeid et al., 1996).

It is not clear by which mechanism excess thyroid hormones may provoke seizures. Thyroxine may potentially cause cortical hyperexcitability by decreasing the number of available benzodiazepine receptors (Go et al., 1988). Thyroid hormones have also been demonstrated experimentally to competitively inhibit neuronal uptake of GABA (Mason et al., 1987). The autoantibody directed against the thyroid stimulating hormone (TSH) receptor on thyroid follicular cells resulting in the hyperthyroidism observed in Graves disease has not been directly associated with neuronal dysfunction.

Systemic lupus erythematosis and epilepsy

Systemic lupus erythematous (SLE) is a multi-organ systemic inflammatory disorder, that may be as prevalent as 1.22 per 1,000 in the U.S, with an incidence rate of 5.56 per 100,000 (Uramoto et al., 1999). There is a female predominance of 3 to 5 times the rate of disease in males. African-Americans and Hispanics are also affected more frequently than Caucasians, and may carry a higher overall morbidity from the disease (Alarcon et al., 1999). Mortality is attributed in most cases to direct end organ damage, vascular causes, or due to complications such as infection.

The estimated prevalence of neuropsychiatric manifestations in patients with SLE varies from 50 to 90% (Brey et al., 2002). Symptoms may include cognitive impairment, dementia, psychosis, anxiety, depression, headache, neuropathy, movement abnormalities, stroke, and seizures. The prevalence of seizures among people with SLE has been reported to be between 8 to 28% (Toubi et al., 1995; Navarrete and Brey, 2000; Brey et al., 2002; Appenzeller et al., 2004; Mikdashi et al., 2005). 5 to 10% of patients experience seizures preceding the diagnosis of lupus, occurring potentially years prior to the onset of other clinical manifestations of the disease (Inzelberg and Korczyn, 1989). Both focal and generalized seizures have been observed in the setting of SLE, as well as status epilepticus. The occurrence of seizures in SLE has been attributed to cerebrovascular thromboembolic events, hypertensive encephalopathy, immune-mediated neuronal damage, and metabolic disturbances secondary to SLE related renal disease (Aarli, 2000; Appenzeller et al., 2004).

The EEG may be normal in the majority of patients who have suffered a single seizure in the setting of SLE. In contrast, interictal epileptiform abnormalities were appreciated in one study, in all lupus patients with a history of recurrent seizures (Appenzeller et al., 2004). Typical findings may include diffuse or asymmetrical slowing, and focal sharp wave activity. When asymmetric slowing occurs, it may preferentially occur over the left hemisphere. In a study of 478 patients with SLE, left hemispheric abnormalities were identified in 79.6% of patients, right hemispheric abnormalities in 7.4%s, and bilateral abnormalities in 13.0% (Glanz et al., 1998).

Epilepsy is significantly more common in SLE patients with lupus associated antiphospholipid antibodies (aPL Abs), and the presence of aPL Abs may be an independent predictor for the development of seizures (Herranz et al., 1994; Liou et al., 1996; Shrivastava et al., 2001; Gibbs and Husain, 2002; Appenzeller et al., 2004; Mikdashi et al., 2005). Although, conflicting data has been presented in at least one study (Formiga et al., 1996). aPL Abs encompass several different antibodies including anticardiolipin antibodies (ACL Abs), β2 glycoprotein 1 antibodies, lupus anticoagulant, and anti-prothrombin. A potential confounder is the high baseline prevalence of these antibodies in patients with SLE. For example, the antibody to cardiolipin, a plasma globulin, is a commonly measured aPL Ab, and has been observed in up to 44% of patients with lupus at baseline (Sebastiani et al., 1991).

Thromboembolic events and thrombocytopenia are also more common in patients with aPL Abs, likely accounting for a higher incidence of focal brain lesions. It is possible that seizures may potentially occur secondary to the occurrence of cerebrovascular compromise, and that the perceived association between aPL Abs and seizures is resultant (Appenzeller et al., 2004; Shoenfeld et al., 2004). In one analysis, the presence of IgG antiphospholipid antibodies in moderate to high titers increased the risk of seizures near onset to nearly 7 times, and seizures during the course of the disease to almost 4 times. The occurrence of stroke in the same study increased the risk of seizures near the onset of SLE by 10 times. Comparatively, nephritis increased the risk of seizures later in the course of the disease by approximately 3 times (Appenzeller et al., 2004). Indeed, some studies of patients with SLE and epilepsy have observed increased aPL Abs in the setting of abnormal neuroimaging (Herranz et al., 1994). Cases where neuroimaging may be normal, may show evidence for microvascular injury on pathological review (Liou et al., 1996).

Experimental data, however, has shown that aPL Abs may bind directly to brain tissue and endothelium (Hess et al., 1993; Kent et al., 2000). Antibodies to aPL may therefore have the ability to disrupt neuronal function directly, potentially accounting for some of the non-thromboembolic CNS manifestations of the anti-phospholipid syndrome. Neuronal hyperexcitability may be increased by aPL Abs through inhibition of the GABA receptor complex (Liou et al., 1994). The antibodies have also been shown to depolarize synaptoneurosomes from rat brainstem (Chapman et al., 1999). Furthermore, aPL Abs may cause neuronal dysfunction by binding to ATP (Chapman et al., 2005). Cimaz et al. have produced a helpful review of the literature, including a discussion in regards to the pathogenetic mechanisms of aPL Abs (Cimaz et al., 2006).

Up to a half of patients who harbor aPL Abs do not have a diagnosis of SLE. They may be seen in association with other primary autoimmune syndromes, in primary antiphospholipid syndrome, or potentially in normal subjects. The antiphospholipid syndrome (APS) is characterized by the presence of aPL Abs, thrombocytopenia, venous and arterial thromboses, and potential obstetrical complications in females. In addition to cardiac, dermatologic, and renal conditions; neurological complications such as stroke and epilepsy have also been reported in association with APS. In a cohort of 1,000 patients with the diagnosis of APS, 7% of patients suffered from epileptic seizures over the course of long term follow up (Cervera et al., 2002).

In another study specifically addressing the risk factors associated with developing epilepsy among 538 patients with APS, the prevalence of epilepsy was reported as 8.6%. Epilepsy was significantly more common in patients with antiphospholipid syndrome secondary to lupus than in patients with primary antiphospholipid syndrome. Patients with CNS thromboembolic events were at four times higher risk for epilepsy than those without. The presence of valvular vegetations increased the risk by 2.9 times, while the diagnosis of SLE raised the risk by 1.4 times. The authors concluded that stroke and SLE may have accounted for, in large part, the observed increased prevalence of epilepsy in patients with APS, although not exclusively (Shoenfeld et al., 2004).

A proportion of patients with epilepsy and aPL Abs, will have no history of stroke or abnormalities on neuroimaging. Some have suggested that in cases where no abnormality is observed on routine imaging, evidence for functional abnormalities potentially indicative of microvascular disease may be observed using other imaging modalities such as PET (Hilker et al., 2000; Shoenfeld et al., 2004). A study of patients with APS found those with persistently positive aPL Abs were at a greater risk for the development of EEG abnormalities. Half of those patients with EEG abnormalities also had a normal MRI, suggesting that EEG may have been more sensitive in detecting subtle regions of cerebral dysfunction (Lampropoulos et al., 2005).

Some studies of unselected groups of patients with epilepsy, with or without a diagnosis of lupus, have reported an increased prevalence of an elevated level of aPL Abs compared to normal subjects, although the data is conflicting (Peltola et al., 2000b; Eriksson et al., 2001). An early study determined IgG ACL Ab positivity in 19% of persons with epilepsy *versus* 3% in controls (Verrot et al., 1997). A follow up study from another group did not confirm these results (Debourdeau et al., 2004). Using various measures of aPL Abs, other investigators have detected antibodies in between 9.7 to 43% of unselected patients with epilepsy (Pardo et al., 2001; Sokol et al., 2004).

In a study of aPL Abs in epilepsy, the frequency of elevated titers was determined for a group of 50 patients with therapy resistant localization related epilepsy, 50 patients with generalized epilepsy syndromes, 52 newly diagnosed patients with seizures, and 82 control subjects. Patients from the newly diagnosed group had significantly elevated IgG ACL titers of 21% *versus* 7% in the control group. IgM ACL was also more prevalent in all study groups in comparison to the control group (Peltola et al., 2000b). A more definitive follow up study from the same investigators, involving a cohort of 960 patients with epilepsy, confirmed elevated anticardiolipin antibodies only in subsets of patients with longstanding or frequent partial seizures of greater than 10 years duration (Ranua et al., 2004). It has been suggested that aPL Abs may be generated in the setting of recent seizures, and over time may be a consequence of poor seizure control (Ranua et al., 2004; Cimaz et al., 2006).

The frequency of aPL Abs in pediatric epilepsy has also been addressed in several studies. As many as 13 to 44% of children with epilepsy may be aPL Ab positive (Angelini et al., 1998; Eriksson et al., 2001; Cimaz et al., 2002; Verrotti et al., 2003). Data is conflicting in regards to which patient characteristics are associated with antibody positivity.

While a lupus like reaction and elevations in lupus associated antibodies in association with antiepileptic drugs has been described, studies have repeatedly shown the lack of an association between epilepsy and the detection of aPL antibodies based solely to the use of antiepileptic medication regimens (Verrot et al., 1997; Peltola et al., 2000b; Eriksson et al., 2001; Cimaz et al., 2002; Ranua et al., 2004).

The association between SLE and epilepsy has been clearly established. While cerebrovascular disease may account for some degree of the presence of epilepsy in SLE, there appear additional contributing factors. The exact contribution of aPL Abs in and out of association with SLE to the pathogenesis of epilepsy remains to be elucidated.

▪ Rasmussen encephalitis

In 1958, Rasmussen published a description of 3 children followed at the Montreal Neurological Institute, with a syndrome characterized by refractory focal seizures due to a chronic localized encephalitis, progressive unilateral brain atrophy, and progressive neurological deterioration (Rasmussen et al., 1958). Rasmussen's own cohort would eventually consist of 51 patients. Patients in the progressive phases of the disease were also described to develop spastic hemiparesis, hemianopsia, sensory loss, ataxia, dysphagia, intellectual deterioration, and aphasia (Rasmussen and Andermann, 1989).

Rasmussen encephalitis (RE) remains relatively uncommon, with an estimated incidence of between 1/500,000 to 1/1,000,000. The disease is sporadic, and classically a disease of children with an average age of onset of 6 years. However, several adult cases have been reported, and adults may comprise as many as 10% of the overall cases (Oguni et al., 1991; Hart et al., 1997; Bien et al., 2005). The oldest reported case in the literature was of a 58 year old female (Hunter et al., 2006).

According to the European consensus statement, the diagnosis of RE is based primarily on clinical, electrographic, and radiographic evidence, and the exclusion of other disease entities. The clinical course of RE has been described in 3 stages (Bien et al., 2002b; Bien et al., 2005).

Stage I may be a relatively nonspecific prodrome, with a median duration of 7 months, and a range of 0 months to 8 years. Symptoms during this time may consist of occasional focal onset seizures and rarely a mild progressive hemiparesis.

Stage II has been described as the acute phase of RE and may be the initial manifestation in a third of patients. The mean duration of this phase is 8 months, with a range of 4 to 8 months (Bien et al., 2005). This acute stage is characterized by frequent medically refractory seizures, and clinical deterioration. Seizures semiology may be variable on initial presentation, and may become polymorphic over time, spreading along the hemisphere (Oguni et al., 1991). Epilepsia partialis continua (EPC) is a classic manifestation of RE and may occur in 56 to 92% of patients (Bien et al., 2005). In one series involving 48 patients, simple partial motor seizures were observed in 77% of patients, somatosensory seizures in 21%, complex partial seizures in 50%, postural seizures in 24%, secondarily generalized seizures in 42% (Oguni et al., 1991). Epilepsy in the context of RE is notoriously difficult to control, particularly EPC, frequently requiring multiple antiepileptic drugs.

Additional manifestations of Stage II may include progressive focal motor deficits developing in parallel to the cortical distribution of seizures. Weakness may initially fluctuate with the severity of seizures, representing a functional deficit in contrast to later fixed deficit due to neuronal loss and cortical atrophy (Chinchilla et al., 1994). Hemianopsia, movement disorders such as hemidystonia and hemichoreathetosis have also been reported (Bhatjiwale et al., 1998; Frucht, 2002). Deterioration in behavior, cognition, attention, memory, and potentially language, if the language dominant hemisphere is involved, may also transpire (Oguni et al., 1991; Bien et al., 2005).

Bihemispheric involvement may become clinically, radiographically, and electrographically evident. EEG may reveal hemispherically independent interictal epileptiform abnormalities, and secondary contralateral spread of focal seizures from the more affected hemisphere. Serial MRIs from a study of 11 RE patients showed progressive atrophy of the "unaffected" hemispheres, but at a significantly lower rate (Larionov *et al.*, 2005). However, cases of true "bilateral RE" with bihemispheric inflammatory lesions are rare comprising less than 5% of reported cases (McLachlan *et al.*, 1993; Chinchilla *et al.*, 1994; DeToledo and Smith, 1994; Tobias *et al.*, 2003).

Stage III has been described as the residual stage. Patients experience stable to slowly progressive hemispheric neurological deficit, hemiparesis, and inevitably, intellectual deterioration. Seizures tend to occur at a lower frequency. Adults tend to have slower deterioration, less residual functional deficit, less prominent brain hemiatrophy, and more occipital regional involvement (Oguni *et al.*, 1991; Hart *et al.*, 1997; Bien *et al.*, 2002b).

MRI studies typically demonstrate unilateral peri-insular enlargement of CSF spaces, with increased parenchymal T2/FLAIR signal, ipsilateral caudate atrophy, with ensuing spread of signal abnormality and atrophy (Tien *et al.*, 1992; Yacubian *et al.*, 1997; Bien *et al.*, 2002b; Chiapparini *et al.*, 2003; Granata *et al.*, 2003b; Bien *et al.*, 2005). Most of the volume loss is observed within the first year. An average rate of atrophy of 29.9 cubic centimeters per year on the more affected side, and 6.8 cubic centimeters per year on the less affected side was measured in 11 immunologically treated patients (Larionov *et al.*, 2005). Rarely neuroimaging may be normal early in the course of the disease, with occasional transient focal edema present early, potentially a consequence of seizure activity. Neuroimaging studies usually do not exhibit substantial amounts of contrast enhancement or calcifications (Bien *et al.*, 2005).

Positron emission tomography (PET) and single photon emission computed tomography (SPECT) studies have shown hypometabolism in affected areas, with focal hypermetabolism on ictal studies (Zupanc *et al.*, 1990; Burke *et al.*, 1992; Tien *et al.*, 1992; Chiapparini *et al.*, 2003). Early metabolic changes are usually more evident in the fronto-temporal lobes, later extending posteriorly. Magnetic resonance spectroscopy studies have shown nonspecific reductions in the NAA/choline ratio consistent with neuronal loss or dysfunction (Adams *et al.*, 1992; Cendes *et al.*, 1995; Chiapparini *et al.*, 2003; Bien *et al.*, 2005).

Electrographic changes including multifocal hemispheric or bihemispheric slowing, unihemispheric attenuation with disruption of the background and sleep architecture, and multifocal epileptiform discharges are commonly observed (So and Gloor, 1991; Andrews *et al.*, 1997; Granata *et al.*, 2003b). Bilateral multiple independent discharges are seen in up to a third of patients, usually more unihemispherically prominent. Bilaterally synchronous epileptiform discharges are seen in up to a half of patients. Seizures are typically lateralized, but may originate from multiple seizure onset zones. Subclinical ictal patterns have been observed. EPC, when present, may not have clearly evident electrographic correlate by scalp recording. Independent ictal patterns over the less affected hemisphere are atypical. Studies with serial EEGs suggests that early in RE, interictal epileptiform abnormalities are localized to the affected hemisphere, with increasingly frequent bilaterally synchronous and contralateral epileptiform activity observed with disease progression. Additionally, immunomodulatory agents may have an effect of diminishing the observed abnormalities.

Routine laboratory testing is generally normal in RE. In the MNI series 50% of patients also had a normal CSF profile. In the remainder lymphocytosis from 16 to 70 cells/uL, elevated CSF protein from 50 to 100 mg/dL, and midzone elevation of the colloidal gold curve was observed (Rasmussen and Andermann, 1989). Oligoclonal bands have been variably reported in 0 to 67% of patients in different series (Dulac, 1996; Granata et al., 2003b; Bien et al., 2005).

Histologically, the early stage of RE is characterized by mild focal inflammation with T-lymphocyte clusters and perivascular cuffing, mild microglial activation with nodule formation, and cortical gliosis with minimal neuronal loss. During the active phase of the disease there is panlaminar inflammation with perivascular and perineuronal lymphocytic cuffing, marked microglial activation, prominent reactive astrocytosis with gliosis, and moderate to severe neuronal loss. Notably, different stages of inflammation may be present simultaneously in different locations of the brain, and that normal and abnormal tissue may be present adjacently, implying a risk of false negatives from small biopsy samples. Biopsies should be obtained from an area with increased T2 abnormalities on MRI, preferably frontal or temporal (Pardo et al., 2004; Bien et al., 2005). During the late phases of the active stage, there is less prominent lymphocytic infiltration with severe panlaminar neuronal loss and cortical necrosis. Finally there is panlaminar cortical cavitation, with only rare neurons, variable microglial activation, and rare lymphocytes (Pardo et al., 2004).

The pathogenesis of RE remains an elusive mystery, and has been an active area of research for decades. Rasmussen postulated an infectious, possibly viral etiology. It is unclear how to account for the predominantly unilateral symptoms and preferential brain hemi-atrophy in RE. It has speculated by some authors that an underlying cerebral lesion may be responsible for precipitating a state of chronic inflammation. A "smoldering effect" has been proposed where there is an initiating underlying excitotoxic lesion such as an infectious, traumatic, or vascular insult producing ongoing seizures, in turn causing breakdown in the blood brain barrier, allowing humoral components to reach and act on neurons, further antigen exposure, and eventual targeting of neurons (Twyman et al., 1995; Andrews et al., 1996; Wise et al., 1996; Bien et al., 2005). Dual pathology has been observed in up to 10% of patients in one case series, with underlying diagnoses including tuberous sclerosis, tumor, cortical dysplasia, vascular abnormalities, and stroke (Hart et al., 1998; Bien et al., 2005). A number infectious etiologies have been postulated including HSV, CMV, EBV, HHV-6 with rare cases showing evidence by PCR or in situ hybridization (Power et al., 1990; McLachlan et al., 1993; Vinters et al., 1993; Jay et al., 1995). Yet, in the majority of pathological studies, no actual evidence of viral particles or inclusions has been identified (Rasmussen, 1978; Atkins et al., 1995).

Both cellular and humoral mechanisms of neuronal injury have been hypothesized. Experiments by Rogers et al. in 1994 with the immunization of rabbits with glutamate receptor subunit 3 antibodies (GluR3 Abs) lead to the observation of clinical seizures and bihemispheric inflammatory CNS histological changes in those animals. An association was made between the phenotype of affected animals and that observed in patients with RE. Further investigation into the presence of GluR3 Abs in 4 RE patients, revealed the presence of GluR3 immunoreactivity in all 3 patients with active disease. The authors hypothesized that seizures or preceding injury prior to the onset of RE, resulted in breakdown in the blood brain barrier, permitting a circulating antibody such as GluR3 to enter the brain, with ensuing immune-mediated neuronal injury. Based on the hypothesis that the GluR3 Abs may be pathogenic in RE, a single seriously ill child was experimentally treated with plasma exchange with transient improvement in symptoms (Rogers et al., 1994).

The glutamate receptor subunit 3 functions as a ligand-gated ion channel receptor in the CNS. The GluR3 Ab binds to neurons and increases glutamate receptor activity, and may lead to excitotoxic complement-independent neuronal damage through glutamate, the dominant excitatory neurotransmitter in the CNS (Rogers et al., 1994; Twyman et al., 1995; Levite et al., 1999; Levite and Hermelin, 1999). GluR3 Abs may additionally function to increase complement activation directed towards neurons and glial cells (He et al., 1998; Whitney and McNamara, 2000; Frassoni et al., 2001). Serum from GluR3 positive RE patients has been shown to cause neuronal death in rat hippocampal cell cultures (Ganor et al., 2004).

The GluR3 Ab, while fairly specific for epilepsy, has not been shown to be exclusive to RE. GluR3 Abs were observed in 7 of 11 RE patients, 60 of 85 patients with epilepsy of other etiology, 7 of 30 patients with other neurological diagnoses, and in 1 of 111 normal subjects (Mantegazza et al., 2002). These results were reiterated by another group who found GluR3 positivity in 2 of 8 RE patients, 13 of 40 patients with non-inflammatory focal epilepsy, 6 of 79 patients with other neurological diagnoses, and in 1 of 41 control subjects (Wiendl et al., 2001). In a different study, the group reported 9 of 11 RE patients to be positive for GluR3 Abs by immunoblot, and 7 of 11 patients with partial epilepsy from another etiology. The authors concluded that the pathogenic mechanism of GluR3 Abs may be shared by different forms of epilepsy (Bernasconi et al., 2002).

The sensitivity of the GluR3 Ab has also been called into question. In a study of 30 patients with RE, GluR3 Abs were detected by ELISA in only 2 of 30 RE patients, and also in 2 of 49 patients with other intractable epilepsies. Only a single patient from this group, one with intractable epilepsy from a cause other than RE, was confirmed by western blot (Watson et al., 2004).

Histopathological evidence suggests a cellular mechanism of injury with the presence of a proportion of CD8 T cells surrounding degenerating neurons in RE (Farrell et al., 1995). Neurons have been shown to express major MHC class I (Bien et al., 2002b). By analysis of T-cell receptors, there appear to be restricted T-cell lineages, likely expanded from precursor T cells responding to discreet antigens (Li et al., 1997). These CD8 T cells have been shown to contain granzyme B (GrB), which may contribute to neuronal death through caspase-mediated apoptosis and further antigen exposure (Gahring et al., 2001; Vezzani and Granata, 2005). GluR3 has been shown to act as an antigen to the immune system only after cleavage by Granzyme B, although this requires the non-glycosylation of a segment of the GluR3 and GrB recognition sequence in order to occur (Gahring et al., 2001).

The additional activation of CD4 T cells may also mobilize B cells to generate the observed autoantibodies (Vezzani and Granata, 2005). In addition to GluR3 Abs, antibodies to Munc-18, a cytosolic presynaptic protein (Yang et al., 2000); and antibodies to NMDA receptor subunit GluRepsilon2 have also been observed in association with RE (Takahashi et al., 2003). Alpha 7 nicotinic acetylcholine receptor antibodies (A7-nAChR Abs) were observed in 2 of 30 patients with RE, while glutamic acid decarboxylase antibodies (GAD Abs) were observed in 3 of 30 RE patients (Watson et al., 2005). Potential antibody mediated activation of the membrane attack complex results in cytotoxic cell death. Sequential infusion of complement components C5b6, C7, C8 and C9 into hippocampi of rats, was shown to result in seizures (Xiong et al., 2003).

In regards to therapy, the existing literature remains difficult to interpret given the low prevalence of the disease, generally a lack of long term patient follow up data, and the absence of a double blinded placebo controlled trial for most of the available treatment options. Additionally, the natural course of the disease may be variable in individuals, with clinical or radiographic outcome measures not clearly defined. The outcome measure of seizure frequency, for example, may decrease in the late progressive stages of RE, with other measures such as hemiparesis, cognitive impairment, and radiographic hemiatrophy may be apparent to a greater degree.

Case reports suggest mild improvement at high doses of steroids early in the active phase of the disease, particularly in the setting of EPC. 10 of 17 RE patients from the MNI series experienced a transient reduction in morbidity and seizure frequency with high dose steroids, although the response was sustained in only 2 of 17 on oral therapy and in 4 of 17 on ongoing intravenous therapy (Hart et al., 1994). Other reports have found relatively comparable findings. 7 of 8 RE patients in another series had similar transient improvements on steroids, with partially sustained effects in 5 (Chinchilla et al., 1994). In another, 6 of 11 RE patients treated with steroids had a transient reduction in seizures and improved neurological status, with long term response uncertain (Granata et al., 2003b).

Experience with other immunomodulating therapies has been modestly encouraging. In one series, 8 of 9 RE patients experienced transient improvement on IVIG, an effect which was sustained in 4 (Hart et al., 1994). In another series, 3 of 11 patients improved on IVIG, with 1 of 11 experiencing sustained results (Granata et al., 2003a). Other case reports have reported improved seizure frequency and neurological function after IVIG, with a prolonged sustained response for up to 4 years (Wise et al., 1996; Leach et al., 1999; Villani et al., 2001; Granata et al., 2003a).

Results have been similar with PE. The girl patient of Rogers et al. experienced at least transient improvement (Rogers et al., 1994). Four patients in another series all experienced transient improvements on plasmapharesis (Andrews et al., 1996). A single patient from a separate case report showed no improvement on PE or steroids, but did respond to IVIG (Villani et al., 2001). Five of 5 patients in a different study experienced neurological improvement on PE, which was sustained in only 1, 2 of 3 patients from the same study also showed transient improvement with Protein A immunoabsorption (Granata et al., 2003a).

The data concerning the use of antivirals is limited and at times conflicting (Bien et al., 2002a). Treatment with zidovidine may have resulted in transient improvement in 1 patient, however treatment was limited by adverse drug effects (DeToledo and Smith, 1994). Gangcyclovir was given to 5 patients with RE. One patient experienced sustained clinical improvement, and two with later onset RE experienced a reduction in seizure frequency. The authors advocated for the consideration of gangcyclovir treatment during the early stages of RE (McLachlan et al., 1996).

Attempted treatment with intraventricular interferon alpha in two separate case reports, resulted in transient neurological improvements (Maria et al., 1993; Dabbagh et al., 1997). A trial of tacrolimus revealed a slower rate of clinical deterioration and hemiatrophy on MRI in 7 RE patients on the drug in comparison to 12 untreated RE patients with an average follow up of 22 months. Tacrolimus did not significantly impact seizure frequency, but also did not have any serious side effects (Bien et al., 2004). Thalidomide was studied as a potential immunosuppressant in RE with improvement in epileptic attacks observed in a single patient (Marjanovic et al., 2003). Cyclophosphamide treatment was attempted in 4 RE patients with no observed improvement after more than 6 months of therapy (Granata et al., 2003a).

Surgical therapy with hemispherectomy carries the highest possibility for seizure freedom in RE. Anatomic resective hemispherectomy carries a complication rate of up to 22% (Vining et al., 1997). Modified procedures including functional disconnection, and subtotal excision are now more typically performed with a complication rate near 4%. Rates of seizure freedom after surgery are reported as high as 63 to 85% (Rasmussen and Andermann, 1989; Vining et al., 1997; Granata et al., 2003b; Delalande et al., 2004a; Bien et al., 2005). Limited resection has been shown to be ineffective in preventing seizures and further eventual neurological deterioration (Rasmussen and Andermann, 1989; Honavar et al., 1992).

The timing of surgical intervention is remains controversial. In children, the brain may display remarkable plasticity. The ability to transition language function between hemispheres is commonly assumed to end around 4 to 6 years of age, but has been documented in the literature to occur up to 16 years of age (Telfeian et al., 2002). The surgical treatment of older patients is limited by potential iatrogenic morbidity. Late-onset cases may also have a more variable course. Some authors advocate for early hemispherectomy, possibly sacrificing neurological function, in the face of disabling seizures and "inevitable" later disability (Vining et al., 1993; Delalande et al., 2004a). Other authors have advocated for hemispherectomy to be performed only after the disease progression has equaled the potential disability from surgery (Rasmussen, 1983; Honavar et al., 1992).

After the diagnosis of RE has been established, depending on the age and hemispheric dominance of the patient, hemispherectomy should be considered in the setting of intractable seizures and severe or impending neurological impairment. The risk of iatrogenic deficits in language and motor function must be factored into the decision. If the risk is deemed too great to proceed with surgery, treatment with immunological therapies is recommended, either up to the point where the patient may experience further deterioration where hemispherectomy should be readdressed, or to the point of clinical plateau consistent with the residual stage of the disease (Bien et al., 2005).

The therapeutic pathway is guided by frequent clinical and radiographic follow up and analysis, and by the essential close involvement of the patient and family in the eventual decision.

■ Celiac disease and epilepsy

Celiac disease (CD) is also known by the terms celiac sprue, non-tropical sprue, and gluten-sensitive enteropathy. It is classified as both an autoimmune disorder and a disease of malabsorption, affecting patients of any age. When exposed to gluten, a protein found in wheat, rye, barley, and oats; the immune system of a patient with CD responds with T-cell mediated antibody production and destruction of the small intestinal villi resulting in malabsorption, and with chronic exposure, malnutrition (Farrell and Kelly, 2002). The treatment of CD involves instituting patient adherence to a gluten-free diet and nutritional supplementation.

Estimates of the prevalence of CD in Americans are as high as 1 in 250 to 1 in 100, although the entity is variable in presentation and frequently underdiagnosed. The disease appears to be genetically determined, with a 70% rate of monozygotic twin concordance (Sollid et al., 2001), and 3 to 17% of first-degree relatives of afflicted persons affected. Approximately 3 to 6% of people with T1D will have also have biopsy confirmed CD. Autoimmune thyroid dysfunction is also more common in patients with concomitant CD. In people with Down syndrome, CD has been observed in 5 to 10%. There is a strong association with genetically determined histocompatibility cell antigens, with the majority of patients with HLA-DQ2 or HLA-DQ8 types (Sollid et al., 1989; Rostom et al., 2004)

Anti-gliadin (AG Abs) and anti-endomysial antibodies (EM Abs) targeting the enzyme tissue transglutaminase (tTG-Abs) are immunological markers of the disease process. EM Abs and tTG Abs have a reported sensitivity in excess of 90% and a specificity of over 95% for the disease. The sensitivity of AG Abs is lower ranging from 70 to 85%, while the specificity is between 70 to 90%. Diagnosis is typically made clinically based on a response to a gluten free diet, by antibody or HLA-type screening, and potentially by serial biopsy of the small intestine while initiating a gluten free diet. While biopsy is not sensitive, a finding of intraepithelial lymphocytosis, crypt hyperplasia, and villous atrophy is highly specific (Rostom et al., 2004; Green et al., 2005).

Signs and symptoms of CD may include: abdominal bloating, pain, chronic diarrhea, weight fluctuations, failure to thrive, fatigue, arthralgia, anemia, ammenorrhea, bone abnormalities, aphthous ulcers, and dermatitis herpetiformis. CD may also potentially remain asymptomatic. Approximately 10% of patients with CD present with neuropsychiatric symptoms, including mood and anxiety issues, cognitive impairment, encephalitis, ataxia, nerve and muscle abnormalities, and migraine (Farrell and Kelly, 2002; Vaknin et al., 2004). White matter abnormalities of unknown significance, as well as cerebral calcifications have been observed in some patients (Kieslich et al., 2001). Between 1 to 5% of patients with CD will also have seizures (Chapman et al., 1978; Hanly et al., 1982; Pengiran Tengah et al., 2004; Vaknin et al., 2004). The reason for neurological dysfunction in CD and a higher propensity towards seizures may be multifactorial with malnutrition, hypocalcemia, hypomagnesemia, vasculitic complications of the disease, and genetic factors playing a role. Altered expression of activated T-cells, cytokines, and tTG might also have direct effects on brain dysfunction in CD (Gobbi, 2005).

A syndrome of celiac disease and epilepsy, in combination with cerebral calcifications, was described in Italy by Sammaritano et al. in 1985, and has been since described by several other groups worldwide (Molteni et al., 1988; Ventura et al., 1991; Ambrosetto et al., 1992; Gobbi et al., 1992a; Gobbi et al., 1992b; Hernandez et al., 1998; Bernasconi et al., 1998; Arroyo et al., 2002). According to a recent review by Gobbi, at least 171 cases have been reported in the literature, mainly from Italy, Argentina, and Spain (Gobbi, 2005). Where data was available for epilepsy classification, partial epilepsy predominated in the large majority of cases, with occipital seizures being the most common. Typical semiology was visual or versive seizures, potentially followed by complex partial or secondarily generalized seizures. Mild cognitive deterioration was described in some patients, with a minority progressing to a severe epileptic encephalopathy.

From a total of 96 cases in the review where electrographic data was available, the majority of patients with abnormalities had revealed unilateral or bilateral occipital spike or sharp wave discharges, which did not necessarily correlate with the presence of occipital calcifications. Focal abnormalities outside the occipital region were described in 4 cases, and generalized abnormalities were described in 11. Diffuse slow spike wave discharges were described in 14 patients, 8 with occipital epilepsy and progression to epileptic encephalopathy (Gobbi, 2005).

Cerebral calcifications tend to be occipital and bilateral, potentially the result of chronic folic acid deficiency or due to chronic immune complex mediated endothelial inflammation. The reason for the predilection of cerebral calcifications and epilepsy for the occipital region has not been explained. It is also unclear whether cerebral calcifications are a result of chronic untreated CD, due to a common genetic association, or coincidental. The exact prevalence of cerebral calcifications in CD is unknown (Gobbi, 2005).

Seizures have in the setting of CD have been shown to be responsive to a gluten free diet, with the response to treatment inversely correlated with the duration of the epilepsy and age at introduction of the diet (Gobbi et al., 1992b; Pratesi et al., 2003).

The data regarding the prevalence of CD related antibodies in unselected patients with epilepsy is conflicting, but does suggest that it is rare. A study screening 177 unselected patients with epilepsy, found 4 patients (2.3%) with biopsy confirmed CD (Cronin et al., 1998). Another screening 199 patients with epilepsy based on AGAb/tTGAb-positivity found 5 patients (2.5%) who also had abnormal gut biopsies, a significantly higher number than the expected prevalence of 0.27% in the study region (Luostarinen et al., 2001). In a larger study of the prevalence of AG Abs, EM Abs, and tTG Abs in 968 unselected patients with epilepsy, no difference was found in comparison with the control group. A significant difference was discovered, however, in the titers of IgA class AG Abs, among patients with primary generalized epilepsy *versus* the reference population, with a relative risk of 1.8. Confirmatory testing for CD was not done. The authors concluded that although there appears to be no increased prevalence of CD associated antibodies among unselected patients with epilepsy, the association between primary generalized epilepsy and CD may reflect a common genetic predisposition among the two diseases (Ranua et al., 2005b). A different study investigating children previously diagnosed with idiopathic partial epilepsy, found 2 out of 25 patients with occipital lobe epilepsy with antibody and histological evidence for clinically silent CD, again raising the possibility of a similar genetic predisposition towards both syndromes (Labate et al., 2001).

The possibility of a link between CD in primarily generalized epilepsy and idiopathic occipital lobe epilepsy is thought provoking, although it is not yet clear in what populations testing would be of highest yield. While screening for CD in unselected patients with epilepsy cannot be recommended based on the existing data, as a potentially treatable entity, it is important to consider CD early particularly in cases with symptoms suggestive of the disease, epilepsy with cerebral calcifications, and when other diagnosis have been excluded.

■ Other autoimmune syndromes and other autoantibodies

Case reports have also described seizures variably occurring in the setting of other autoimmune diseases including sarcoidosis (Sponsler et al., 2005), Sjogren syndrome (Delalande et al., 2004b), Bechet disease (Aykutlu et al., 2002), Wegener granulomatosis (Nishino et al., 1993), dermatomyositis (Elst et al., 2003), and inflammatory bowel disease (Akhan et al., 2002). Seizures have been reported both as a result of acute neurological exacerbation and secondary to disease or medication related toxic-metabolic derangements.

The presence of a number of other antibodies in patients with epilepsy is an ongoing active area of research. Disruption of ion channel function is a known mechanism for seizures, rendering ion channels or receptors a potential target in autoimmune mediated epilepsy syndromes (McKnight et al., 2005). Antibodies to voltage-gated potassium channels (VGKC Abs) have been reported to occur in the setting of limbic encephalitis and seizures (Vincent et al., 2004). Spontaneous clinical improvement or response in association with variable regimens of steroids, IVIG, and PE have been described in small case series (Vincent et al., 2004; McKnight et al., 2005). Increased titers of VGKC Abs were detected in 16 of 139 (11%) patients with seizures but in only 1 control (0.5%). Eight VGKC positive patients presented with an acute or subacute encephalopathic process, 3 patients improved spontaneously, and 5 patients responded to immunomotherapy. The other eight all had epilepsy of long duration (McKnight et al., 2005). A follow up study of 106 female patients with epilepsy found VGKC Abs raised in 6 (5.7%), who were clinically indistinct from the rest of the subjects (Majoie et al., 2006).

Anti-GM1 ganglioside antibodies (GM1 Abs) have been shown to be epileptogenic in rats (Karpiak et al., 1981). Gangliosides are components of the synaptic membrane, and antibodies directed towards them may inhibit the synaptic binding of GABA, and modulate calcium channel mediated GABA release (Frieder and Rapport, 1987; Palace and Lang, 2000). In a study of 64 patients with various types of epilepsy, 4 patients (6.25%) had elevated titers of GM1 Abs. All 4 had medically refractory partial epilepsy, normal neuroimaging, and psychiatric complications. Two of these patients were treated successfully with IVIG (Bartolomei *et al.*, 1996). Another anecdotal case of a patient with focal motor status, normal imaging, Waldenstrom macroglobinemia, and response to immunomodulatory therapy has been reported (Guillon *et al.*, 1997). GM1 Abs were observed in 1 of 96 patients studied with JME, and in 1 of 25 healthy controls, and were decidedly not associated with JME or medically refractory disease (Aykutlu *et al.*, 2005). Interestingly, in light of the association between lupus and epilepsy, GM1 Abs have also been observed in up to 15.5% of patients with SLE (Galeazzi *et al.*, 2000).

In a study of 968 patients with epilepsy, antimitochondrial antibodies (AM Abs) were detected in 3.9% of patients *versus* 1.9% of controls, a significantly higher rate. The presence of AM Abs was weakly associated with longer disease duration and older age at onset, and had no correlation with other cormorbidities or medications. AM Abs have previously been described in association with primary biliary sclerosis, bacterial infections, certain medications, myocardial infarction, and graft *versus* host disease. The authors concluded that seizures may have played a potential role in immunological activation and the formation of nonspecific AM Abs, which were of limited clinical significance (Ranua *et al.*, 2005a).

Seizure improvement in the setting of infantile spasms (West syndrome) and less consistently with Lennox-Gastaut syndrome has been observed in association with the administration of corticotropin (ACTH) and steroids. West syndrome and Lennox-Gastaut syndrome are heterogeneous and of uncertain pathogenesis. They may potentially arise from a number of different etiologies. It is unclear why steroids or ACTH produce a positive effect in these syndromes, and the cause may be independent of an immune suppressive effect (Aarli, 2000). Likewise, steroids (Marescaux *et al.*, 1990; Sinclair and Snyder, 2005) and IVIG therapy (Fayad *et al.*, 1997; Mikati and Shamseddine, 2005) have been used successfully in some cases of acquired epileptic aphasia (Landau-Kleffner syndrome) (Hirsch *et al.*, 2006). Anti-endomesial antibodies, myelin basic protein antibodies (MBP Abs), anti-neural antibodies, and brain derived neurotrophic factor antibodies (BDNF Abs) have been described in association with this syndrome (Connolly *et al.*, 1999; Connolly *et al.*, 2006). Although, due to the coexistence of some of these autoantibodies in other syndromes such as autism and other epilepsy types, they are believed to be nonspecific and a secondary marker of disease rather than directly pathogenic (Connolly *et al.*, 2006).

References

Aarli JA. Epilepsy and the immune system. *Arch Neurol* 2000; 57: 1689-92.

Adams C, Hwang PA, Gilday DL, Armstrong DC, Becker LE, Hoffman HJ. Comparison of SPECT, EEG, CT, MRI, and pathology in partial epilepsy. *Pediatr Neurol* 1992; 8: 97-103.

Aiello DP, DuPlessis AJ, Pattishall EG, 3rd, Kulin HE. Thyroid storm. Presenting with coma and seizures. In a 3-year-old girl. *Clin Pediatr (Phila)* 1989; 28: 571-4.

Akhan G, Andermann F, Gotman MJ. Ulcerative colitis, status epilepticus and intractable temporal seizures. *Epileptic Disord* 2002; 4: 135-7.

Alarcon GS, Friedman AW, Straaton KV, Moulds JM, Lisse J, Bastian HM, *et al.* Systemic lupus erythematosus in three ethnic groups: III. A comparison of characteristics early in the natural history of the LUMINA cohort. LUpus in MInority populations: NAture *vs* Nurture. *Lupus* 1999; 8: 197-209.

Ambrosetto G, Antonini L, Tassinari CA. Occipital lobe seizures related to clinically asymptomatic celiac disease in adulthood. *Epilepsia* 1992; 33: 476-81.

American Association of Clinical Endocrinologists. Medical guidelines for clinical practice for the evaluation and treatment of hyperthyroidism and hypothyroidism. *Endocr Pract* 2002; 8: 457-69.

Andrews PI, Dichter MA, Berkovic SF, Newton MR, McNamara JO. Plasmapheresis in Rasmussen's encephalitis. *Neurology* 1996; 46: 242-6.

Andrews PI, McNamara JO, Lewis DV. Clinical and electroencephalographic correlates in Rasmussen's encephalitis. *Epilepsia* 1997; 38: 189-94.

Angelini L, Granata T, Zibordi F, Binelli S, Zorzi G, Besana C. Partial seizures associated with anti-phospholipid antibodies in childhood. *Neuropediatrics* 1998; 29: 249-53.

Appenzeller S, Cendes F, Costallat LT. Epileptic seizures in systemic lupus erythematosus. *Neurology* 2004; 63: 1808-12.

Arain A, Abou-Khalil B, Moses H. Hashimoto's encephalopathy: documentation of mesial temporal seizure origin by ictal EEG. *Seizure* 2001; 10: 438-41.

Arroyo HA, De Rosa S, Ruggieri V, de Davila MT, Fejerman N. Epilepsy, occipital calcifications, and oligosymptomatic celiac disease in childhood. *J Child Neurol* 2002; 17: 800-6.

Atkins MR, Terrell W, Hulette CM. Rasmussen's syndrome: a study of potential viral etiology. *Clin Neuropathol* 1995; 14: 7-12.

Aydin A, Cemeroglu AP, Baklan B. Thyroxine-induced hypermotor seizure. *Seizure* 2004; 13: 61-5.

Aykutlu E, Baykan B, Serdaroglu P, Gokyigit A, Akman-Demir G. Epileptic seizures in Behcet disease. *Epilepsia* 2002; 43: 832-5.

Aykutlu E, Baykan B, Gurses C, Gokyigit A, Saruhan-Direskeneli G. No association of anti-GM1 and anti-GAD antibodies with juvenile myoclonic epilepsy: a pilot study. *Seizure* 2005; 14: 362-6.

Baekkeskov S, Nielsen JH, Marner B, Bilde T, Ludvigsson J, Lernmark A. Autoantibodies in newly diagnosed diabetic children immunoprecipitate human pancreatic islet cell proteins. *Nature* 1982; 298: 167-9.

Baekkeskov S, Aanstoot HJ, Christgau S, Reetz A, Solimena M, Cascalho M, *et al.* Identification of the 64K autoantigen in insulin-dependent diabetes as the GABA-synthesizing enzyme glutamic acid decarboxylase. *Nature* 1990; 347: 151-6.

Barker JM. Clinical review: Type 1 diabetes-associated autoimmunity: natural history, genetic associations, and screening. *J Clin Endocrinol Metab* 2006; 91: 1210-7.

Barker RA, Revesz T, Thom M, Marsden CD, Brown P (1998). Review of 23 patients affected by the stiff man syndrome: clinical subdivision into stiff trunk (man) syndrome, stiff limb syndrome, and progressive encephalomyelitis with rigidity. **65**: 633-640.

Bartolomei F, Boucraut J, Barrie M, Kok J, Dravet C, Viallat D, *et al.* Cryptogenic partial epilepsies with anti-GM1 antibodies: a new form of immune-mediated epilepsy? *Epilepsia* 1996; 37: 922-6.

Bernasconi A, Bernasconi N, Andermann F, Dubeau F, Guberman A, Gobbi G, *et al.* Celiac disease, bilateral occipital calcifications and intractable epilepsy: mechanisms of seizure origin. *Epilepsia* 1998; 39: 300-6.

Bernasconi P, Cipelletti B, Passerini L, Granata T, Antozzi C, Mantegazza R, *et al.* Similar binding to glutamate receptors by Rasmussen and partial epilepsy patients' sera. *Neurology* 2002; 59: 1998-2001.

Bhatjiwale MG, Polkey C, Cox TC, Dean A, Deasy N. Rasmussen's encephalitis: neuroimaging findings in 21 patients with a closer look at the basal ganglia. *Pediatr Neurosurg* 1998; 29: 142-8.

Bien CG, Elger CE, Wiendl H. Advances in pathogenic concepts and therapeutic agents in Rasmussen's encephalitis. *Expert Opin Investig Drugs* 2002a; 11: 981-9.

Bien CG, Widman G, Urbach H, Sassen R, Kuczaty S, Wiestler OD, et al. The natural history of Rasmussen's encephalitis. *Brain* 2002b; 125: 1751-9.

Bien CG, Gleissner U, Sassen R, Widman G, Urbach H, Elger CE. An open study of tacrolimus therapy in Rasmussen encephalitis. *Neurology* 2004; 62: 2106-9.

Bien CG, Granata T, Antozzi C, Cross JH, Dulac O, Kurthen M, et al. Pathogenesis, diagnosis and treatment of Rasmussen encephalitis: a European consensus statement. *Brain* 2005; 128: 454-71.

Bjorgaas M, Sand T, Gimse R. Quantitative EEG in type 1 diabetic children with and without episodes of severe hypoglycemia: a controlled, blind study. *Acta Neurol Scand* 1996; 93: 398-402.

Boers PM and Colebatch JG. Hashimoto's encephalopathy responding to plasmapheresis. *J Neurol Neurosurg Psychiatry* 2001; 70: 132.

Bohnen NI, Parnell KJ, Harper CM. Reversible MRI findings in a patient with Hashimoto's encephalopathy. *Neurology* 1997; 49: 246-7.

Brain L, Jellinek EH, Ball K. Hashimoto's disease and encephalopathy. *Lancet* 1966; 2: 512-4.

Brey RL, Holliday SL, Saklad AR, Navarrete MG, Hermosillo-Romo D, Stallworth CL, et al. Neuropsychiatric syndromes in lupus: prevalence using standardized definitions. *Neurology* 2002; 58: 1214-20.

Brismar T, Hyllienmark L, Ekberg K, Johansson BL. Loss of temporal lobe beta power in young adults with type 1 diabetes mellitus. *Neuroreport* 2002; 13: 2469-73.

Burke GJ, Fifer SA, Yoder J. Early detection of Rasmussen's syndrome by brain SPECT imaging. *Clin Nucl Med* 1992; 17: 730-1.

Butler MH, Solimena M, Dirkx R, Jr., Hayday A, De Camilli P. Identification of a dominant epitope of glutamic acid decarboxylase (GAD-65) recognized by autoantibodies in stiff-man syndrome. *J Exp Med* 1993; 178: 2097-106.

Canton A, de Fabregas O, Tintore M, Mesa J, Codina A, Simo R. Encephalopathy associated to autoimmune thyroid disease: a more appropriate term for an underestimated condition? *J Neurol Sci* 2000; 176: 65-9.

Castillo P, Woodruff B, Caselli R, Vernino S, Lucchinetti C, Swanson J, et al. Steroid-responsive encephalopathy associated with autoimmune thyroiditis. *Arch Neurol* 2006; 63: 197-202.

Cendes F, Andermann F, Silver K, Arnold DL. Imaging of axonal damage *in vivo* in Rasmussen's syndrome. *Brain* 1995; 118 (Pt 3): 753-8.

Cervera R, Piette JC, Font J, Khamashta MA, Shoenfeld Y, Camps MT, et al. Antiphospholipid syndrome: clinical and immunologic manifestations and patterns of disease expression in a cohort of 1,000 patients. *Arthritis Rheum* 2002; 46: 1019-27.

Chang BS and Lowenstein DH. Epilepsy. *N Engl J Med* 2003; 349: 1257-66.

Chapman EM and Maloof F. Bizarre clinical manifestations of hyperthyroidism. *N Engl J Med* 1956; 254: 1-5.

Chapman J, Cohen-Armon M, Shoenfeld Y, Korczyn AD. Antiphospholipid antibodies permeabilize and depolarize brain synaptoneurosomes. *Lupus* 1999; 8: 127-33.

Chapman J, Soloveichick L, Shavit S, Shoenfeld Y, Korczyn AD. Antiphospholipid antibodies bind ATP: a putative mechanism for the pathogenesis of neuronal dysfunction. *Clin Dev Immunol* 2005; 12: 175-80.

Chapman RW, Laidlow JM, Colin-Jones D, Eade OE, Smith CL. Increased prevalence of epilepsy in coeliac disease. *Br Med J* 1978; 2: 250-1.

Chiapparini L, Granata T, Farina L, Ciceri E, Erbetta A, Ragona F, et al. Diagnostic imaging in 13 cases of Rasmussen's encephalitis: can early MRI suggest the diagnosis? *Neuroradiology* 2003; 45: 171-83.

Chinchilla D, Dulac O, Robain O, Plouin P, Ponsot G, Pinel JF, et al. Reappraisal of Rasmussen's syndrome with special emphasis on treatment with high doses of steroids. *J Neurol Neurosurg Psychiatry* 1994; 57: 1325-33.

Chong JY, Rowland LP, Utiger RD. Hashimoto encephalopathy: syndrome or myth? *Arch Neurol* 2003; 60: 164-71.

Cimaz R, Romeo A, Scarano A, Avcin T, Viri M, Veggiotti P, et al. Prevalence of anti-cardiolipin, anti-beta2 glycoprotein I, and anti-prothrombin antibodies in young patients with epilepsy. Epilepsia 2002; 43: 52-9.

Cimaz R, Meroni PL, Shoenfeld Y. Epilepsy as part of systemic lupus erythematosus and systemic antiphospholipid syndrome (Hughes syndrome). Lupus 2006; 15: 191-7.

Connolly AM, Chez MG, Pestronk A, Arnold ST, Mehta S, Deuel RK. Serum autoantibodies to brain in Landau-Kleffner variant, autism, and other neurologic disorders. J Pediatr 1999; 134: 607-13.

Connolly AM, Chez M, Streif EM, Keeling RM, Golumbek PT, Kwon JM, et al. Brain-derived neurotrophic factor and autoantibodies to neural antigens in sera of children with autistic spectrum disorders, Landau-Kleffner syndrome, and epilepsy. Biol Psychiatry 2006; 59: 354-63.

Cronin CC, Jackson LM, Feighery C, Shanahan F, Abuzakouk M, Ryder DQ, et al. Coeliac disease and epilepsy. Qjm 1998; 91: 303-8.

Dabbagh O, Gascon G, Crowell J, Bamoggadam F. Intraventricular interferon-alpha stops seizures in Rasmussen's encephalitis: a case report. Epilepsia 1997; 38: 1045-9.

Daw K, Ujihara N, Atkinson M, Powers AC. Glutamic acid decarboxylase autoantibodies in stiff-man syndrome and insulin-dependent diabetes mellitus exhibit similarities and differences in epitope recognition. J Immunol 1996; 156: 818-25.

De Aizpurua HJ, Wilson YM, Harrison LC. Glutamic acid decarboxylase autoantibodies in preclinical insulin-dependent diabetes. Proc Natl Acad Sci U S A 1992; 89: 9841-5.

Debourdeau P, Gerome P, Zammit C, Saillol A, Aletti M, Bargues L, et al. Frequency of anticardiolipin, antinuclear and anti beta2GP1 antibodies is not increased in unselected epileptic patients: a case-control study. Seizure 2004; 13: 205-7.

Delalande O, Fohlen M, Bulteau C, Jalin C. [Surgery for intractable focal epilepsy in children]. Rev Neurol (Paris) 2004a; 160 Spec No 1: 5S195-202.

Delalande S, de Seze J, Fauchais AL, Hachulla E, Stojkovic T, Ferriby D, et al. Neurologic manifestations in primary Sjogren syndrome: a study of 82 patients. Medicine (Baltimore) 2004b; 83: 280-91.

DeToledo JC and Smith DB. Partially successful treatment of Rasmussen's encephalitis with zidovudine: symptomatic improvement followed by involvement of the contralateral hemisphere. Epilepsia 1994; 35: 352-5.

The Diabetes Control and Complications Trial Research Group. Hypoglycemia in the Diabetes Control and Complications Trial.. Diabetes 1997; 46: 271-86.

Duffey P, Yee S, Reid IN, Bridges LR. Hashimoto's encephalopathy: postmortem findings after fatal status epilepticus. Neurology 2003; 61: 1124-6.

Dulac O. Rasmussen's syndrome. Curr Opin Neurol 1996; 9: 75-7.

Eeg-Olofsson O. Hypoglycemia and neurological disturbances in children with diabetes mellitus. Acta Paediatr Scand Suppl 1977: 91-6.

Ellis TM and Atkinson MA. The clinical significance of an autoimmune response against glutamic acid decarboxylase. Nat Med 1996; 2: 148-53.

Elst EF, Kamphuis SS, Prakken BJ, Wulffraat NM, van der Net J, Peters AC, et al. Case report: severe central nervous system involvement in juvenile dermatomyositis. J Rheumatol 2003; 30: 2059-63.

Erdo SL and Wolff JR. gamma-Aminobutyric acid outside the mammalian brain. J Neurochem 1990; 54: 363-72.

Eriksson K, Peltola J, Keranen T, Haapala AM, Koivikko M. High prevalence of antiphospholipid antibodies in children with epilepsy: a controlled study of 50 cases. Epilepsy Res 2001; 46: 129-37.

Esclapez M, Tillakaratne NJ, Kaufman DL, Tobin AJ, Houser CR. Comparative localization of two forms of glutamic acid decarboxylase and their mRNAs in rat brain supports the concept of functional differences between the forms. J Neurosci 1994; 14: 1834-55.

Evans EC. Neurologic complications of myxedema: convulsions. Ann Intern Med 1960; 52: 434-44.

Expert Committee on the Diagnosis and Classification of Diabetes Mellitus. Report of the expert committee on the diagnosis and classification of diabetes mellitus. *Diabetes Care* 2003; 26 (suppl 1): S5-20.

Farrell MA, Droogan O, Secor DL, Poukens V, Quinn B, Vinters HV. Chronic encephalitis associated with epilepsy: immunohistochemical and ultrastructural studies. *Acta Neuropathol (Berl)* 1995; 89: 313-21.

Farrell RJ and Kelly CP. Celiac sprue. *N Engl J Med* 2002; 346: 180-8.

Fayad MN, Choueiri R, Mikati M. Landau-Kleffner syndrome: consistent response to repeated intravenous gamma-globulin doses: a case report. *Epilepsia* 1997; 38: 489-94.

Ferlazzo E, Raffaele M, Mazzu I, Pisani F. Recurrent status epilepticus as the main feature of Hashimoto's encephalopathy. *Epilepsy Behav* 2006; 8: 328-30.

Ferracci F, Moretto G, Candeago RM, Cimini N, Conte F, Gentile M, et al. Antithyroid antibodies in the CSF: their role in the pathogenesis of Hashimoto's encephalopathy. *Neurology* 2003; 60: 712-4.

Ferracci F, Bertiato G, Moretto G. Hashimoto's encephalopathy: epidemiologic data and pathogenetic considerations. *J Neurol Sci* 2004; 217: 165-8.

Ferracci F and Carnevale A. The neurological disorder associated with thyroid autoimmunity. *J Neurol* 2006; 253: 975-84.

Fliers E and Wiersinga WM. Myxedema coma. *Rev Endocr Metab Disord* 2003; 4: 137-41.

Forchetti CM, Katsamakis G, Garron DC. Autoimmune thyroiditis and a rapidly progressive dementia: global hypoperfusion on SPECT scanning suggests a possible mechanism. *Neurology* 1997; 49: 623-6.

Formiga F, Moga I, Canet R, Pac M, Mitjavila F, Pujol R. [Antiphospholipid antibodies and epilepsy in patients with systemic lupus erythematosus]. *Rev Clin Esp* 1996; 196: 734-6.

Frassoni C, Spreafico R, Franceschetti S, Aurisano N, Bernasconi P, Garbelli R, et al. Labeling of rat neurons by anti-GluR3 IgG from patients with Rasmussen encephalitis. *Neurology* 2001; 57: 324-7.

Frieder B and Rapport MM. The effect of antibodies to gangliosides on Ca2+ channel-linked release of gamma-aminobutyric acid in rat brain slices. *J Neurochem* 1987; 48: 1048-52.

Frucht S. Dystonia, athetosis, and epilepsia partialis continua in a patient with late-onset Rasmussen's encephalitis. *Mov Disord* 2002; 17: 609-12.

Gahring L, Carlson NG, Meyer EL, Rogers SW. Granzyme B proteolysis of a neuronal glutamate receptor generates an autoantigen and is modulated by glycosylation. *J Immunol* 2001; 166: 1433-8.

Galeazzi M, Annunziata P, Sebastiani GD, Bellisai F, Campanella V, Ferrara GB, et al. Anti-ganglioside antibodies in a large cohort of European patients with systemic lupus erythematosus: clinical, serological, and HLA class II gene associations. European Concerted Action on the Immunogenetics of SLE. *J Rheumatol* 2000; 27: 135-41.

Ganor Y, Goldberg-Stern H, Amromd D, Lerman-Sagie T, Teichberg VI, Pelled D, et al. Autoimmune epilepsy: some epilepsy patients harbor autoantibodies to glutamate receptors and dsDNA on both sides of the blood-brain barrier, which may kill neurons and decrease in brain fluids after hemispherotomy. *Clin Dev Immunol* 2004; 11: 241-52.

Gibbs JW, 3rd and Husain AM. Epilepsy associated with lupus anticoagulant. *Seizure* 2002; 11: 207-9.

Giometto B, Nicolao P, Macucci M, Tavolato B, Foxon R, Bottazzo GF. Temporal-lobe epilepsy associated with glutamic-acid-decarboxylase autoantibodies. *Lancet* 1998; 352: 457.

Glanz BI, Schur PH, Khoshbin S. EEG abnormalities in systemic lupus erythematosus. *Clin Electroencephalogr* 1998; 29: 128-31.

Go T, Ito M, Okuno T, Mikawa H. Effect of thyroid hormones on benzodiazepine receptors in neuron-enriched primary cultures. *J Neurochem* 1988; 51: 1497-500.

Gobbi G, Ambrosetto P, Zaniboni MG, Lambertini A, Ambrosioni G, Tassinari CA. Celiac disease, posterior cerebral calcifications and epilepsy. *Brain Dev* 1992a; 14: 23-9.

Gobbi G, Bouquet F, Greco L, Lambertini A, Tassinari CA, Ventura A, et al. Coeliac disease, epilepsy, and cerebral calcifications. The Italian Working Group on Coeliac Disease and Epilepsy. *Lancet* 1992b; 340: 439-43.

Gobbi G. Coeliac disease, epilepsy and cerebral calcifications. *Brain Dev* 2005; 27: 189-200.

Granata T, Fusco L, Gobbi G, Freri E, Ragona F, Broggi G, et al. Experience with immunomodulatory treatments in Rasmussen's encephalitis. *Neurology* 2003a; 61: 1807-10.

Granata T, Gobbi G, Spreafico R, Vigevano F, Capovilla G, Ragona F, et al. Rasmussen's encephalitis: early characteristics allow diagnosis. *Neurology* 2003b; 60: 422-5.

Green PH, Rostami K, Marsh MN. Diagnosis of coeliac disease. *Best Pract Res Clin Gastroenterol* 2005; 19: 389-400.

Guillon B, de Ferron E, Feve JR, Honnorat J, Caudie C, Nogues B, et al. Simple partial status epilepticus and antiglycolipid IgM antibodies: possible epilepsy of autoimmune origin. *Arch Neurol* 1997; 54: 1194-6.

Hagopian WA, Karlsen AE, Gottsater A, Landin-Olsson M, Grubin CE, Sundkvist G, et al. Quantitative assay using recombinant human islet glutamic acid decarboxylase (GAD65) shows that 64K autoantibody positivity at onset predicts diabetes type. *J Clin Invest* 1993; 91: 368-74.

Halonen H, Hiekkala H, Huupponen T, Hakkinen VK. A follow-up EEG study in diabetic children. *Ann Clin Res* 1983; 15: 167-72.

Hanly JG, Stassen W, Whelton M, Callaghan N. Epilepsy and coeliac disease. *J Neurol Neurosurg Psychiatry* 1982; 45: 729-30.

Hart YM, Cortez M, Andermann F, Hwang P, Fish DR, Dulac O, et al. Medical treatment of Rasmussen's syndrome (chronic encephalitis and epilepsy): effect of high-dose steroids or immunoglobulins in 19 patients. *Neurology* 1994; 44: 1030-6.

Hart YM, Andermann F, Fish DR, Dubeau F, Robitaille Y, Rasmussen T, et al. Chronic encephalitis and epilepsy in adults and adolescents: a variant of Rasmussen's syndrome? *Neurology* 1997; 48: 418-24.

Hart YM, Andermann F, Robitaille Y, Laxer KD, Rasmussen T, Davis R. Double pathology in Rasmussen's syndrome: a window on the etiology? *Neurology* 1998; 50: 731-5.

He XP, Patel M, Whitney KD, Janumpalli S, Tenner A, McNamara JO. Glutamate receptor GluR3 antibodies and death of cortical cells. *Neuron* 1998; 20: 153-63.

Henchey R, Cibula J, Helveston W, Malone J, Gilmore RL. Electroencephalographic findings in Hashimoto's encephalopathy. *Neurology* 1995; 45: 977-81.

Hernandez MA, Colina G, Ortigosa L. Epilepsy, cerebral calcifications and clinical or subclinical coeliac disease. Course and follow up with gluten-free diet. *Seizure* 1998; 7: 49-54.

Herranz MT, Rivier G, Khamashta MA, Blaser KU, Hughes GR. Association between antiphospholipid antibodies and epilepsy in patients with systemic lupus erythematosus. *Arthritis Rheum* 1994; 37: 568-71.

Hess DC, Sheppard JC, Adams RJ. Increased immunoglobulin binding to cerebral endothelium in patients with antiphospholipid antibodies. *Stroke* 1993; 24: 994-9.

Hilker R, Thiel A, Geisen C, Rudolf J. Cerebral blood flow and glucose metabolism in multi-infarct-dementia related to primary antiphospholipid antibody syndrome. *Lupus* 2000; 9: 311-6.

Hirsch E, Valenti MP, Rudolf G, Seegmuller C, de Saint Martin A, Maquet P, et al. Landau-Kleffner syndrome is not an eponymic badge of ignorance. *Epilepsy Res* 2006; 70 (suppl 1): S239-47.

Honavar M, Janota I, Polkey CE. Rasmussen's encephalitis in surgery for epilepsy. *Dev Med Child Neurol* 1992; 34: 3-14.

Honnorat J, Trouillas P, Thivolet C, Aguera M, Belin MF. Autoantibodies to glutamate decarboxylase in a patient with cerebellar cortical atrophy, peripheral neuropathy, and slow eye movements. *Arch Neurol* 1995; 52: 462-8.

Howorka K, Pumprla J, Saletu B, Anderer P, Krieger M, Schabmann A. Decrease of vigilance assessed by EEG-mapping in type I diabetic patients with history of recurrent severe hypoglycaemia. *Psychoneuroendocrinology* 2000; 25: 85-105.

Hunter GR, Donat J, Pryse-Phillips W, Harder S, Robinson CA. Rasmussen's encephalitis in a 58-year-old female: still a variant? *Can J Neurol Sci* 2006; 33: 302-5.

Hyllienmark L, Maltez J, Dandenell A, Ludvigsson J, Brismar T. EEG abnormalities with and without relation to severe hypoglycaemia in adolescents with type 1 diabetes. *Diabetologia* 2005; 48: 412-9.

Inzelberg R and Korczyn AD. Lupus anticoagulant and late onset seizures. *Acta Neurol Scand* 1989; 79: 114-8.

Jabbari B and Huott AD. Seizures in thyrotoxicosis. *Epilepsia* 1980; 21: 91-6.

Jansen HJ, Doebe SR, Louwerse ES, van der Linden JC, Netten PM. Status epilepticus caused by a myxoedema coma. *Neth J Med* 2006; 64: 202-5.

Jay V, Becker LE, Otsubo H, Cortez M, Hwang P, Hoffman HJ, et al. Chronic encephalitis and epilepsy (Rasmussen's encephalitis): detection of cytomegalovirus and herpes simplex virus 1 by the polymerase chain reaction and in situ hybridization. *Neurology* 1995; 45: 108-17.

Jellinek EH. Fits, faints, coma, and dementia in myxoedema. *Lancet* 1962; 2: 1010-2.

Karpiak SE, Mahadik SP, Graf L, Rapport MM. An immunological model of epilepsy: seizures induced by antibodies to GM1 ganglioside. *Epilepsia* 1981; 22: 189-96.

Kash SF, Johnson RS, Tecott LH, Noebels JL, Mayfield RD, Hanahan D, et al. Epilepsy in mice deficient in the 65-kDa isoform of glutamic acid decarboxylase. *Proc Natl Acad Sci U S A* 1997; 94: 14060-5.

Kent MN, Alvarez FJ, Ng AK, Rote NS. Ultrastructural localization of monoclonal antiphospholipid antibody binding to rat brain. *Exp Neurol* 2000; 163: 173-9.

Kieslich M, Errazuriz G, Posselt HG, Moeller-Hartmann W, Zanella F, Boehles H. Brain white-matter lesions in celiac disease: a prospective study of 75 diet-treated patients. *Pediatrics* 2001; 108: E21.

Kim J, Namchuk M, Bugawan T, Fu Q, Jaffe M, Shi Y, et al. Higher autoantibody levels and recognition of a linear NH2-terminal epitope in the autoantigen GAD65, distinguish stiff-man syndrome from insulin-dependent diabetes mellitus. *J Exp Med* 1994; 180: 595-606.

Korczyn AD and Bechar M. Convulsive fits in thyrotoxicosis. *Epilepsia* 1976; 17: 33-4.

Kothbauer-Margreiter I, Sturzenegger M, Komor J, Baumgartner R, Hess CW. Encephalopathy associated with Hashimoto thyroiditis: diagnosis and treatment. *J Neurol* 1996; 243: 585-93.

Kwan P, Sills GJ, Kelly K, Butler E, Brodie MJ. Glutamic acid decarboxylase autoantibodies in controlled and uncontrolled epilepsy: a pilot study. *Epilepsy Res* 2000; 42: 191-5.

Labate A, Gambardella A, Messina D, Tammaro S, Le Piane E, Pirritano D, et al. Silent celiac disease in patients with childhood localization-related epilepsies. *Epilepsia* 2001; 42: 1153-5.

Lampropoulos CE, Koutroumanidis M, Reynolds PP, Manidakis I, Hughes GR, D'Cruz DP. Electroencephalography in the assessment of neuropsychiatric manifestations in antiphospholipid syndrome and systemic lupus erythematosus. *Arthritis Rheum* 2005; 52: 841-6.

Larionov S, Konig R, Urbach H, Sassen R, Elger CE, Bien CG. MRI brain volumetry in Rasmussen encephalitis: the fate of affected and "unaffected" hemispheres. *Neurology* 2005; 64: 885-7.

Leach JP, Chadwick DW, Miles JB, Hart IK. Improvement in adult-onset Rasmussen's encephalitis with long-term immunomodulatory therapy. *Neurology* 1999; 52: 738-42.

Levin ME and Daughaday WH. Fatal coma due to myxedema. *Am J Med* 1955; 18: 1017-21.

Levite M, Fleidervish IA, Schwarz A, Pelled D, Futerman AH. Autoantibodies to the glutamate receptor kill neurons via activation of the receptor ion channel. *J Autoimmun* 1999; 13: 61-72.

Levite M and Hermelin A. Autoimmunity to the glutamate receptor in mice – a model for Rasmussen's encephalitis? *J Autoimmun* 1999; 13: 73-82.

Li Y, Uccelli A, Laxer KD, Jeong MC, Vinters HV, Tourtellotte WW, et al. Local-clonal expansion of infiltrating T lymphocytes in chronic encephalitis of Rasmussen. *J Immunol* 1997; 158: 1428-37.

Liou HH, Wang CR, Chou HC, Arvanov VL, Chen RC, Chang YC, et al. Anticardiolipin antisera from lupus patients with seizures reduce a GABA receptor-mediated chloride current in snail neurons. *Life Sci* 1994; 54: 1119-25.

Liou HH, Wang CR, Chen CJ, Chen RC, Chuang CY, Chiang IP, et al. Elevated levels of anticardiolipin antibodies and epilepsy in lupus patients. Lupus 1996; 5: 307-12.

Luostarinen L, Dastidar P, Collin P, Peraaho M, Maki M, Erila T, et al. Association between coeliac disease, epilepsy and brain atrophy. Eur Neurol 2001; 46: 187-91.

Majoie HJ, de Baets M, Renier W, Lang B, Vincent A. Antibodies to voltage-gated potassium and calcium channels in epilepsy. Epilepsy Res 2006; 71: 135-41.

Mantegazza R, Bernasconi P, Baggi F, Spreafico R, Ragona F, Antozzi C, et al. Antibodies against GluR3 peptides are not specific for Rasmussen's encephalitis but are also present in epilepsy patients with severe, early onset disease and intractable seizures. J Neuroimmunol 2002; 131: 179-85.

Marescaux C, Hirsch E, Finck S, Maquet P, Schlumberger E, Sellal F, et al. Landau-Kleffner syndrome: a pharmacologic study of five cases. Epilepsia 1990; 31: 768-77.

Maria BL, Ringdahl DM, Mickle JP, Smith LJ, Reuman PD, Gilmore RL, et al. Intraventricular alpha interferon therapy for Rasmussen's syndrome. Can J Neurol Sci 1993; 20: 333-6.

Marjanovic BD, Stojanov LM, Zdravkovic DS, Kravljanac RM, Djordjevic MS. Rasmussen syndrome and long-term response to thalidomide. Pediatr Neurol 2003; 29: 151-6.

Martinelli P, Pazzaglia P, Montagna P, Coccagna G, Rizzuto N, Simonati S, et al. Stiff-man syndrome associated with nocturnal myoclonus and epilepsy. J Neurol Neurosurg Psychiatry 1978; 41: 458-62.

Mason GA, Walker CH, Prange AJ, Jr., Bondy SC. GABA uptake is inhibited by thyroid hormones: implications for depression. Psychoneuroendocrinology 1987; 12: 53-9.

McCorry D, Nicolson A, Smith D, Marson A, Feltbower RG, Chadwick DW. An association between type 1 diabetes and idiopathic generalized epilepsy. Ann Neurol 2006; 59: 204-6.

McKeon A, McNamara B, Sweeney B. Hashimoto's encephalopathy presenting with psychosis and generalized absence status. J Neurol 2004; 251: 1025-7.

McKnight K, Jiang Y, Hart Y, Cavey A, Wroe S, Blank M, et al. Serum antibodies in epilepsy and seizure-associated disorders. Neurology 2005; 65: 1730-6.

McLachlan RS, Girvin JP, Blume WT, Reichman H. Rasmussen's chronic encephalitis in adults. Arch Neurol 1993; 50: 269-74.

McLachlan RS, Levin S, Blume WT. Treatment of Rasmussen's syndrome with ganciclovir. Neurology 1996; 47: 925-8.

Mikati MA and Shamseddine AN. Management of Landau-Kleffner syndrome. Paediatr Drugs 2005; 7: 377-89.

Mikdashi J, Krumholz A, Handwerger B (2005). Factors at diagnosis predict subsequent occurrence of seizures in systemic lupus erythematosus. **64:** 2102-2107.

Molteni N, Bardella MT, Baldassarri AR, Bianchi PA. Celiac disease associated with epilepsy and intracranial calcifications: report of two patients. Am J Gastroenterol 1988; 83: 992-4.

National Institute of Diabetes and Digestive and Kidney Diseases. National Diabetes Statistics fact sheet: general information and national estimates on diabetes in the United States. 2005

Navarrete MG and Brey RL. Neuropsychiatric Systemic Lupus Erythematosus. Curr Treat Options Neurol 2000; 2: 473-485.

Nemni R, Braghi S, Natali-Sora MG, Lampasona V, Bonifacio E, Comi G, et al. Autoantibodies to glutamic acid decarboxylase in palatal myoclonus and epilepsy. Ann Neurol 1994; 36: 665-7.

Nielsen PE and Ranlov P. Myxoedema Coma. Two Case Reports and a Review. Acta Endocrinol (Copenh) 1964; 45: 353-64.

Nishino H, Rubino FA, DeRemee RA, Swanson JW, Parisi JE. Neurological involvement in Wegener's granulomatosis: an analysis of 324 consecutive patients at the Mayo Clinic. Ann Neurol 1993; 33: 4-9.

Nolte KW, Unbehaun A, Sieker H, Kloss TM, Paulus W. Hashimoto encephalopathy: a brainstem vasculitis? Neurology 2000; 54: 769-70.

Obeid T, Awada A, al Rajeh S, Chaballout A. Thyroxine exacerbates absence seizures in juvenile myoclonic epilepsy. Neurology 1996; 47: 605-6.

Oguni H, Andermann F, Rasmussen TB The natural history of the syndrome of chronic encephalitis and epilepsy: a study of the MNI series of fortyeight cases. In: A. F, ed. *Chronic encephalitis and epilepsy. Rasmussen's syndrome*. Boston: Butterworth-Heinemann, 1991: 7-35.

Olson JA, Olson DM, Sandborg C, Alexander S, Buckingham B. Type 1 diabetes mellitus and epilepsia partialis continua in a 6-year-old boy with elevated anti-GAD65 antibodies. *Pediatrics* 2002; 109: E50.

Palace J and Lang B. Epilepsy: an autoimmune disease? *J Neurol Neurosurg Psychiatry* 2000; 69: 711-4.

Pardo A, Gonzalez-Porque P, Gobernado JM, Jimenez-Escrig A, Lousa M. Study of antiphospholipid antibodies in patients treated with antiepileptic drugs. *Neurologia* 2001; 16: 7-10.

Pardo CA, Vining EP, Guo L, Skolasky RL, Carson BS, Freeman JM. The pathology of Rasmussen syndrome: stages of cortical involvement and neuropathological studies in 45 hemispherectomies. *Epilepsia* 2004; 45: 516-26.

Pearce DA, Atkinson M, Tagle DA. Glutamic acid decarboxylase autoimmunity in Batten disease and other disorders. *Neurology* 2004; 63: 2001-5.

Peltola J, Kulmala P, Isojarvi J, Saiz A, Latvala K, Palmio J, et al. Autoantibodies to glutamic acid decarboxylase in patients with therapy-resistant epilepsy. *Neurology* 2000a; 55: 46-50.

Peltola JT, Haapala A, Isojarvi JI, Auvinen A, Palmio J, Latvala K, et al. Antiphospholipid and antinuclear antibodies in patients with epilepsy or new-onset seizure disorders. *Am J Med* 2000b; 109: 712-7.

Pengiran Tengah DS, Holmes GK, Wills AJ. The prevalence of epilepsy in patients with celiac disease. *Epilepsia* 2004; 45: 1291-3.

Piga M, Serra A, Deiana L, Loi GL, Satta L, Di Liberto M, et al. Brain perfusion abnormalities in patients with euthyroid autoimmune thyroiditis. *Eur J Nucl Med Mol Imaging* 2004; 31: 1639-44.

Power C, Poland SD, Blume WT, Girvin JP, Rice GP. Cytomegalovirus and Rasmussen's encephalitis. *Lancet* 1990; 336: 1282-4.

Pratesi R, Modelli IC, Martins RC, Almeida PL, Gandolfi L. Celiac disease and epilepsy: favorable outcome in a child with difficult to control seizures. *Acta Neurol Scand* 2003; 108: 290-3.

Primavera A, Brusa G, Novello P. Thyrotoxic encephalopathy and recurrent seizures. *Eur Neurol* 1990; 30: 186-8.

Radetti G, Dordi B, Mengarda G, Biscaldi I, Larizza D, Severi F. Thyrotoxicosis presenting with seizures and coma in two children. *Am J Dis Child* 1993; 147: 925-7.

Ramirez-Montealegre D, Chattopadhyay S, Curran TM, Wasserfall C, Pritchard L, Schatz D, et al. Autoimmunity to glutamic acid decarboxylase in the neurodegenerative disorder Batten disease. *Neurology* 2005; 64: 743-5.

Rantala H, Kulmala P, Savola K, Knip M. Absence of glutamic acid decarboxylase antibodies in childhood epilepsies. *Pediatr Neurol* 1999; 21: 794-6.

Ranua J, Luoma K, Peltola J, Haapala AM, Raitanen J, Auvinen A, et al. Anticardiolipin and antinuclear antibodies in epilepsy – a population-based cross-sectional study. *Epilepsy Res* 2004; 58: 13-8.

Ranua J, Luoma K, Auvinen A, Haapala AM, Maki M, Peltola J, et al. Antimitochondrial antibodies in patients with epilepsy. *Epilepsy Behav* 2005a; 7: 95-7.

Ranua J, Luoma K, Auvinen A, Maki M, Haapala AM, Peltola J, et al. Celiac disease-related antibodies in an epilepsy cohort and matched reference population. *Epilepsy Behav* 2005b; 6: 388-92.

Rasmussen T, Olszewski J, Lloydsmith D. Focal seizures due to chronic localized encephalitis. *Neurology* 1958; 8: 435-45.

Rasmussen T. Further observations on the syndrome of chronic encephalitis and epilepsy. *Appl Neurophysiol* 1978; 41: 1-12.

Rasmussen T. Hemispherectomy for seizures revisited. *Can J Neurol Sci* 1983; 10: 71-8.

Rasmussen T and Andermann F. Update on the syndrome of "chronic encephalitis" and epilepsy. *Cleve Clin J Med* 1989; 56 (suppl Pt 2): S181-4.

Roberts CG and Ladenson PW. Hypothyroidism. *Lancet* 2004; 363: 793-803.

Rodriguez AJ, Jicha GA, Steeves TD, Benarroch EE, Westmoreland BF. EEG changes in a patient with steroid-responsive encephalopathy associated with antibodies to thyroperoxidase (SREAT, Hashimoto's encephalopathy). *J Clin Neurophysiol* 2006; 23: 371-3.

Rogers SW, Andrews PI, Gahring LC, Whisenand T, Cauley K, Crain B, et al. Autoantibodies to glutamate receptor GluR3 in Rasmussen's encephalitis. *Science* 1994; 265: 648-51.

Rostom A, Dubé C, Cranney A, Saloojee N, Sy R, Garritty C, et al. Celiac Disease. Evidence Report/ Technology Assessment No. 104. (Prepared by the University of Ottawa Evidence-based Practice Center, under Contract No. 290-02-0021.) AHRQ. Publication No. 04-E029-2. 2004

Ruegg S. Anti-glutamic acid decarboxylase anti-bodies – the missing link between epilepsy and diabetes. *Ann Neurol* 2006; 59: 728-9.

Saiz A, Arpa J, Sagasta A, Casamitjana R, Zarranz JJ, Tolosa E, et al. Autoantibodies to glutamic acid decarboxylase in three patients with cerebellar ataxia, late-onset insulin-dependent diabetes mellitus, and polyendocrine autoimmunity. *Neurology* 1997; 49: 1026-30.

Sawka AM, Fatourechi V, Boeve BF, Mokri B. Rarity of encephalopathy associated with autoimmune thyroiditis: a case series from Mayo Clinic from 1950 to 1996. *Thyroid* 2002; 12: 393-8.

Schauble B, Castillo PR, Boeve BF, Westmoreland BF. EEG findings in steroid-responsive encephalopathy associated with autoimmune thyroiditis. *Clin Neurophysiol* 2003; 114: 32-7.

Sebastiani GD, Passiu G, Galeazzi M, Porzio F, Carcassi U. Prevalence and clinical associations of anticardiolipin antibodies in systemic lupus erythematosus: a prospective study. *Clin Rheumatol* 1991; 10: 289-93.

Seyfried TN, Glaser GH, Yu RK. Thyroid hormone can restore the audiogenic seizure susceptibility of hypothyroid DBA/2J mice. *Exp Neurol* 1981; 71: 220-5.

Shaw PJ, Walls TJ, Newman PK, Cleland PG, Cartlidge NE. Hashimoto's encephalopathy: a steroid-responsive disorder associated with high anti-thyroid antibody titers – report of 5 cases. *Neurology* 1991; 41: 228-33.

She JX. Susceptibility to type I diabetes: HLA-DQ and DR revisited. *Immunol Today* 1996; 17: 323-9.

Shi Y, Kanaani J, Menard-Rose V, Ma YH, Chang PY, Hanahan D, et al. Increased expression of GAD65 and GABA in pancreatic beta-cells impairs first-phase insulin secretion. *Am J Physiol Endocrinol Metab* 2000; 279: E684-94.

Shibata N, Yamamoto Y, Sunami N, Suga M, Yamashita Y. [Isolated angiitis of the CNS associated with Hashimoto's disease]. *Rinsho Shinkeigaku* 1992; 32: 191-8.

Shoenfeld Y, Lev S, Blatt I, Blank M, Font J, von Landenberg P, et al. Features associated with epilepsy in the antiphospholipid syndrome. *J Rheumatol* 2004; 31: 1344-8.

Shrivastava A, Dwivedi S, Aggarwal A, Misra R. Anti-cardiolipin and anti-beta2 glycoprotein I antibodies in Indian patients with systemic lupus erythematosus: association with the presence of seizures. *Lupus* 2001; 10: 45-50.

Sinclair DB and Snyder TJ. Corticosteroids for the treatment of Landau-kleffner syndrome and continuous spike-wave discharge during sleep. *Pediatr Neurol* 2005; 32: 300-6.

Singh BM and Strobos RJ. Epilepsia partialis continua associated with nonketotic hyperglycemia: clinical and biochemical profile of 21 patients. *Ann Neurol* 1980; 8: 155-60.

Skanse B and Nyman GE. Thyrotoxicosis as a cause of cerebral dysrhythmia and convulsive seizures. *Acta Endocrinol (Copenh)* 1956; 22: 246-63.

Sloviter RS, Dichter MA, Rachinsky TL, Dean E, Goodman JH, Sollas AL, et al. Basal expression and induction of glutamate decarboxylase and GABA in excitatory granule cells of the rat and monkey hippocampal dentate gyrus. *J Comp Neurol* 1996; 373: 593-618.

Smith DL and Looney TJ. Seizures secondary to thyrotoxicosis and high-dosage propranolol therapy. *Arch Neurol* 1983; 40: 457-8.

So NK and Gloor P Electroencephalographic and electrocorticographic findings in chronic encephalitis of the Rasmussen type.. In: A. F, ed. *Chronic encephalitis and epilepsy: Rasmussen's syndrome.* Boston: Butterworth-Heinemann, 1991: 37-45.

Soghomonian JJ and Martin DL. Two isoforms of glutamate decarboxylase: why? *Trends Pharmacol Sci* 1998; 19: 500-5.

Sokol DK, McIntyre JA, Wagenknecht DR, Dropcho EJ, Patel H, Salanova V, et al. Antiphospholipid and glutamic acid decarboxylase antibodies in patients with focal epilepsy. *Neurology* 2004; 62: 517-8.

Solimena M, Folli F, Denis-Donini S, Comi GC, Pozza G, De Camilli P, et al. Autoantibodies to glutamic acid decarboxylase in a patient with stiff-man syndrome, epilepsy, and type I diabetes mellitus. *N Engl J Med* 1988; 318: 1012-20.

Solimena M, Folli F, Aparisi R, Pozza G, De Camilli P. Autoantibodies to GABA-ergic neurons and pancreatic beta cells in stiff-man syndrome. *N Engl J Med* 1990; 322: 1555-60.

Sollid LM, Markussen G, Ek J, Gjerde H, Vartdal F, Thorsby E. Evidence for a primary association of celiac disease to a particular HLA-DQ alpha/beta heterodimer. *J Exp Med* 1989; 169: 345-50.

Sollid LM, McAdam SN, Molberg O, Quarsten H, Arentz-Hansen H, Louka AS, et al. Genes and environment in celiac disease. *Acta Odontol Scand* 2001; 59: 183-6.

Sponsler JL, Werz MA, Maciunas R, Cohen M. Neurosarcoidosis presenting with simple partial seizures and solitary enhancing mass: case reports and review of the literature. *Epilepsy Behav* 2005; 6: 623-30.

Steinhoff BJ. Optimizing therapy of seizures in patients with endocrine disorders. *Neurology* 2006; 67: S23-7.

Striano P, Pagliuca M, Andreone V, Zara F, Coppola A, Striano S. Unfavourable outcome of Hashimoto encephalopathy due to status epilepticus. One autopsy case. *J Neurol* 2006; 253: 248-9.

Su YH, Izumi T, Kitsu M, Fukuyama Y. Seizure threshold in juvenile myoclonic epilepsy with Graves disease. *Epilepsia* 1993; 34: 488-92.

Sundaram MB, Hill A, Lowry N. Thyroxine-induced petit mal status epilepticus. *Neurology* 1985; 35: 1792-3.

Takahashi Y, Mori H, Mishina M, Watanabe M, Fujiwara T, Shimomura J, et al. Autoantibodies to NMDA receptor in patients with chronic forms of epilepsia partialis continua. *Neurology* 2003; 61: 891-6.

Telfeian AE, Berqvist C, Danielak C, Simon SL, Duhaime AC. Recovery of language after left hemispherectomy in a sixteen-year-old girl with late-onset seizures. *Pediatr Neurosurg* 2002; 37: 19-21.

Thrush DC and Boddie HG. Episodic encephalopathy associated with thyroid disorders. *J Neurol Neurosurg Psychiatry* 1974; 37: 696-700.

Tien RD, Ashdown BC, Lewis DV, Jr., Atkins MR, Burger PC. Rasmussen's encephalitis: neuroimaging findings in four patients. *AJR Am J Roentgenol* 1992; 158: 1329-32.

Timiras PS and Woodbury DM. Effect of thyroid activity on brain function and brain electrolyte distribution in rats. *Endocrinology* 1956; 58: 181-92.

Tisch R and McDevitt H. Insulin-dependent diabetes mellitus. *Cell* 1996; 85: 291-7.

Tobias SM, Robitaille Y, Hickey WF, Rhodes CH, Nordgren R, Andermann F. Bilateral Rasmussen encephalitis: postmortem documentation in a five-year-old. *Epilepsia* 2003; 44: 127-30.

Toubi E, Khamashta MA, Panarra A, Hughes GR. Association of antiphospholipid antibodies with central nervous system disease in systemic lupus erythematosus. *Am J Med* 1995; 99: 397-401.

Twyman RE, Gahring LC, Spiess J, Rogers SW. Glutamate receptor antibodies activate a subset of receptors and reveal an agonist binding site. *Neuron* 1995; 14: 755-62.

Uramoto KM, Michet CJ, Jr., Thumboo J, Sunku J, O'Fallon WM, Gabriel SE. Trends in the incidence and mortality of systemic lupus erythematosus, 1950-1992. *Arthritis Rheum* 1999; 42: 46-50.

Vaknin A, Eliakim R, Ackerman Z, Steiner I. Neurological abnormalities associated with celiac disease. *J Neurol* 2004; 251: 1393-7.

Vasconcellos E, Pina-Garza JE, Fakhoury T, Fenichel GM. Pediatric manifestations of Hashimoto's encephalopathy. *Pediatr Neurol* 1999; 20: 394-8.

Ventura A, Bouquet F, Sartorelli C, Barbi E, Torre G, Tommasini G. Coeliac disease, folic acid deficiency and epilepsy with cerebral calcifications. *Acta Paediatr Scand* 1991; 80: 559-62.

Verrot D, San-Marco M, Dravet C, Genton P, Disdier P, Bolla G, et al. Prevalence and signification of antinuclear and anticardiolipin antibodies in patients with epilepsy. Am J Med 1997; 103: 33-7.

Verrotti A, Greco R, Altobelli E, Latini G, Morgese G, Chiarelli F. Anticardiolipin, glutamic acid decarboxylase, and antinuclear antibodies in epileptic patients. Clin Exp Med 2003; 3: 32-6.

Vezzani A and Granata T. Brain inflammation in epilepsy: experimental and clinical evidence. Epilepsia 2005; 46: 1724-43.

Vianello M, Tavolato B, Giometto B. Glutamic acid decarboxylase autoantibodies and neurological disorders. Neurol Sci 2002; 23: 145-51.

Vianello M, Keir G, Giometto B, Betterle C, Tavolato B, Thompson EJ. Antigenic differences between neurological and diabetic patients with anti-glutamic acid decarboxylase antibodies. Eur J Neurol 2005; 12: 294-9.

Vianello M, Giometto B, Vassanelli S, Canato M, Betterle C, Mucignat C. Peculiar labeling of cultured hippocampal neurons by different sera harboring anti-glutamic acid decarboxylase autoantibodies (GAD-Ab). Exp Neurol 2006; 202: 514-8.

Villani F, Spreafico R, Farina L, Giovagnoli AR, Bernasconi P, Granata T, et al. Positive response to immunomodulatory therapy in an adult patient with Rasmussen's encephalitis. Neurology 2001; 56: 248-50.

Vincent A, Buckley C, Schott JM, Baker I, Dewar BK, Detert N, et al. Potassium channel antibody-associated encephalopathy: a potentially immunotherapy-responsive form of limbic encephalitis. Brain 2004; 127: 701-12.

Vining EP, Freeman JM, Brandt J, Carson BS, Uematsu S. Progressive unilateral encephalopathy of childhood (Rasmussen's syndrome): a reappraisal. Epilepsia 1993; 34: 639-50.

Vining EP, Freeman JM, Pillas DJ, Uematsu S, Carson BS, Brandt J, et al. Why would you remove half a brain? The outcome of 58 children after hemispherectomy-the Johns Hopkins experience: 1968 to 1996. Pediatrics 1997; 100: 163-71.

Vinters HV, Wang R, Wiley CA. Herpesviruses in chronic encephalitis associated with intractable childhood epilepsy. Hum Pathol 1993; 24: 871-9.

Vulliemoz S and Seeck M. An association between type 1 diabetes and idiopathic generalized epilepsy. Ann Neurol 2006; 59: 728.

Wall CR. Myxedema coma: diagnosis and treatment. Am Fam Physician 2000; 62: 2485-90.

Wasserfall CH and Atkinson MA. Autoantibody markers for the diagnosis and prediction of type 1 diabetes. Autoimmun Rev 2006; 5: 424-8.

Watson R, Jiang Y, Bermudez I, Houlihan L, Clover L, McKnight K, et al. Absence of antibodies to glutamate receptor type 3 (GluR3) in Rasmussen encephalitis. Neurology 2004; 63: 43-50.

Watson R, Jepson JE, Bermudez I, Alexander S, Hart Y, McKnight K, et al. Alpha7-acetylcholine receptor antibodies in two patients with Rasmussen encephalitis. Neurology 2005; 65: 1802-4.

Whitney KD and McNamara JO. GluR3 autoantibodies destroy neural cells in a complement-dependent manner modulated by complement regulatory proteins. J Neurosci 2000; 20: 7307-16.

Wiendl H, Bien CG, Bernasconi P, Fleckenstein B, Elger CE, Dichgans J, et al. GluR3 antibodies: prevalence in focal epilepsy but no specificity for Rasmussen's encephalitis. Neurology 2001; 57: 1511-4.

Wilson WP, Johnson JE, Feist FW. Thyroid Hormone and Brain Function. Ii. Changes in Photically Elicited Eeg Responses Following the Administration of Triiodothyronine to Normal Subjects. Electroencephalogr Clin Neurophysiol 1964; 16: 329-31.

Wise MS, Rutledge SL, Kuzniecky RI. Rasmussen syndrome and long-term response to gamma globulin. Pediatr Neurol 1996; 14: 149-52.

Xiong ZQ, Qian W, Suzuki K, McNamara JO. Formation of complement membrane attack complex in mammalian cerebral cortex evokes seizures and neurodegeneration. J Neurosci 2003; 23: 955-60.

Yacubian EM, Marie SK, Valerio RM, Jorge CL, Yamaga L, Buchpiguel CA. Neuroimaging findings in Rasmussen's syndrome. J Neuroimaging 1997; 7: 16-22.

Yamamoto T, Fukuyama J, Fujiyoshi A. Factors associated with mortality of myxedema coma: report of eight cases and literature survey. *Thyroid* 1999; 9: 1167-74.

Yang R, Puranam RS, Butler LS, Qian WH, He XP, Moyer MB, *et al*. Autoimmunity to munc-18 in Rasmussen's encephalitis. *Neuron* 2000; 28: 375-83.

Yoshimoto T, Doi M, Fukai N, Izumiyama H, Wago T, Minami I, *et al*. Type 1 diabetes mellitus and drug-resistant epilepsy: presence of high titer of anti-glutamic acid decarboxylase autoantibodies in serum and cerebrospinal fluid. *Intern Med* 2005; 44: 1174-7.

Zupanc ML, Handler EG, Levine RL, Jahn TW, ZuRhein GM, Rozental JM, *et al*. Rasmussen encephalitis: epilepsia partialis continua secondary to chronic encephalitis. *Pediatr Neurol* 1990; 6: 397-401.

Section V:
From randomized controlled trials to patient-oriented decision making

From randomised controlled trials to patient-oriented therapy: *methodology and clinical issues*

Philippe Ryvlin

Department of Functional Neurology and Epileptology, CTRS-IDEE, Hospices Civils de Lyon, INSERM U821, Lyon, France

The complex path that links drug trials to clinical practice include four main components *(Figure 1)* that all offer opportunities to illustrate a number of issues raised by the treatment of newly diagnosed epilepsy. Randomised controlled trials (RCTs) represent the first component, and supposedly the foundation of evidence-based decisions, including guidelines and practice parameters that represent the second component. These guidelines primarily target physicians involved in the field (the third component), and are expected to help optimising the care of the general population of patients with epilepsy (the fourth component).

All these four aspects of the therapeutic equation are primarily concerned by specific outcomes that seem to differ from one component to another. RCTs favor indicators of the efficacy or effectiveness of antiepileptic drugs (AEDs) that facilitate statistical analysis, such as time to treatment failure. This type of outcome measure might not be readily translated by patients into their own therapeutic expectations. Guidelines usually refer to the same clinical endpoints than those measured in RCTs, but also often place more emphasis than RCTs on cost-effectiveness. Whereas both RCTs and guidelines are primarily interested in population outcomes, physicians and patients focus on individual results. Still, an important gap might distinguish physicians and patients perspectives regarding the most disabling aspects of chronic diseases, as illustrated in multiple sclerosis (Rothwell *et al.*, 1997). In this condition, patients were primarily concerned by mental health and emotional role limitation, whereas their treating physicians placed more emphasis on physical role limitation and function (Rothwell *et al.*, 1997).

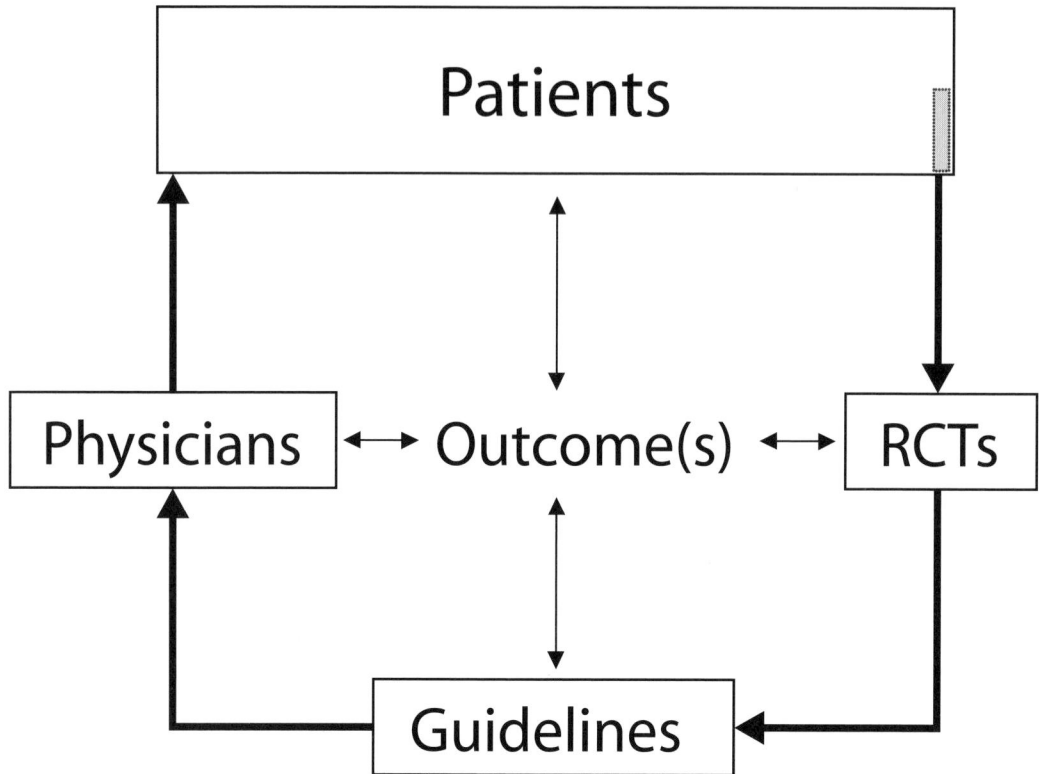

Figure 1. Methodological and clinical issues

■ Issues in clinical practice: physician's bias and evidence-based patient information

More generally, it is wise to acknowledge that physician's assumption of their patient expectations regarding the most relevant treatment outcome might be wrong, unless properly discussed at the individual level. Accordingly, the American Academy of Neurology (AAN) together with the Child Neurology Society have edited practice parameters for the treatment of a first unprovoked seizure stressing that *"the decision should be individualized and take into account patient and family preference"* (Hirtz et al., 2003).

However, patient and family preference must be based on appropriate information regarding the risks and benefits associated with the various treatment options. For instance, the discussion as to whether or not to initiate AED therapy following a single or two unprovoked seizures require that the patient and his family receive detailed information regarding the risk of another seizure, with or without treatment, as well as the potential harm of such seizure *versus* that of AED-related side effect. But the classic and simplistic notions that a single seizure is not epilepsy and should not be treated, whereas two unprovoked seizures more than 24 hours apart require anti-epileptic therapy, is far from reflecting current epidemiological data. In a long term prospective study of 407 children with a single unprovoked seizure, the risk of a second attack at five years was 43%, whereas the subsequent risk of a third seizure, in the subset of patients who seized twice, was 72% at five years (Shinnar et al., 2000). In a patient highly reluctant to start AED therapy, the two above risks of another seizure without treatment might be judged as equally acceptable, whereas conversely, these risks might be perceived as equally unacceptable in a patient who feels extremely anxious of suffering from another seizure. In other words, the objective difference between a 43% and 72% risk of recurrence is far from representing an all or nothing situation, and can be translated in very diffrent ways by individual patients. This example stresses the value of providing detailed information for allowing "evidence-based" patient and family preference. Such information should take into account the well established risk factors of seizure recurrence that have been recently elegantly implemented into an easy to use prognostic index algorithm, derived from the MESS trial (Kim et al., 2006), and detailed in another chapter of this book (Beghi, 2007). Similarly, the risk of seizure-related serious injury or death in patients with a single unprovoked seizure or a newly diagnosed epilepsy should be commented upon, thanks to recently published very reassuring data (Ryvlin, 2006). Finally, we would hope that a precise and unbiased information regarding the effectiveness of AEDs is offered to the patient. This issue is in our view much more difficult to address, due to the lack of cleacut consensus among experts and guidelines, as illustrated farther. At the present time, we believe that the majority of physicians involved in the primary care of patients with single unprovoked seizure or newly diagnosed epilepsy do not master the essential pieces of information discussed above and that continuous medical education in the field should be a priority.

■ Limitations of guidelines

A general limitation of clinical guidelines across diseases and health issues, is their limited impact upon physician's practice patterns (Søndergaard et al., 2003). In striking contrast with the very strict criteria that apply to the selection of data used to established guidelines (primarily deriving from double blind RCTs), no such systematic assessment has been proposed to evaluate the utility of guidelines. It is indeed peculiar that a process that put so much emphasis on the methodology used by others to generate informative data, ignores the same basic rules of objective testing for evaluating its own relevance. In fact, only a few randomised controlled trials have tested the impact of guidelines in various clinical settings, such as prescription by general practionner (GP) of narrow-spectrum penicillins or of inhaled steroids in asthma (Søndergaard et al., 2003; Søndergaard et al., 2002). These rare RTCs found no significant impact of disseminating guidelines on GP practice patterns, even when associated with detailed postal feedback of the physician prescriptions.

Several factors might explain guidelines failure to modify clinical practice, including reluctance to change prescription patterns and lack of time or lack of interest on the part of the physician, as well as sub-optimal educational values of guidelines.

For intance, the National Institute for Clinical Excellence (NICE) and Scottish Intercollegiate Guidelines Network (SIGN) have undertaken comprehensive reviews of epilepsy care, including recommendations regarding AED therapy. While the scientific value of these documents is remarkable, their format, and in particular their length and complexity, make these guidelines unlikely to be red and endorsed by a large number of neurologists.

The educational impact of guidelines is further hampered by significant discrepancies across the various recommendation edited by the AAN (French et al., 2006), the NICE and SIGN organisations, and the International League Against Epilepsy (ILAE) (Glauser et al., 2006) (Tables I and II). For example, the AAN recommends established AEDs (carbamazepine, phenytoin, valproate and divalproate) as well as newer AEDs (lamotrigine, topiramate and oxcarbazepine) as first-line drugs of choice for the treatment of partial/mix generalized tonic-clonic seizures (French et al., 2006), whereas the NICE guidelines propose a tiered approach to the use of the newer AEDs in this indication, recommending that they be employed only when the patient does not respond adequately to the established drugs used in first-line therapy. The SIGN guidelines offer intermediate recommendations with a selection of only two old and two new generation AEDs as first line monotherapy (carbamazepine, valproate, lamotrigine and oxcarbazepine). Finally, the ILAE systematic review concludes that the best available evidence was not conclusive enough to be used in the development of recommendations for diagnosing, monitoring, and treating patients with epilepsy (Glauser et al., 2006). Accordingly, a paper evaluating guidelines for the management of breast cancer showed a higher level of full agreement between guideline recommendations when the sources of evidence used to support decisions were of high quality (Cruse et al., 2002). With better medical data and international collaborative efforts it may be possible to develop a set of guidelines with a more wide-reaching application.

Table I. Guidelines recommendations for the treatment of partial epilepsies

AEDs	AAN	NICE	SIGN	ILAE
Phenobarbital	1st			Level C
Phenytoin	1st			Level A
Carbamazepine	1st	1st	1st	Level A
Valproate	1st	1st	1st	Level A
Vigabatrin				Level C
Gabapentin	1st			Level C (A*)
Lamotrigine	1st	2nd	1st	Level C (A*)
Oxcarbazepine	1st	2nd	1st	Level C (A*)
Topiramate	1st	2nd		Level C
Levetiracetam	–	–	–	Level A**

Level A*: Level A evidence for either elderly patients or children only (level C for non elderly adults)
Level A**: Level A according to criteria edited by the ILAE guidelines (Glauser et al., Epilepsia 2006), but not mentioned in these guidelines since the later were published prior to the publication of the levetiracetam versus controlled-release carbamazepine monotherapy trial (Brodie et al., Neurology 2007)

Table II. Main conclusions extracted from guidelines for partial epilepsies

ILAE: The absence of rigorous comprehensive adverse-effects data makes it impossible to develop an evidence-based guideline aimed at identifying the overall optimal recommended initial-monotherapy AED.

AAN: Patients with newly diagnosed epilepsy who require treatment can be initiated on standard AEDs such as carbamazepine, phenytoin, valproate, phenobarbital or on the new AEDs: lamotrigine, gabapentin, oxcarbazepine, or topiramate.

SIGN: Carbamazepine, valproate, lamotrigine, and oxcarbazepine can all be regarded as first-line treatments for partial and secondary generalized seizures.

NICE: First-line monotherapy should be initiated with one of the older AEDs such as carbamazepine or valproate unless these drugs are not suitable because there are contraindications or the potential for interactions with other drugs the person is taking, because they have been poorly tolerated by the person in the past, or because the person is a woman of childbearing potential.

Limitations of RCTs

As illustrated in *Table II*, the ILAE guidelines have emphasized the low levels of evidence available for the majority of AEDs. This is further detailed in *Table III* for partial epilepsies across the different age groups, as well as for idiopathic generalised epilepsies.

As a matter of fact, only four class I and two class II RCTs, all performed in partial epilepsy, were identified at the time of the ILAE guidelines publication, as listed below:

Class I RCTs

– Carbamazepine/Phenytoin/Phenobarbital/Primidone in adults (Mattson *et al.*, 1985).

– Carbamazepine/Vigabatrin in adults (Chadwick *et al.*, 1999).

– Oxcarbazepine/Phenytoin in children (Guerreiro *et al.*, 1997).

– Lamotrigine/Gabapentin/Carbamazepine in elderly (Rowan *et al.*, 2005).

Class II RCTs

– Carbamazepine/Valproate in adults (Mattson *et al.*, 1992).

– Lamotrigine/Carbamazepine in elderly (Brodie *et al.*, 1999).

The first of these two RCTs did not meet class I criteria because of a non detectable inferior boundary that exceeded 20% (23%), whereas the second had a too short duration.

Another RCT fulfilling class I study criteria was more recently published, and compared Levetiracetam and controlled-release Carbamazepine in aduls with partial epilepsy (Brodie *et al.* 2007).

Overall, lamotrigine and gabapentin proved more effective than carbamazepine in elderly (Brodie *et al.*, 1999; Rowan *et al.*, 2005), whereas oxcarbazepine proved more effective than phenytoin in children (Guerreiro *et al.*, 1997). In non elderly adults, carbamazepine proved more effective then phenobarbital, primidone, and vigabatrin

Table III. Levels of evidence for AEDs first line monotherapy *(adapted from Glauser et al., Epilepsia 2006)*

AEDs	Partial Epilepsies			Idiopathic Generalised Epilepsies		
	Adults	Elderly	Children	CAE	JME	GTCS
Phenobarbital	C		C			
Phenytoin	A		C			
Carbamazepine	A	C	C			
Valproate	B	D	C	C	D	C
Ethosuximide				C		
Primidone	D					
Clonazepam	D					
Vigabatrin	C		D			
Gabapentin		A				
Lamotrigine	C	A	D	C	D	C
Oxcarbazepine	C		A			
Topiramate	C	D	C		D	C
Levetiracetam	A*				D	
Zonisamide					D	

A*: Level A according to criteria edited by the ILAE guidelines (Glauser *et al.*, *Epilepsia* 2006), but not mentionned in these guidelines since the later were published prior to the publication of the levetiracetam *versus* controlled-release carbamazepine monotherapy trial (Brodie *et al.*, *Neurology* 2007)

(Mattson *et al.*, 1985; Chadwick *et al.*, *Lancet* 1999), whereas valproate showed comparable effectiveness than carbamazepine, and levetiracetam, comparable effectiveness than controlled-release carbamazepine (Mattson *et al.*, 1992; Brodie *et al.*, 2007).

It thus appears that a number of well designed head to head comparison between AEDs are lacking in the different age groups and epilepsy syndromes. As a response to this limitation, a recent pragmatic and large scale open-label randomised trial has compared carbamazepine, lamotrigine, gabapentine, oxcarbazepine, and topiramate in partial epilepsy, as well as valproate, lamotrigine and topiramate in generalised and unclassified epilepsies (Marson *et al.*, 2007). This study concluded that lamotrigine was more effective than carbamazepine, gabapentine and topiramate as first line monotherapy in partial epilepsy (Marson *et al.*, 2007), and that valproate was more effective than topiramate and more efficacious than lamotrigine in generalised or unclassified epilepsies (Marson *et al.*, 2007). However, due to its open-label design, this study is classified as a class III RCT and urges us to consider the potential impact of an investigator bias towards some of the tested AEDs. In particular, the criteria used to define drug failure, either related to insufficient efficacy or adverse events, stricly held upon the investigators personal judgment.

Class I and II double blind RCTs also suffer important limitations. Exclusion criteria are stringent and only allow to investigate sub-populations that are not representative of the general population of patients with epilepsy. Important aspects of AEDs, such as their teratogenicity, interaction with other drugs including oral contraception and chronic treatment of symptomatic epilepsies (chemotherapies, antiretroviral or antiparasitic agents, anticoagulants), pharmacokinetic properties in patients with renal or hepatic dysfunction, or tolerability in patients with severe psychiatric comorbidity, can hardly be addressed in ethically designed double-blind RCTs. In a recent review of treatment issues in major specific clinical situations encountered in epilepsy, and rarely or never assessed in RCTs, such as brain tumor, HIV, cysticercosis, metabolic dysfunctions, mental retardation, ADHD, psychiatric comorbidity and women of child bearing potential, it was concluded that the regrouping of all these "minorities" eventually represented a majority of patients with epilepsy (Ryvlin, 2007). Even in stroke, a condition that represents up to 11% of all etiologies in adult epilepsy, no RCT is available (Ryvlin *et al.*, 2007).

The great majority of double-blind RCTs are sponsored by the industry, and primarily performed for regulatory purposes. These are two potential limitations to the relevance of trial design with respect to clinical practice, and probably explain why most of these trials are class III RCTs. However, about half of the class I and II RCTs were performed by the veterans administration, and aimed to address relevant clinical issues (Mattson *et al.*, 1985; Mattson *et al.*, 1992; Rowan *et al.*, 2005).

Still, the veterans trials (as well as most other RCTs) failed to take into account an important aspect of AEDs characteristics, specifically the galenic of carbamazepine. Indeed, except for two recent studies (Brodie *et al.*, 2007; Saetre *et al.*, 2006), only immediate-release carbamazepine (IR-CBZ) was used in previous comparative monotherapy trials, including those performed by the veterans administration (Mattson *et al.*, 1985; Mattson *et al.*, 1992; Rowan *et al.*, 2005). Controlled-release carbamazepine (CR-CBZ) was found to be better tolerated than IR-CBZ (Persson *et al.*, 1990; Ficker *et al.*, 2005). It is therefore possible that the significantly better tolerability of lamotrigine and gabapentin over IR-CBZ in elderly patients (Brodie *et al.*, 1999; Rowan *et al.*, 2005), would not be observed if CR-CBZ would have been used as a comparator. In fact, a recent european study has compared lamotrigine with CR-CBZ in newly diagnosed epilepsy in elderlies, and found no significant difference in tolerability (Saetre *et al.*, 2006). Similarly, levetiracetam was compared to CR-CBZ in a large double blind RCT that fulfills the class I criteria published by the ILAE. Though levetiracetam was associated with less adverse events leading to discontinuation of treatment, difference between the two drugs was not significant (Brodie *et al.*, 2007). Both the above studies also used a low first target dose of CR-CBZ (400 mg) that probaly contributed to the favorable tolerability of the drug. In line with previous observations (Kwan and Brodie, 2000), the majority of patients that eventually proved to be controlled by CR-CBZ did so at 400 mg daily (Brodie *et al.*, 2007), highly suggesting that this dosage of CR-CBZ represents the most appropriate comparator for evaluating new AEDs as first line monotherapy. At the present time, however, only the levetiracetam study in adults (Brodie *et al.*, 2007), and the european lamotrigine trial in the elderly (Saetre *et al.*, 2006) have asserted such a comparison.

The duration of RCTs is another important issue. A minimum of one year of follow-up is required for class I monotherapy trials (Glauser et al., 2006). This is still probably suboptimal, when compared to the duration of treament recommended before considering tappering off AED in seizure free-patient (at least two years). Open-label pragmatic trials can organise longer duration of follow-up, as for the SANAD study that lasted an average of three years (Marson et al., 2007). However, despite longer follow-up, the primary efficacy endpoint of this trial was calculated as the time to achieve a 12 months seizure free period, thus not assessing the likelihood of achieving longer period of seizure freedom.

Finally, an important issue raised by epilepsy monotherapy RCTs is the so-called detectable non-inferiority boundary (DNIB). When comparing the efficacy of two AEDs in a population sample, with the aim to show non inferiority of a new drug as compared to whatever the gold standard, confidence intervals are provided indicating that the true difference between the two drugs has a 95% likelihood to lie within this interval. At the present time, the acceptable lower limit of this difference is 20% relative (Glauser et al., 2006). This is an empirical value, that was primarily agreed upon in order to qualify at least a few existing RCTs as class I study (Glauser et al., 2006). However, one could argue that a 20% difference is clinically significant, and that a more conservative approach, such as a 10% DNIB, would be more appropriate. This would need to perform much larger trials than those conducted so far. This effort might be justified by some hints suggesting that CBZ might be slightly more efficacious than modern AEDs such as lamotrigine and gabapentin (Rowan et al., 2005; Gamble et al., 2006; Saetre et al., 2006).

In conclusion, a number of issues questionned most of the conclusions derived from the numerous RCTs perfomed in epilepsy during the last 20 years. It is therefore not surprising that guidelines remain unable to provide precise and consensual practice parameters for the choice of a first line monotherapy. According to the great difficulty observed in other fields of medicine for translating trivial guidelines into effective changes in prescription patterns, we are clearly facing huge challenges in epilepsy care. A first mandatory step will be that experts in AEDs trials agree on a roadmap that address all above issues.

References

Brodie MJ, Overstall PW, Giorgi L. Multicentre, double-blind, randomised comparison between lamotrigine and carbamazepine in elderly patients with newly diagnosed epilepsy. The UK Lamotrigine Elderly Study Group. *Epilepsy Res* 1999; 37: 81-7.

Brodie MJ, Perucca E, Ryvlin P, Ben-Menachem E, Meencke HJ; Levetiracetam Monotherapy Study Group. Comparison of levetiracetam and controlled-release carbamazepine in newly diagnosed epilepsy. *Neurology* 2007; 68: 402-8.

Chadwick D. Safety and efficacy of vigabatrin and carbamazepine in newly diagnosed epilepsy: a multicentre randomised double-blind study. Vigabatrin European Monotherapy Study Group. *Lancet* 1999; 354: 13-9.

Cruse H, Winiarek M, Marshburn J, Clark O, Djulbegovic B. Quality and methods of developing practice guidelines. *BMC Health Services Research* 2002; 2: 1.

Ficker DM, Privitera M, Krauss G, Kanner A, Moore JL, Glauser T. Improved tolerability and efficacy in epilepsy patients with extended-release carbamazepine. *Neurology* 2005; 65: 593-5.

French J, Kanner AM, Bautista J, Abou-Khalil B, Browne T, Harden CL, Theodore WH et al. Efficacy and tolerability of the new antiepileptic drugs I: treatment of new onset. *Neurology* 2006; 62: 1252-60.

Gamble C, Williamson PR, Chadwick DW, Marson AG. A meta-analysis of individual patient responses to lamotrigine or carbamazepine monotherapy. *Neurology* 2006; 66: 1310-7.

Glauser T, Ben-Menachem E, Bourgeois B, Cnaan A, Chadwick D, Guerreiro C, Kalviainen R et al. ILAE treatment guidelines: evidence-based analysis of antiepileptic drug efficacy and effectiveness as initial monotherapy for epileptic seizures and syndromes. *Epilepsia* 2006; 47: 1094-120.

Guerreiro MM, Vigonius U, Pohlmann H, de Manreza ML, Fejerman N, Antoniuk SA, Moore A. A double-blind controlled clinical trial of oxcarbazepine *versus* phenytoin in children and adolescents with epilepsy. *Epilepsy Res* 1997; 27: 205-13.

Hirtz D, Berg A, Bettis D, Camfield C, Camfield P, Crumrine P, Gaillard WD, Schneider S, Shinnar S; Quality Standards Subcommittee of the American Academy of Neurology; Practice Committee of the Child Neurology Society. Practice parameter: treatment of the child with a first unprovoked seizure: Report of the Quality Standards Subcommittee of the American Academy of Neurology and the Practice Committee of the Child Neurology Society. *Neurology* 2003; 60: 166-75.

Kim LG, Johnson TL, Marson AG, Chadwick DW; MRC MESS Study group. Prediction of risk of seizure recurrence after a single seizure and early epilepsy: further results from the MESS trial. *Lancet Neurol* 2006; 5: 317-22.

Kwan P, Brodie MJ. Early identification of refractory epilepsy. *N Engl J Med* 2000; 342: 314-9.

Marson AG, Al-Kharusi AM, Alwaidh M, Appleton R, Baker GA, Chadwick DW et al. The SANAD study of effectiveness of carbamazepine, gabapentin, lamotrigine, oxcarbazepine, or topiramate for treatment of partial epilepsy: an unblinded randomised controlled trial. *Lancet* 2007a; 369: 1000-15.

Marson AG, Al-Kharusi AM, Alwaidh M, Appleton R, Baker GA, Chadwick DW et al. The SANAD study of effectiveness of valproate, lamotrigine, or topiramate for generalised and unclassifiable epilepsy: an unblinded randomised controlled trial. *Lancet* 2007b; 369: 1016-26.

Mattson RH, Cramer JA, Collins JF, Smith DB, Delgado-Escueta AV, Browne TR, Williamson PD, Treiman DM, McNamara JO, McCutchen CB et al. Comparison of carbamazepine, phenobarbital, phenytoin, and primidone in partial and secondarily generalized tonic-clonic seizures. *N Engl J Med* 1985; 313: 145-51.

Mattson RH, Cramer JA, Collins JF. A comparison of valproate with carbamazepine for the treatment of complex partial seizures and secondarily generalized tonic-clonic seizures in adults. The Department of Veterans Affairs Epilepsy Cooperative Study No. 264 Group. *N Engl J Med* 1992; 327: 765-71.

NICE. The epilepsies: the diagnosis and management of the epilepsies in adults and children in primary and secondary care. (www.nice.org.uk/CG020NICEguideline) 2006. Accessed 3-11-2006.

Payakachat N, Summers K, Barbuto J. A comparison of clinical practice guidelines in the initial pharmacological management of new-onset epilepsy in adults. *Journal of Managed Care Pharmacy* 2006; 12: 55-60.

Persson LI, Ben-Menachem E, Bengtsson E, Heinonen E. Differences in side effects between a conventional carbamazepine preparation and a slow-release preparation of carbamazepine. *Epilepsy Res* 1990; 6: 134-40.

Rothwell PM, McDowell Z, Wong CK, Dorman PJ. Doctors and patients don't agree: cross sectional study of patients' and doctors' perceptions and assessments of disability in multiple sclerosis. *BMJ* 1997; 314: 1580-3.

Rowan AJ, Ramsay RE, Collins JF, Pryor F, Boardman KD, Uthman BM, Spitz M, Frederick T, Towne A, Carter GS, Marks W, Felicetta J, Tomyanovich ML; VA Cooperative Study 428 Group. New onset geriatric epilepsy: a randomized study of gabapentin, lamotrigine, and carbamazepine. *Neurology* 2005; 64: 1868-73.

Ryvlin P, Montavont A, Nighoghossian N. Optimizing therapy of seizures in stroke patients. *Neurology* 2006; 67 (suppl 4): S3-9.

Ryvlin P. Optimizing therapy in specific clinical situations: The rule rather the exceptions. *Neurology* 2006; 67 (suppl 4): S1-2.

Ryvlin P. When to start antiepileptic drug treatment: seize twice might not harm. *Curr Opin Neurol* 2006; 19: 154-6.

Saetre *et al*. An international multicenter randomized double blind controlled trial of lamotrigine and sustained-release carbamazepine in the treatment of newly diagnosed epilepsy in the elderly. *Epilepsia* 2007 (in press).

Shinnar S, Berg AT, O'Dell C, Newstein D, Moshe SL, Hauser WA. Predictors of multiple seizures in a cohort of children prospectively followed from the time of their first unprovoked seizure. *Ann Neurol* 2000; 48: 140-7.

SIGN. Diagnosis and management of epilepsy in adults: a national clinical guideline. 2006. Ref Type: Statute.

Sondergaard J, Andersen M, Stovring H, Kragstrup J. Mailed prescriber feedback in addition to a clinical guideline has no impact: a randomised, controlled trial. *Scandinavian Journal of Primary Health Care* 2003; 21: 47-51.

Sondergaard J, Andersen M, Vach K, Kragstrup J, Maclure M, Gram L. Detailed postal feedback about prescribing to asthma patients combined with a guideline statement showed no impact: a randomised controlled trial. *European Journal of Clinical Pharmacology* 2002; 58: 127-32.

Treatment of first unprovoked seizure

Ettore Beghi

Centro per l'Epilessia e Clinica Neurologica, Ospedale "San Gerardo", Monza, and Istituto di Ricerche Farmacologiche "Mario Negri," Milan, Italy

The problems posed by the management of a first epileptic seizure are largely defined by the peculiarities of this condition. First of all, epileptic seizures are episodic manifestations which tend to recur with similar characteristics in the same patient, to occur at any age, and to be unpredictable in the large majority of cases. Second, even though seizures are rarely life-threatening, they expose the patient to environmental risks and limit his/her autonomy and socio-economic efficiency. Third, seizures are caused by several different causes and may disappear when the underlying clinical condition is removed. Fourth, in many patients seizures tend to persist, sometimes for a lifetime, and require chronic treatment with drugs which are not always effective, cause significant adverse effects and, for the most recent compounds, have a high cost. Fifth, seizures may interfere with several personal choices (school, professional activities, pregnancy, etc.). Sixth, seizures may represent a medical emergency, or at least they are perceived as such, and trigger emergency interventions involving many health care professionals. Last, seizures may occur in patients with comorbidities, who are treated with drugs potentially interfering with antiepileptic medication.

When a patient presents with a first seizure, the caring physician has to address several clinical questions. These include: (a) the diagnosis and the definitions of an epileptic seizure; (b) the relationship between a seizure and any underlying epileptogenic condition; (c) the risk of recurrence of the seizure; (d) the impact of treatment on this risk and on the long-term prognosis of epilepsy; (e) the risk:benefit ratio of pharmacological treatment; and (f) the sociocultural, emotional and legal implications of seizure recurrence compared with the tolerability and acceptance of chronic therapy. The questions a through c have been addressed elsewhere in this book. Only the seizure definitions will be reported here for clarity and completeness. The rationale, advantages and limitations of the treatment of the first unprovoked seizure will be discussed in detail.

Definitions

By definition, epilepsy is considered as two or more unprovoked seizures occurring at least 24 hours apart (Commission, 1993). Thus, the patient who presents with a first unprovoked seizure (or cluster of seizures within 24 hours) does not yet qualify for the diagnosis. An epileptic seizure is a transient occurrence of signs and/or symptoms due to abnormal excessive or synchronous neuronal activity in the brain (Fisher et al., 2005). Status epilepticus is a seizure lasting at least 30 minutes or a series of seizures occurring over at least a 30-minute period during which the patient never fully regains consciousness. Patients presenting with multiple seizures are no more likely to have seizure recurrence, irrespective of etiology or treatment (Kho et al., 2006). Seizures should be also defined as *acute symptomatic*, *progressive symptomatic* or *unprovoked*, with reference to the presence or absence of known precipitants. Known seizure precipitants include fever, head injury, alcohol and drug abuse (including withdrawal), metabolic/toxic disturbances, infection, stroke, and epileptogenic drugs. As opposed to *acute symptomatic seizures*, defined as "seizures occurring in the course or after a known or suspected cerebral insult," *unprovoked seizures* occur in the absence of a presumed acute precipitating insult. Unprovoked seizures may be classified symptomatic or idiopathic/cryptogenic. Idiopathic or cryptogenic unprovoked seizures are seizures for which no clear antecedent etiology can be detected. Symptomatic unprovoked seizures (also called *remote symptomatic seizures*) may occur in individuals with documented, fairly stable antecedent conditions, including strokes, traumatic head injuries, cerebral palsy, mental retardation, and malformations of the central nervous system. *Progressive symptomatic seizures* are seizures occurring in the context of a progressive CNS disease (like tumors, Alzheimer's disease and other degenerative conditions). All these factors are associated with a substantially higher risk of epileptic seizures.

Although acute symptomatic seizures are a risk factor for unprovoked seizures and epilepsy, they may not necessarily relapse, provided that the underlying epileptogenic condition is properly diagnosed and treated.

Rationale for the use of AEDs for the prevention of seizures and epilepsy

The epileptogenic process is characterized by a number of morphologic abnormalities, including neuron loss, gliosis, axonal and dendritic plasticity, inflammation, neurogenesis, and molecular reorganization (Jutila et al., 2002). The clinical manifestations are spontaneous seizures and cognitive decline, which in some patients may be part of a worsening condition, as shown by biochemical, imaging, and neuropsychological studies (Pitkanen and Sutula, 2002).

More than 70% of patients with newly diagnosed epilepsy will achieve complete seizure control with the available AEDs and about 50% will enter terminal remission (Kwan and Brodie, 2000; Annegers et al., 1979). As several observational studies report a significant correlation between number of seizures before treatment, multiple recurrences and chance of long-term remission (Collaborative Group, 1988; Shinnar et al., 2000; MacDonald et al., 2000), early treatment may be followed by a better long-term prognosis of epilepsy. Although randomized clinical trials comparing the long-term effects of treatment of the first unprovoked seizure and the treatment of the relapse show similar rates of remission of epilepsy (see below), this is not evidence against an antiepileptogenic action of AEDs, because at the time of the first seizure the cascade of events characterizing epileptogenesis may have already occurred at least in part. In addition, although timing, speed, and characteristics of the neurobiological changes may differ depending on the pathophysiology of the CNS insult, timely treatment of epileptogenic conditions with AEDs may halt or at least slow the process leading to irreversible neuronal death, thus preventing the occurrence of seizures and epilepsy.

■ The impact of treatment on the recurrence of a first seizure and on the long-term prognosis of epilepsy

A number of randomized studies have consistently shown the positive effects of treatment of the first unprovoked seizure on the risk of recurrence (Marson et al., 2005; Das et al., 2000; Gilad et al., 1996; FIRST Group, 1993; Chandra et al., 1992; Camfield et al., 1989) *(Table I)*. Among these, a large multicenter open trial (the FIRST study) was conducted to assess the treatment of the first seizure on the risk of relapse and the long-term prognosis of epilepsy in 397 children and adults (FIRST Group 1993). Overall, 36 of 204 treated patients and 75 of 193 untreated patients were referred for seizure relapse. The cumulative time-dependent risk of relapse among treated individuals was 4% at 1 month, 7% at 3 months, 9% at 6 months, 17% at 12 months, and 25% at 24 months. The figures for untreated individuals were 8, 18, 28, 41, and 51%. The hazard ratio of relapse for untreated patients was 2.8 (95% CI, 1.9-4.2). The efficacy of treatment was maintained despite the fact that 41 (20%) of treated patients discontinued the AED at some point. The results of this study were confirmed by an even larger pragmatic open multicenter randomized trial (the MESS study) comparing immediate and deferred treatment for early epilepsy and single seizures in children and adults (Marson et al., 2005). Patients were randomized if both the clinician and the patient were uncertain whether to start or withhold treatment. In this trial, 722 patients were randomized to immediate treatment and 721 to deferred treatment. Of these, 404 and 408 had a single seizure. Immediate treatment prolonged the time to the first relapse (RR 1.5; 95% CI 1.2-1.8) and increased the proportion of patients achieving immediate 2-year remission (64 vs 52%) (p = 0.023). These studies support the assumption that treatment of the first unprovoked epileptic seizure significantly affects the short-term prognosis of a first seizure by reducing the risk of further seizure relapse. However, they also show that the long-term prognosis of epilepsy is virtually unaffected by the treatment of the first seizure. In the FIRST study, the chance of 2-year remission at two and four years after randomization was 68 and 72% in the immediate treatment group and 60 and 67% in the deferred treatment group (Musicco et al., 1997). At ten years, the probability of 2-year remission was 85% in patients on immediate treatment and 86% in those treated only after seizure recurrence (Leone et al., 2006). In the MESS study, the chance of 2-year remission at two, five and eight years was 69, 92, and 95% with immediate treatment and 61, 92, and 96% with the deferred treatment (Marson et al., 2005).

A prognostic model was developed from the MESS study to enable identification of patients at low, medium, or high risk of recurrence (Kim et al., 2006). Number of seizures at presentation, presence of a neurological disorder, and an abnormal EEG were indicators of future seizures. Individuals with two or three seizures, a neurological disorder, or an abnormal EEG, were identified as the medium-risk group, those with two of these features or more than three seizures as the high-risk group, and those with a single seizure only as the low-risk group.

The long-term outcome of epilepsy was also unchanged by treatment of the first seizure in children enrolled in a small Canadian randomized trial and followed for 15 years (Camfield et al., 2002) (Table I). These findings are in keeping with studies conducted in developing countries, where patients are left untreated or receive drugs only after a prolonged disease course and repeated seizures. In these studies, untreated patients from developing countries tend to achieve seizure remission in proportions similar to those of patients under treatment (Watts 1992), and the delayed start of treatment equals in efficacy the early treatment of developed countries (Feksi et al., 1991). In addition, population-based studies in developing countries show high spontaneous remission rates, even without AEDs (Placencia et al., 1992 and 1994; Osuntokun et al., 1987).

In summary, treatment of the first unprovoked epileptic seizure seems to reduce the risk of recurrence during the active phase of the disease but does not influence the long-term prognosis of epilepsy. A clear demonstration of the symptomatic rather than curative role of AEDs also comes from the results of meta-analyses of studies on their prophylactic use following head trauma (Schierhout and Roberts, 2004), brain tumor (Glantz et al., 2000), craniotomy (Kuijlen et al., 1996) and other clinical conditions (Temkin, 2001). The results of the clinical investigations are in keeping with animal studies and support the concept that none of the drugs currently in use for the treatment of epilepsy can prevent the establishment of a chronic seizure disorder (Pitkanen and Sutula, 2002).

■ Safety and tolerability of antiepileptic drugs

Treatment of the first unprovoked seizure should be guided by the goal of complete seizure control without intolerable adverse reactions. Although dose-related adverse effects of AEDs are frequent components of the pharmacologic effects of drugs, idiosyncratic side effects are of particular concern. All the older and some of the newer drugs have caused serious idiosyncratic drug reactions (Glauser, 2000). Although clinical monitoring of drug safety is useful, especially when viewed in the context of the incidence of serious adverse reactions, presymptomatic blood studies fail to predict disease development. For example, test abnormalities such as benign leucopenia or transient hepatic enzyme elevations do not predict the occurrence of life-threatening reactions.

Chronic adverse drug reactions have been reported in about a third of ambulatory patients receiving chronic therapy with "older" AEDs, 22% of whom on monotherapy (Collaborative Group, 1986). The incidence of adverse drug reactions tends to increase with increasing dosage, even when plasma levels are maintained within the

Table I. Randomized clinical trials on the treatment of the first unprovoked seizure

Author(s), year	Setting	Population (N)	Drug and Comparator (N)	12-month Recurrence (%)	1-yr remission (%)	2-yr remission (%)	5-yr remission (%)	Notes
Camfield, 1989	Population-based pediatric neurology service	31 children	CBZ 10-20 mg/kg/d (14) No meds (17)	CBZ (14) No meds (53)	–	Treated (80) No meds (88)	–	CBZ stopped for adverse events in 4 patients Somnolence (14%) Rash (14%)
Chandra, 1992	University and private hospitals	228 adults	VPA 1,200 mg (115) Placebo (113)	Placebo (4) VPA (56)	–	–	–	VPA adverse events: **gastrointes-tinal** (3%) **weight gain** (4%) **hair loss** (2%)
FIRST, 1993 Musicco et al., 1997 Leone et al., 2007	University and general hospitals	387 aged 2-70 years	PB 15-40 mg/ml (103) CBZ 4-10 mg/ml (63) VPA 50-100 mg/ml (33) PHT 10-20 mg/ml (5) No meds (193)	Treated (17) No meds (28)	Treated (93) No meds (90)	Treated (81) No meds (78)	Treated (64) No meds (63)	Treatment stopped for adverse events in 14 patients
Gilad et al., 1996	Hospital emergency department	91 aged 18-50 years	CBZ **10mg/kg/d** (46) No meds (45)	Treated (13) No meds (59)	–	–	–	20% switched to VPA
Das et al., 2000	Neurology outpatient service	76 children and adults	Treated (36) No meds (40)	Treated (11) No meds (45)	–	–	–	–
Marson et al., 2005	UK and non UK centers	812 children and adults	CBZ (328) VPA (325) PHT (25) LTG (19)	Treated (27)* No meds (34)*	–	Treated (95) No meds (96)	–	Adverse events: **immediate** treatment (39%) **deferred** treatment (35%)

CBZ = Carbamazepine; LTG = Lamotrigine; PB = Phenobarbital; PHT = Phenytoin; VPA = Valproate.
(*) Estimated with approximation from Figure 2; Meds = medications.

so-called therapeutic range (Mattson et al., 1985 and 1992). Although the newer AEDs seem to offer some advantages in terms of tolerability, fewer drug interactions and simpler pharmacokinetics (Perucca, 2005), our knowledge concerning their safety profiles cannot yet considered adequate due to the relatively short time of exposure to some of them and to the limited number of exposed individuals.

The prevalence of adverse drug effects may be even higher when an active search is made, as with the assessment of behavioral and cognitive functions. It is also known that the currently available AEDs have an adverse influence on mental and behavioral functions, increased by higher plasma levels and polypharmacy (Glauser, 2004; Loring and Meador, 2001).

There are individuals having greater susceptibility to the adverse effects of drugs. These include infants and the elderly, in whom drug metabolism might be inefficient because of the presence of immature or aging metabolic pathways; pregnant women, who are exposed to the teratogenic effects of AEDs and have an increased liver metabolic capacity; and patients with hematologic, hepatic, and renal disturbances, in whom drug metabolism may be defective (Levy et al., 2002). The risk:benefit ratio of the anticonvulsant drug treatment must be carefully assessed in patients at their first epileptic seizure, as even a modest risk might not be accepted and might affect compliance with the proposed therapeutic regimens.

In the FIRST study (FIRST Group, 1993), adverse events were reasons for drug withdrawal in 7% of cases (14/204). In the MESS study (Marson et al., 2005), patients in the immediate treatment group were more likely to report at least one adverse event than those in the deferred group (difference 8.6%; 95%CI 3.6-13.6).

■ Other factors

The decision to treat a first epileptic seizure must be also based on legal, emotional and sociocultural factors, which are pertinent to the individual patient's situation (Berg and Chadwick, 2000). One legal factor influencing the decision to treat a first epileptic seizure is the need for the patient to drive in line with the national licensing regulations on epilepsy and driving (Beghi and Sander, 2005). Another factor that may encourage treatment after a first seizure is the local health insurance system. In countries with public health insurance coverage, no pressures are made on the therapeutic decisions; however, in countries such as the US, the risk of recurrence must be minimized to prevent financial complications to the patient. Compliance is also influential in deciding whether to treat a patient after a first seizure. Although it may be difficult to assess compliance in a newly diagnosed patient, poor compliers should be identified, as failure to adhere to the proposed treatment regimen is one of the most common causes of treatment failure (Leppik and Schmidt, 1988). There are also sociocultural and emotional factors for each patient, to be considered when deciding whether the complications of a recurrence outweigh the risk of acute or chronic drug toxicity. These factors must be carefully evaluated on an individual basis, regardless of any general recommendation.

■ Withholding treatment after a first seizure

Given the high potential for misdiagnosis among epileptic seizures and nonepileptic events (Chadwick, 1994; Kapoor, 2002), treatment should be generally deferred in patients in whom the diagnosis of a first epileptic seizure is uncertain. This is also the case for individuals in whom the recurrence of the seizure does not pose significant physical and psychological problems or who might be unduly exposed to the adverse effects of the AED.

Patients withholding treatment should consider restriction of dangerous jobs, non-commercial driving and recreational activities.

■ Starting treatment after a first seizure

Commercial and professional drivers with a first unprovoked seizure should be subject to restrictive rules and receive treatment after a first seizure. Patients at higher risk of recurrence (see chapter by Sheryl Haut *et al.*) might be also considered for treatment after a single unprovoked seizure. In adults holding a driving license, the risk:benefit analysis must be individualized. Any treatable epileptogenic condition must be identified and given specific therapy. The treatment of the first unprovoked seizure might be indicated in patients with a documented etiology and/or an abnormal EEG. Individuals with a first seizure associated with a neurological deficit present from birth, progressive neurological disease, or gross structural lesion might be also candidates of immediate treatment. Status epilepticus, although not strongly associated with an increased risk of seizure recurrence, should be treated as it may increase the risk of subsequent status in children (Berg *et al.*, 2004). The social complications (eg, loss of employment) and the emotional reflections of a relapse should be also strongly considered.

■ Drug choice and daily dose

If AED treatment is considered after a first seizure, the chosen AED should have high efficacy, long-term safety, good tolerability, low interaction potential and allow a good quality of life, since half of all patients would never have another seizure without treatment. The starting dose should be in the lower range.

The evidence-based ILAE treatment guidelines focused on AED efficacy and effectiveness as initial monotherapy for patients with newly diagnosed or untreated epilepsy (Glauser *et al.*, 2006) can be adopted also in patients with a first unprovoked seizure. This issue is being discussed in more details by AT Marson in this book.

However, the choice of AED should be also subjected to factors such as teratogenicity, the patient's cognitive abilities, drug interactions, physician familiarity with the drug and cost.

■ Duration of treatment

In childhood epilepsy drug treatment must be usually continued until the child has been seizure-free for 1-2 years. If children start treatment after a first seizure, there is little justification for continuing treatment beyond one year seizure-free, except for a few epilepsy syndromes (such as juvenile myoclonic epilepsy), which usually require long term medication.

There are no precise recommendations on the length of treatment after a first seizure in adults. An individual decision is thus required and should consider the medical and social consequences of an additional seizure. EEG and neuroimaging could be used to help with this decision because persistent EEG abnormalities and a documented etiology are associated with a higher risk of relapse when AED treatment is withdrawn after several years of remission (Berg and Shinnar, 1994). If medication is started after a first seizure in adults, we suggest at least one year of treatment, except for those at low risk for recurrence, when 6 months of seizure freedom may be sufficient.

■ Guidelines for the treatment of a first unprovoked seizure

According to the Italian League **Against** Epilepsy **(LICE)** guidelines for the diagnosis and treatment of the first epileptic seizure (Beghi et al., 2006), two distinct settings must be identified, which require separate management: the acute and the long-term treatment of the seizure. For each setting, the levels of evidence are outlined along with the strength of the recommendations *(Table II)*.

Acute treatment of the seizure

Levels of evidence. Etiological treatment of acute symptomatic seizures has strong biological plausibility, although there is no evidence from adequately controlled studies that treating the etiology of a first acute symptomatic seizure is followed by a lower risk of relapse. In one randomized study (Solari et al., 1997) treatment with benzodiazepines of a first unprovoked generalized tonic-clonic seizure was followed by a significant decrease in the risk of relapse (evidence level 2).

Recommendations. In the presence of a first acute symptomatic seizure (metabolic encephalopathy, acute CNS injury in patients with an underlying treatable condition), treatment of the cause is recommended. Symptomatic therapy of a first unprovoked seizure is not justified unless the seizure has the characteristics of status epilepticus.

Long-term treatment of the seizure

Levels of evidence. The decision to treat a first seizure with AEDs is largely determined by the risk of relapse. Even if this risk may vary from case to case, the highest rates of recurrence are found in patients with an abnormal EEG and a documented brain lesion (Berg and Shinnar, 1991) (level of evidence 1). In general, the risk of recurrence is highest in the first 12 months and is almost reduced to zero 2 years after the seizure (Beghi and Ciccone, 1993). Evidence level 1 and 2 studies have consistently shown that treatment of a first unprovoked seizure decreases the risk of relapse in the following two years, but it does not affect the probability of long-term remission both in children and in adults (Musicco et al., 1997; Hirtz et al., 2003; Marson et al., 2005).

Recommendations. Indiscriminate treatment of the first unprovoked seizure with AEDs is not recommended. Treatment may be considered in patients in whom electrophysiological and imaging data indicate an increased risk of relapse (presence of structural

Table II. Levels of evidence and strength of recommendations (*) (Beghi et al. 2006)

Levels of evidence

Level 1. Evidence obtained from prospective cohort studies with adequate design; includes also evidence obtained from meta-analyses of randomized clinical trials and from at least one randomized clinical trial

Level 2. Evidence obtained from cohort studies with suboptimal design or from case-control studies; includes also evidence obtained from at least one controlled non randomized trial and evidence obtained from at least one other well-designed, quasi-experimental study

Level 3. Evidence obtained from other observational non-experimental studies

Level 4. Evidence obtained from expert opinions (including commissions of experts and single authoritative experts. Indicates the absence of good quality studies

Strength of recommendations

Grade A. The intervention (whether diagnostic or therapeutic) is to be recommended because it is clearly effective, or to be discouraged because it is ineffective or harmful. The recommendation is based on evidence level 1.

Grade B. The intervention is probably effective, ineffective or harmful. The intervention may be recommended to specific subgroups of patients. The recommendation is based on evidence levels 2 and 3.

Grade C. The intervention is possibly effective, ineffective or harmful. The intervention deserves further evaluation before being recommended or discouraged. The recommendation is based on evidence level 4.

(*) The definitions of the levels of evidence and the strength of the recommendations used in this guideline are based on the scheme adopted by the *U.S. Agency for Health Care and Policy Research*. According to this scheme, each diagnostic and therapeutic intervention is recommended according to the level of scientific evidence. The efficacy of each diagnostic intervention (for example, the use of a laboratory test) is measured by its ability to modify the *a priori* diagnostic hypothesis. The efficacy of each therapeutic intervention is measured by its ability to modify the prognosis (*i.e.*, the tendency of seizures to relapse). However, correlations between levels of evidence and strength of recommendations should be interpreted flexibly and within the context of the individual's clinical, social, emotional, and personal situation. The levels of evidence and the strength of the recommendations are generally indicated at the beginning of each set of procedures being discussed; other indications requiring different diagnostic or therapeutic management are noted in parentheses within the text.

CNS abnormalities and/or EEG abnormalities) and in those in whom the risks and the benefits of treatment are in favor of the latter, after consideration of the social, emotional and personal implications of seizure relapse and of treatment itself. There are situations which may indicate deferral of treatment (*e.g.*, pregnancy) while others, for example patients performing potentially dangerous activities, may favor initiation of treatment. In either case, the patient should be involved in the decision process. Treatment modalities (choice of drug, drug dosages and duration of treatment) are the same as for the treatment of patients who had recurrent seizures and their discussion is beyond the scope of the present guideline.

■ Other recommendations and conclusions

The Quality Standards Subcommittee of the American Academy of Neurology (**AAN**) and the Practice Committee of the Child Neurology Society have developed the following recommendations for children and adolescents (Hirtz *et al.*, 2003): 1. Treatment with **AEDs** is not indicated for the prevention of the development of epilepsy; 2. Treatment with **AEDs** may be considered in circumstances where the benefits of reducing the risk of a second seizure outweigh the risk of pharmacological and psychosocial side effects. In the absence of official AAN guidelines for the adults (which are awaited), these recommendations can be also applied for the adults.

In line with these requirements, Bernd Pohlmann-Eden and co-workers (2006) defined a few steps to be taken by the family doctor (and the neurologist) for the management of the first seizure, among which: 1. Assurance that the event was a first seizure, based on history and physical examination; 2. Exclusion of acute provoking factors; 3. Arrangement of EEG and (if available) MRI; 4. Calculation on an individual basis of the recurrence risk and the social and psychological consequences of a recurrent seizure; 5. Review of the restrictions of the patient's activities, with special reference to driving; 6. Discussion of the (abstention from) AED treatment prescription.

References

Annegers JF, Hauser WA, Elvebalk LR. Remission of seizures and relapse in patients with epilepsy. *Epilepsia* 1979; 30: 729-37.

Beghi E, Sander JWAS. Epilepsy and driving. *BMJ* 2005; 331: 60-1.

Beghi E, Ciccone A, and the First Seizure Trial Group (FIRST). Recurrence after a first unprovoked seizure. Is it still a controversial issue? *Seizure* 1993; 2: 5-10.

Beghi E, De Maria G, Gobbi G, Veneselli E. Diagnosis and treatment of the first epileptic seizure: guidelines of the Italian League against Epilepsy. *Epilepsia* 2006; 47 (suppl 5): 2-8.

Berg AT, Chadwick DW. Starting artiepileptic drugs. In: Schmidt D, Schachter S, eds. *Epilepsy: Problem solving and clinical practice*. London, UK: Martin Dunitz Ltd, 2000: 207-19.

Berg AT, Shinnar S. The risk of seizure recurrence following a first unprovoked seizure: A quantitative review. *Neurology* 1991; 41: 965-72.

Berg AT, Shinnar S, Testa FM et al. Status epilepticus after the initial diagnosis of epilepsy in children. *Neurology* 2004; 63: 1027-34.

Camfield P, Camfield C, Dooley J, Smith E, Garner B. A randomized study of carbamazepine *versus* no medication after a first unprovoked seizure in childhood. *Neurology* 1989; 39: 851-2.

Camfield P, Camfield C, Smith S, Dooley J, Smith E. Long-term outcome is unchanged by antiepileptic drug treatment after a first seizure: a 15-year follow-up from a randomized trial in childhood. *Epilepsia* 2002; 43: 662-3.

Chadwick D. Epilepsy. *J Neurol Neurosurg Psychiatry* 1994; 57: 264-77.

Chandra B. First seizure in adults: to treat or not to treat. *Clin Neurol Neurosurg* 1992; 94 (suppl): S61-S63.

Collaborative Group for Epidemiology of Epilepsy. Adverse reactions to antiepileptic drugs: a multicenter survey of clinical practice. *Epilepsia* 1986; 27: 323-30.

Collaborative Group for the Study of Epilepsy. Prognosis of epilepsy in newly referred patients: a multicenter prospective study. *Epilepsia* 1988; 29: 236-43.

Commission on Epidemiology and Prognosis, International League Against Epilepsy. Guidelines for epidemiologic studies on epilepsy. *Epilepsia* 1993; 34: 592-6.

Das CP, Sawhney IM, Lal V, Prabhakar S. Risk of recurrence of seizures following single unprovoked idiopathic seizure. *Neurol India* 2000; 48: 357-60.

Feksi AT, Kaamugisha J, Sander JWAS, Gatiti S, Shorvon SD. Comprehensive primary health care antiepileptic drug treatment programme in rural and semi-urban Kenya. *Lancet* 1991; 337: 406-9.

First Seizure Trial Group. Randomized clinical trial on the efficacy of antiepileptic drugs in reducing the risk of relapse after a first unprovoked tonic-clonic seizure. *Neurology* 1993; 43: 478-83.

Fisher RS, van Emde Boas W, Blume W *et al*. Epileptic seizures and epilepsy: definitions proposed by the International League Against Epilepsy (ILAE) and the International Bureau for Epilepsy (IBE). *Epilepsia* 2005; 46: 470-2.

Gilad R, Lampl Y, Gabbay U, Eshel Y, Sarova-Pinhas I. Early treatment of a single generalized tonic-clonic seizure to prevent recurrence. *Arch Neurol* 1996; 53: 1149-52.

Glantz MJ, Cole BF, Forsyth PA *et al*. Practice parameter: anticonvulsant prophylaxis in patients with newly diagnosed brain tumors. *Neurology* 2000; 54: 1886-93.

Glauser TA. Idiosyncratic reactions: new methods of identifying high-risk patients. *Epilepsia* 2000;41 (suppl 8): S16-S29.

Glauser TA. Behavioral and psychiatric adverse events associated with antiepileptic drugs commonly used in pediatric patients. *J Child Neurol* 2004; 19 (suppl 1): S25-S38.

Glauser T, Ben-Menachem E, Bourgeois B *et al*. ILAE treatment guidelines: evidence-based analysis of antiepileptic drug efficacy and effectivenss as initial monotherapy for epileptic seizures and syndromes. *Epilepsia* 2006; 47: 1094-120.

Hirtz D, Berg A, Bettis D *et al*. Practice Parameter: treatment of the child with a first unprovoked seizure: Report of the QSS of the AAN and the Practice Committee of the CNS. *Neurology* 2003; 60: 166-75.

Kapoor WN. Current evaluation and management of syncope. *Circulation* 2002; 106: 1606-9.

Jutila L, Immonen A, Partanen K *et al*. Neurobiology of epileptogenesis in the temporal lobe. *Adv Technical Standards Neurosurg* 2002; 27: 3-22.

Kho K, Lawn ND, Dunne JW, Linto J. First seizure presentation: Do multiple seizures within 24 hours predict recurrence? *Neurology* 2006; 67: 1047-9.

Kim LG, Johnson TL, Marson AG, Chadwick DW on behalf of the MESS Study. Prediction of risk of seizure recurrence after a single seizure and early epilepsy: Further results from the MESS trial. *Lancet Neurol* 2006; 5: 317-22.

Kuijlen JMA, Teernstra OPM, Kessels AGH *et al*. Effectiveness of antiepileptic prophylaxis used with supratentorial craniotomies: a meta-analysis. *Seizure* 1996; 5: 291-8.

Kwan P, Brodie MJ. Early identification of refractory epilepsy. *N Engl J Med* 2000; 342: 314-9.

Leone MA, Solari A, Beghi E; for the FIRST Group. Treatment of the first tonic-clonic seizure does not affect long-term remission of epilepsy. *Neurology* 2006; 67: 2227-9.

Leppik IE, Schmidt D. Consensus statement on compliance in epilepsy. In: Schmidt D, Leppik IE, ed. *Compliance in Epilepsy*. Amsterdam-New York-Oxford: Elsevier, 1988: 179-182.

Levy RH, Mattson RH, Melbrum BS, Perucca E. *AED* (5th Ed): Philadelphia: Lippincott Williams and Wilkins, 2002.

Loring DW, Meador KJ. Cognitive and behavioral effects of epilepsy treatment. *Epilepsia* 2001; 42 (suppl 8): 24-32.

MacDonald BK, Johnson AL, Goodridge DM *et al*. Factors predicting prognosis of epilepsy after presentation with seizures. *Ann Neurol* 2000; 48: 833-41.

Marson A, Jacoby A, Johnson A, Kim L, Gamble C, Chadwick D. Immediate *versus* deferred antiepileptic drug treatment for early epilepsy and single seizures: a randomised controlled trial. *Lancet* 2005; 365: 2007-13.

Mattson RM, Cramer JA, Collins JF, and the Department of Veterans Affairs Epilepsy Cooperative Study No. 264 Group. A comparison of valproate with carbamazepine for the treatment of complex partial seizures and secondarily generalized tonic-clonic seizures in adults. *N Engl J Med* 1992; 327: 765-71.

Mattson RH, Cramer JA, Collins JF et al. Comparison of carbamazepine, phenobarbital, phenytoin and primidone in partial and secondarily generalized tonic-clonic seizures. *N Engl J Med* 1985; 313: 145-51.

Musicco M, Beghi E, Solari A, Viani F, and the First Seizure Trial Group. Treatment of first tonic-clonic seizure does not improve the prognosis of epilepsy. *Neurology* 1997; 49: 991-8.

Osuntokun BO, Adeuja AOG, Nottidge VA et al. Prevalence of the epilepsies in Nigerian Africans: a community based study. *Epilepsia* 1987; 28: 272-9.

Perucca E. An introduction to antiepileptic drugs. *Epilepsia* 2005; 46 (suppl 4): 31-7.

Pitkanen A. Efficacy of current antiepileptics to prevent neurodegeneration in epilepsy models. *Epilepsy Res* 2002; 50: 141-60.

Pitkanen A, Sutula T. Is epilepsy a progressive disorder? Prospects for new therapeutic approaches in temporal lobe epilepsy. *Lancet Neurol* 2002; 1: 173-81.

Placencia M, Shorvon SD, Paredes V, Bimos C, Sander JWAS, Suarez J. Cascante SM. Epileptic seizures in an Andean region of Ecuador. *Brain* 1992; 115: 771-82.

Placencia M, Sander JW, Roman M, Madera A, Crespo F, Cascante SM, Shorvon SD. The characteristics of epilepsy in a largely untreated population in rural Ecuador. *J Neurol Neurosurg Psychiatry* 1994; 57: 320-5.

Pohlmann-Eden B, Beghi E, Camfield C, Camfield P. The first seizure and its management in adults and children. *BMJ* 2006; 332: 339-42.

Schierhout G, Roberts I. Anti-epileptic drugs for preventing seizures following acute traumatic brain injury. The Cochrane Library, Issue 3, 2004.

Shinnar S, Berg AT, O'Dell C et al. Predictors of multiple seizures in a cohort of children prospectively followed from the time of their first unprovoked seizure. *Ann Neurol* 2000; 48: 140-7.

Solari A, Musicco M, BEGHI E, for the First Seizure Trial Group (FIRST). Acute antiepileptic treatment at a first unprovoked tonic-clonic seizure and the risk of subsequent seizures. *Neurology* 1997; 48: A44-A45.

Temkin NR. Antiepileptogenesis and seizure prevention trials with antiepileptic drugs: meta-analysis of controlled trials. *Epilepsia* 2001; 42: 515-24.

Watts AE. The natural history of untreated epilepsy in a rural community in Africa. *Epilepsia* 1992; 33: 464-8.

Treatment of newly diagnosed epilepsy

Anthony G. Marson

The University of Liverpool and The Walton Centre NHS Trust, Liverpool, UK

For the patient with newly diagnosed epilepsy, there are an increasing number of antiepileptic drugs (AEDs) to choose from; this includes drugs often referred to as "standard AEDs" including carbamazepine phenytoin, phenobarbital and valproate as well as drugs that are often referred to as "new AEDs". Of the new AEDS, at the time of writing, lamotrigine (Gamble et al., 2006; Brodie et al., 1995; 1999; Reunanen et al., 1996), levetiracetam (Brodie et al., 2007), oxcarbazepine (Christe et al., 1997, Dam et al., 1989) and topiramate (Sachdeo et al., 1997; Privitera et al., 2003) have a license in at least one country for use as monotherapy, whilst gabapentin, pregabalin and vigabatrin do not, although vigabatrin is licensed as monotherapy for infantile spasms in tuberous sclerosis.

Any decision regarding the most appropriate treatment for an individual patient will need to take a number of factors into account. This will include information about a drugs efficacy and tolerability compared to other treatments, and may also involve a discussion about trade offs between these outcomes. One group for whom this trade off is particularly important is women of child bearing age whose offspring may be exposed to the teratogenic effects of AEDs. The ultimate aim of AED treatment is to improve the quality of life of patients and the information about the relative effects of AEDs on quality of life is also important, as is the cost associated with any improvement, most commonly measured as cost effectiveness. Almost all health care systems are subject to some form of rationing as budgets for health care are not infinite, and policy makers and managers have to make choices about which health care interventions to make available, and such decisions are increasingly informed by information about cost effectiveness of differing technologies. In the UK, the National Institute for Health and Clinical Excellence decides which treatments should be available through the UK National Health Service and its decisions are based primarily upon cost effectiveness.

Reliable evidence about the relative effects of AEDs will come from studies with designs that minimise bias, and there is an established hierarchy of evidence with systematic reviews of randomized controlled trials and randomized controlled trials at the top, followed by observational studies, case reports and finally expert opinion.

RCTs are the most appropriate methodology to assess efficacy, adverse effects that are common and occur in the short to medium term, quality of life and cost effectiveness. RCTs are not however the appropriate methodology to assess the risk of rare but life threatening events (*e.g.* Stevens Johnson syndrome), teratogenic effects, or adverse effects occurring many years after starting treatment. Similarly, even adverse events that are common and serious may be missed in RCTs if the events are not expected and not measured, the best example of which is vigabatrin-associated visual field defects. Evidence about these adverse effects will come from studies that have used observational designs. Thus any decision or policy about the choice of AED may require an appraisal of evidence from both RCTs and observational studies.

In recent years a number of evidence based guidelines for treating epilepsy have been published. This includes those published by the ILAE and NICE (NICE Epilepsy Guidelines 2004). The guidelines produced by NICE represent the most comprehensive attempt to both appraise existing evidence and provide guidance to health care workers and policy makers regarding the management of patients with epilepsy. Both the ILAE and NICE guidelines highlight inadequacies of existing data about antiepileptic drug monotherapy with respect to informing clinical practice and policy.

■ Which outcomes in monotherapy RCTs

Epilepsy is a longer term condition with many patients taking antiepileptic drug treatment for many years, most commonly as monotherapy, with the majority of patients remaining on the first AED to which they are exposed. The choice of first AED for a patient is arguably therefore the most important treatment decision that they will make. This decision must be informed by data that reflects longer term outcomes, and those outcomes must be relevant to patients. In 1998 the ILAE commission on antiepileptic drugs made recommendations on the outcomes that should be assessed in AED monotherapy RCTs (Commission on antiepileptic drugs, 1998b). This commission primarily had representation from physicians and from industry, but people with epilepsy were not represented. The recommended primary outcomes were time to treatment failure (retention time) and time to achieve a 12 month remission from seizures, whilst secondary outcomes included time to a first or Nth seizure and adverse effects.

The ultimate aim of medical treatments is to improve quality of life, and quality of life measures are increasingly used as outcome measures in clinical trials. These measures capture the impact of seizure control and adverse effects upon an individual, but also capture information about many other domains relevant to the individual. At present however there is no consensus on the QOL measures that should be used in AED monotherapy trials but a number of batteries exist including the QOLIE 89 (Cramer *et al.*, 1999) and the Liverpool battery (Baker *et al.*, 1994).

Policy makers and health care providers will usually have limited budgets to spend on health care and will need information regarding cost and benefit to help them decide which treatments to provide, preferably those that provide the greatest benefit for the minimum cost. This information will come from a health economic evaluation, one form of which is a cost effectiveness analysis where benefit is measured as quality adjusted life years (QALYs), and cost/benefit is measured as cost per QALY. The most reliable way to compare the cost effectiveness of two or more treatment alternatives is to collect cost and effectiveness data (QALY's) in the context of an RCT. At present there is no consensus on the best tool for measuring QOLYs. Generic measures to assess QALY's including the EQ-5D can be used (Brooks 1996), but no epilepsy specific tool has been developed.

■ Comparisons of standard AEDs as monotherapy

Numerous RCTs have been undertaken that compare one or more of our standard drugs as monotherapy, most of which have been summarised in Cochrane systematic reviews that have used an individual patient data approach to meta-analysis. This includes a comparison of carbamazepine vs valproate (Marson et al., 2000), phenytoin vs valproate (Tudur Smith et al., 2001), carbamazepine vs phenytoin (Tudur Smith et al., 2002), phenytoin vs phenobarbitone (Taylor et al., 2001), carbamazepine vs phenobarbitone (Tudur Smith et al., 2003 ; de Silva M et al., 1996; Mattson et al., 1992; Richens et al., 1994; Verity et al., 1995) (1,195 patients). For the analysis patients were separated into two subgroups, those classified as having partial onset seizures and those classified as having generalized onset tonic clonic seizures. *Figure 1* shows results for time to treatment failure, with results expressed as hazard ratios with 95% confidence intervals (CIs) (*Figure 1*).

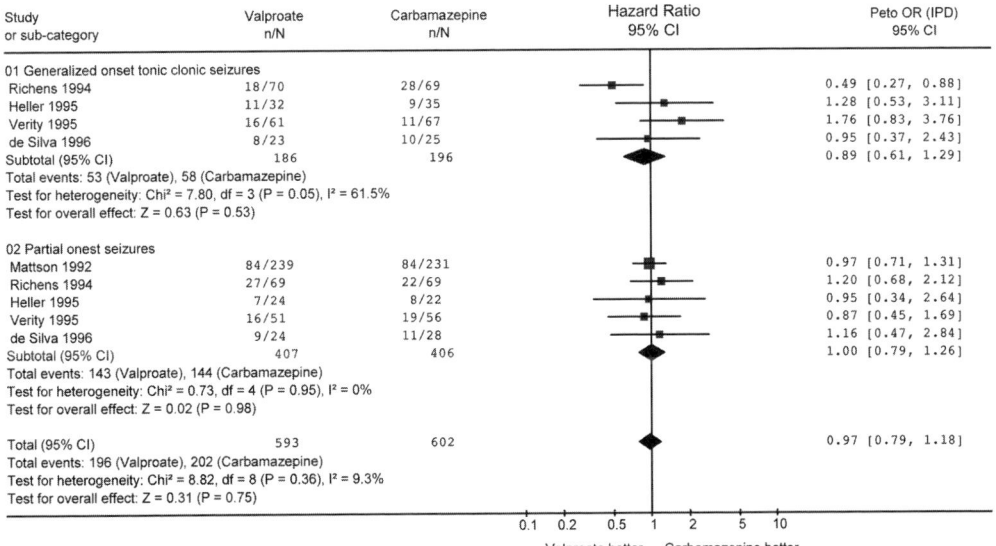

Figure 1. Carbamazemine *versus* valproate: time to treatment withdrawal.

For patients with generalized onset tonic clonic seizures the summary estimate suggests an advantage for valproate (HR = 0.89), but the confidence intervals are wide (0.61 to 1.29) and no significant difference is found and in fact the possibility of an advantage for either drug is not excluded. For the subgroup with partial onset seizures the estimate suggests no difference between the two drugs (HR = 1.00), but the confidence intervals are wide (0.79 to 1.26), and again we are unable to exclude the possibility of an important advantage for either drug.

Figure 2 shows results for time to a 12 month remission from seizures. For patients with generalized onset tonic clonic seizures, the trials included in the meta-analysis did not collect data on other seizure types during follow up (e.g. absence or myoclonus), hence results only apply to generalized onset tonic clonic seizures. For that subgroup the estimate suggests no difference between the two drugs (HR = 0.96) with wide confidence intervals (0.75 to 1.24) which do not exclude the possibility of an important advantage for either drug *(Figure 2)*.

For the subgroup with partial onset seizures the estimate suggests an advantage for carbamazepine (HR = 0.87) with confidence intervals just suggesting a statistically significant difference of borderline statistical significance (0.74 to 1.02).

The results of this meta-analysis therefore provide some evidence to support current guidelines (NICE Epilepsy Guidelines 2004) that recommend carbamazepine as a first choice for patients with partial onset seizures. Results do not however provide evidence to support recommendations that valproate is a first choice for patients with generalized onset seizures.

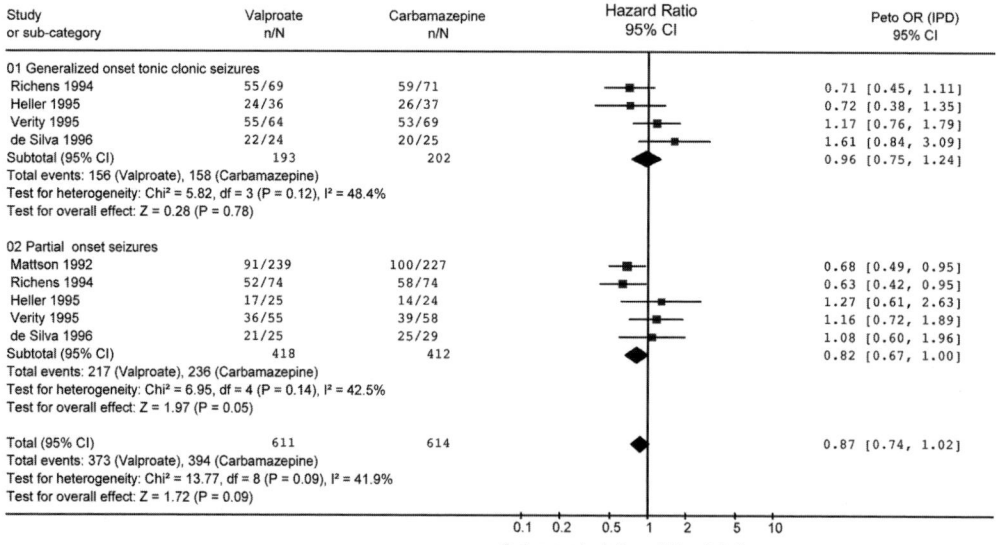

Figure 2. Carbamazemine *versus* valproate: time to 12 month remission.

Closer inspection of the trials included in this meta-analysis reveals a number of reasons why a difference between valproate and carbamazepine was not found for patients with generalised onset seizures. This includes the misclassification of epilepsy and seizure types. For example around 30% of patients classified as having generalised onset seizures had seizure onset after the age of 30 which would be extremely unlikely for patients with an idiopathic generalized epilepsy. Also, the failure to measure other seizure types such as myoclonus or absence may be important, as the main difference between carbamazepine and valproate for patients with an idiopathic generalized epilepsy may be in the effect upon these seizures types. Future monotherapy trials must be designed to avoid these short falls.

Table I summarises results form other meta-analyses of trials comparing standard AEDs as monotherapy where subgroup results are given for patients with partial onset vs generalized onset seizures are given. Results show that phenobarbitone is significantly worse for time to treatment withdrawal than either carbamazepine or phenytoin whilst no difference is found for time to 12 month remission, consistent with a higher failure rate of phenobarbitone due to poorer tolerability. The comparison of valproate and phenytoin fails to find a difference between these two drugs and again confidence intervals are wide and we are unable to exclude an important advantage for either drug.

In summary, existing trials comparing standard treatments have largely failed to find convincing evidence of differences between treatments and their ability to do so has been limited by inadequate power, misclassification of patients' seizures and a failure to collect data on generalized seizure types other than tonic clonic seizures during follow-up. Trials have also failed to examine quality of life or health economic outcomes (Table I).

Table I. Summary hazard ratios from meta-analysis of trials comparing standard antiepileptic drugs

Comparison/subgroup	Time to treatment withdrawal[$]	Time to 12 month remission[*]
Carbamazepine vs valproate		
Generalised onset tonic clonic seizures	0.81 (0.62 to 1.29)	0.96 (0.75 to 1.24)
Partial onset seizures	1.00 (0.79 to 1.26)	0.82 (0.67 to 1.00)**
Valproate vs phenytoin		
Generalised onset tonic clonic seizures	0.98 (0.60 to 1.58)	1.06 (0.71 to 1.57)
Partial onset seizures	1.23 (0.77 to 1.98)	1.02 (0.68 to 1.54)
Carbamazepine versus phenobarbital		
Generalised onset tonic clonic seizures	1.78 (0.87 to 3.62)	0.61 (0.36 to 1.03)
Partial onset seizures	1.60 (1.18 to 2.17)**	1.03 (0.72 to 1.49)
Phenytoin vs phenobarbital		
Generalised onset tonic clonic seizures	4.32 (1.77 to 10.6)**	0.77 (0.46 to 1.28)
Partial onset seizures	1.47 (1.09 to 1.97)**	0.98 (0.69 to 1.39)

$ HR > 1 favours first drug, * HR > 1 favours second drug, ** significant difference.

■ New versus standard antiepileptic drug monotherapy

The last decade and a half has seen the licensing and introduction of a number of new antiepileptic drugs. According to guidelines for antiepileptic drug development (Commission on antiepileptic drugs of the International League Against Epilepsy, 1989a) these have all been licensed initially on the basis of placebo-controlled add-on clinical trials in patients with refractory partial epilepsy. An aggregate data meta-analysis of these studies (Marson et al., 1996) indicated by indirect comparisons that some agents may be more effective than others, though no statistically significant differences were found.

Once a drug has a license for use as an add-on treatment, industry will usually embark upon a monotherapy trial programme in order to gain a license for use as monotherapy. The majority of such trials have been RCTs comparing a new AED with a standard AED such as carbamazepine or phenytoin (Bill et al., 1997; Brodie et al., 1995; Christe et al., 1997 ; Chadwick et al., 1998 ; Guerreiro et al., 1997 ; Dam et al., 1989 ; Reunanen et al., 1996; Kalviainen et al., 1995; Sachdeo et al., 1997; Steiner et al., 1999 ; Chadwick, 1999 ; Brodie et al., 1999 : Brodie et al., 1997; Brodie et al., 2002 ; Anhut et al., 1995 ; Privitera et al., 2003). It must be borne in mind that the primary focus of these trials is to meet the drug regulatory authorities such as the FDA or EMEA, and these trials have significant limitations for informing clinical practice and treatment policies.

Some of these limitations are illustrated by the trials comparing lamotrigine and carbamazepine which have been summarised in an individual patient data meta-analysis that included data from 5 RCTs (1384) patients (Gamble et al., 2006). Some of the strengths of these trials in terms of internal validity may in fact limit their ability to inform clinical practice. For example these trial have fixed dosing and titration policies and strict inclusion and exclusion criteria, the former limiting the ability of clinicians to tailor treatment for the patient as they feel appropriate and the latter resulting in the recruitment of a selected population which limit's the external validity of the trial.

For the meta-analysis, data were available for time to treatment withdrawal, but all of the trials were of less than 12 months duration, hence time to 12 month remission could not be investigated as an outcome, although time to 6 month remission and time to first seizure could be investigated. The overall results of this meta-analysis are summarised in *table II*.

For time to treatment withdrawal results indicate a significant advantage for lamotrigine. The two main reasons for treatment withdrawal are adverse effects and inadequate seizure control. Failure for these events tend to occur at different time points with treatment withdrawal for adverse effects occurring early following the initiation of treatment, and treatment withdrawal for inadequate seizure control occurring later. Trials of too short duration will fail to capture treatment withdrawal events due to inadequate seizure control and may thus be biased towards finding and advantage for a well tolerated drug that may be less effective. One could argue that trials of less than 12 months duration would be subject to such a bias. When the seizure control outcomes are examined, for time to a first seizure there are no significant differences,

Table II. Summary of results of meta-analysis comparing lamotrigine and carbamazepine monotherapy

Subgroup	Time to treatment failure*	Time to 6 month remission$	Time to first seizure*
Partial onset seizures	0.62 (0.45 to 0.86)**	0.72 (0.54 to 0.97)**	1.28 (0.98 to 1.66)
Generalized onset seizures	0.48 (0.26 to 0.89)**	1.37 (0.74 to 2.56)	0.96 (0.62 to 1.47)
Overall	0.59 (0.44 to 0.78)**	0.82 (0.62 to 1.06)	1.18 (0.94 to 1.48)

* HR > 1 favours carbamazepine, $ HR > 1 favours lamotrigine, ** statistically significant.

but the estimate for partial onset seizure favours carbamazepine. For time to a 6 month remission from seizures there is a statistically significant advantage for patients with partial onset seizures. Thus, lamotrigine has a clear advantage for time to treatment withdrawal, and it was largely upon the basis of this data that lamotrigine has granted a monotherapy license. However the relatively short duration of the trials do not allow an adequate examination of treatment failure for inadequate seizure control and these data cannot exclude the possibility of lamotrigine being inferior in terms of seizure control.

■ Equivalence and non-inferiority

As demonstrated above, despite being designed to find differences between AEDs, few monotherapy RCTs have actually done so, and it is likely that differences in efficacy between AEDs may be small. More recently, clinicians and regulatory authorities have given consideration to designing trials to show equivalence or non-inferiority, particularly for studies of new treatments (Commission on antiepileptic drugs, 1998a; Jones et al., 1996). For example the ILAE commission on antiepileptic drugs in 1998 suggested that a new AED could be considered as a first line treatment if trials comparing it with a standard AED demonstrate that the new AED has equivalent efficacy and superior tolerability.

The protocol for any equivalence trial should state an a priori definition of equivalence, which will usually be based upon the definition of a statistic commonly referred to as "delta (Δ)". In this context,? represents the smallest important clinical difference that it would be worthwhile to detect between two treatments for a particular outcome. For example, by 12 months, one might expect 50% of patients given a standard treatment to have a seizure recurrence. If it was agreed that there would be no important difference if on a new treatment 40% (or 60%) of patients had a recurrence, then Δ would be set at 10%. Clearly, assigning a value to Δ requires a clinical judgement.

Having agreed upon a value of Δ, attention can be turned to the point estimate of effect and its associated 95% confidence interval. In order to show equivalence, the confidence interval for the difference in outcome between two study arms will need to lie within the boundaries defined by $\pm\Delta$, as illustrated in *Figure 3*.

For non-inferiority trials the focus is primarily upon the lower limit of the confidence interval *(Figure 3)*. The name of such trials is somewhat of a misnomer as they are not designed to demonstrate that a new treatment is not inferior to a standard

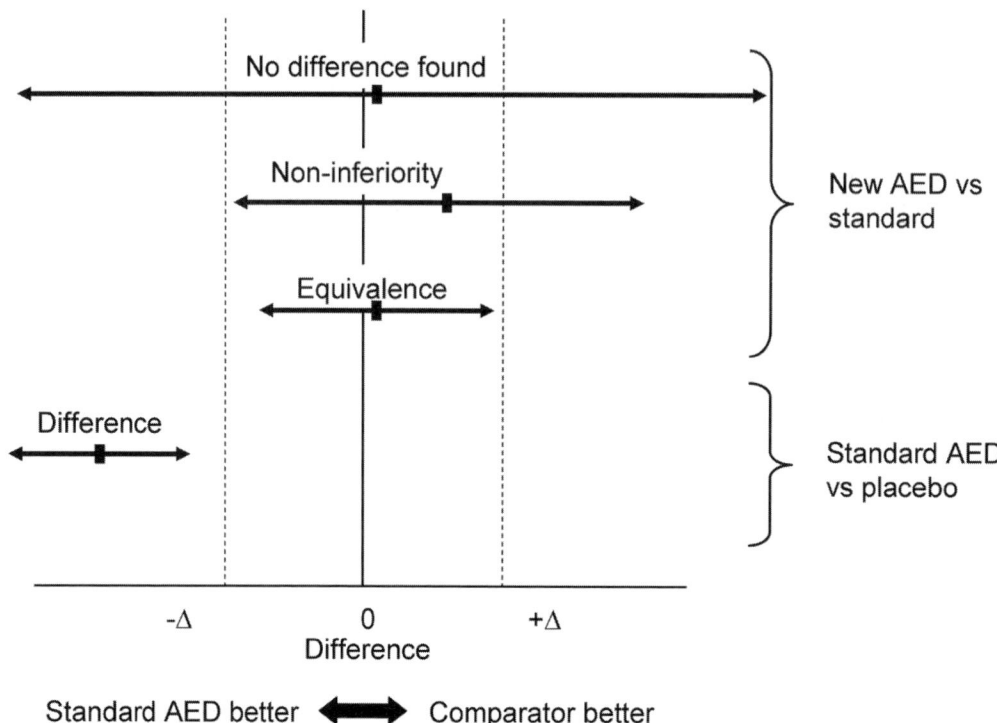

Figure 3. Estimates and 95% confidence intervals for a hypothetical outcome, illustrating equivalence and non-inferiority.

treatment. They are designed to demonstrate that when compared to a standard treatment, a new treatment is no worse than a pre-specified amount (Δ). At this point in time, there is no consensus view as to appropriate values of Δ for monotherapy AED trials. In addition, no systematic research has been undertaken in which the views of patients and clinicians have been sought, in an attempt to underpin and ensure the relevance of judgements made about the values of Δ in AED monotherapy trials. This deficit must be resolved if we are to undertake further equivalence or non-inferiority trials in epilepsy.

■ The SANAD trial – a randomized controlled trial comparing monotherapy with standard and new antiepileptic drugs

In view of the lack of reliable evidence to inform practice and policy regarding the use of new AEDs as monotherapy, in 1998 the NHS Health Technology Assessment Programme in the UK commissioned the SANAD trial to assess the longer term effectiveness and cost effectiveness of standard *versus* new antiepileptic drugs.

SANAD was effectively two trials, referred to below as arm A (Marson et al., 2007b) and arm B (Marson et al. 2007a). Patients were entered into arm A if the clinician thought that the carbamazepine was the standard drug of first choice and patients were randomized to treatment with carbamazepine, gabapentin, lamotrigine, or topiramate. Part way through the trial oxcarbazepine was added to the randomization scheme. To try and compensate for the loss of power by adding another treatment group to the randomization the duration of follow-up extended was by 12 months to increase power. Patients entered arm B if the clinician thought that valproate was the standard treatment and patients were randomized to treatment with valproate, lamotrigine or topiramate.

The design of SANAD was "pragmatic" and intended to inform every day clinical practice. Inclusion criteria were broad, with patients entered if they were aged 5 and over and had had two or more epileptic seizures and AED monotherapy was considered the best option. Patients were excluded if they had acute symptomatic seizures (including febrile seizures) or a known progressive brain pathology. SANAD was un-blinded, as blinding would have required a double dummy approach which would depart form routine clinical practice, would have significantly increased the cost of the trial and would have been impractical in the context of a trial with longer term follow-up. There was no fixed dosing in SANAD, there were guidelines for AED dosing and titration, but clinicians were able to follow their usual practice, making judgements about the most appropriate dose and titration for individual patients

SANAD had two primary outcomes: time to treatment failure (retention time) and time to 12 month remission. Other outcomes included time to a first seizure, adverse effects, quality of life outcomes and health economic outcomes. SANAD was powered to find equivalence between standard and new antiepileptic drugs for the primary outcomes with? set at 10% on an absolute scale.

Recruitment started in 1999 and was completed in 2004 with all patients followed up for a further 12 month. A total of 2,437 were recruited, and a total of 7,800 patient years of data collected making SANAD the largest epilepsy trial undertaken to date.

■ SANAD arm A

Arm A recruited 1,721 patients, 88% of whom were classified as having a cryptogenic or symptomatic partial epilepsy, 10% as having an unclassified epilepsy, 1% with an idiopathic partial epilepsy and 1% with an idiopathic generalized epilepsy. As oxcarbazepine was added to the randomization part way through the trial, fewer patients were allocated to this drug. As a result comparisons with oxcarbazepine have less power.

For time to treatment failure lamotrigine was significantly superior to carbamazepine, gabapentin and topiramate *(Figure 4)*. Compared to oxcarbazepine, the estimate suggests that lamotrigine is superior but the confidence intervals are too wide to infer a statistically significant difference. When the reasons for treatment failure are examined, lamotrigine is superior to carbamazepine due to better tolerability, but failure rates due to lack of efficacy are similar. Topiramate has a higher failure rate due to poorer tolerability whilst gabapentin has a higher failure rate due to lack of efficacy *(Figure 4)*.

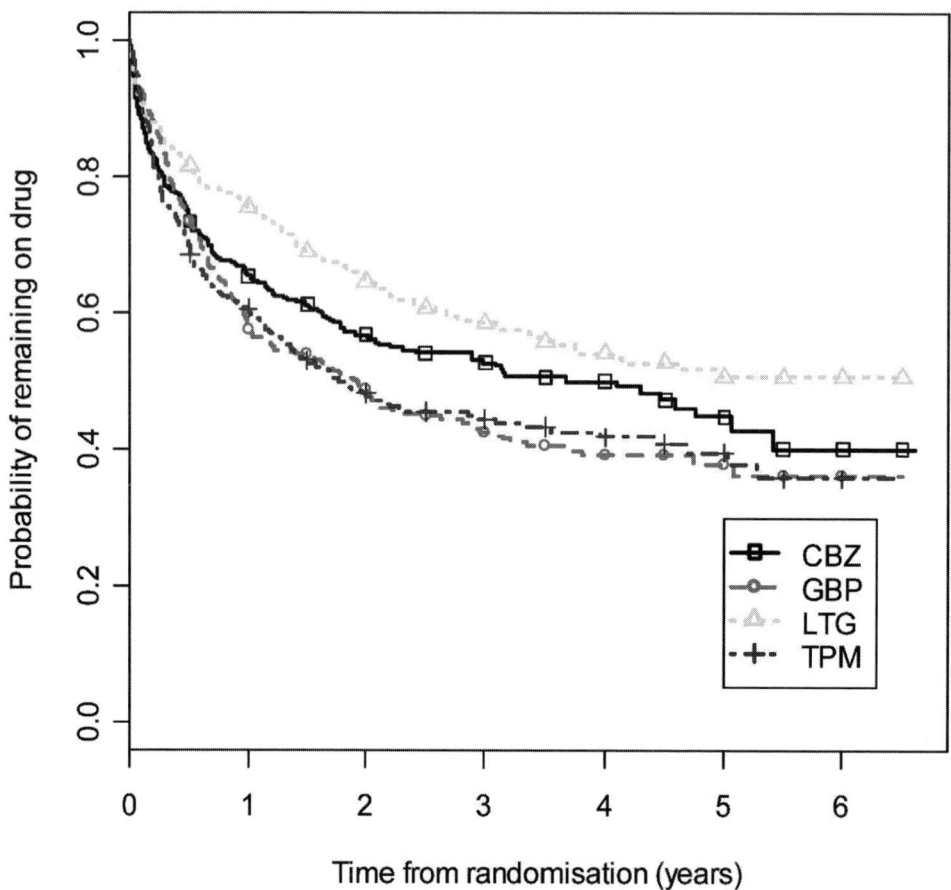

Figure 4. Time to treatment failure SANAD arm A.

For time to 12 moth remission estimates suggest that lamotrigine and carbamazepine are similar for this outcome, and superior to both gabapentin and topiramate. *Table III* summarises results for an intention to treat and per protocol analysis. In the intention to treat analysis all patients are included in the analysis, irrespective of the treatment they actually receive, even if they never received the randomized treatment or switch from the randomized treatment and achieve a remission on another drug. An intention to treat analysis thus compared the policy of starting one treatment compared with another, and minimises the risk of finding a false positive difference between two treatments. An intention to treat analysis is however biased towards finding equivalence or non-inferiority between two drugs. A per protocol analysis censors patients at the time that the randomized treatment is withdrawn and it is the conservative analysis when examining equivalence or non-inferiority *(Table III)*.

Table III. Time to 12 month remission for lamotrigine and carbamazepine

		Year					
		1	2	3	4	5	6
Intention to treat							
Carbamazepine	% with a 12 month remission (95% CI)	36 (31,41)	60 (55,66)	69 (63,74)	77 (72,82)	82 (77,87)	85 (79,91)
Lamotrigine	Difference (95% CI)	−7 (−13,0)	−3 (−11,4)	3 (−4,11)	−1 (−8,7)	−3 (−10,5)	−2 (−11,7)
Per protocol							
Carbamazepine	% with a 12 month remission (95% CI)	29 (24, 34)	44 (39, 50)	48 (42, 53)	50 (44, 55)	53 (47, 58)	*
Lamotrigine	Difference (95% CI)	−4 (−11, 3)	0 (−8, 7)	4 (−4, 12)	5 (−3, 12)	3 (−5, 11)	*

* too few data.
Adapted from Marson *et al.* 2007b.

For the per protocol analyses, the annual point estimates range from suggesting a 4% advantage for carbamazepine at 1 year to a 5% advantage for lamotrigine at 4 years. The lower confidence intervals around the estimates of a difference between lamotrigine and carbamazepine is − 11% at 1 year and thereafter ranges from − 8% to − 5%, which would been in keeping with the a priori equivalence/non-inferiority boundary of − 10%.

The quality of life battery found no important difference between the treatment policies, the reasons for which are not clear and are being further investigated. The health economic analysis suggests an 84% probability that lamotrigine would be cost effective at a cost per QALY in the UK of £30,000, a ceiling that is often used in decisions regarding cost effectiveness in the UK. The strength of estimating QALY's from generic QOL questionnaires such as the EQ-5D (as used in SANAD) is that the cost per QALY estimates are generic and can be across health care domains such as cardiology or nephrology, thus allowing policy makers to make finding decisions across the breadth of healthcare. However, such generic measures may be insensitive to QOL benefits in some diseases. A further supplementary cost effectiveness analysis estimated cost per seizure avoided and suggests that lamotrigine has a 70% chance of being cost effective at a cost per seizure avoided of £160, and an 82% chance of being cost effective at £800 per seizure avoided. Although this latter measure is more specific to epilepsy in that it measures costs associated with avoiding seizures, it is not a measure that can be compared across other areas of health care. These health economic results do however suggest that lamotrigine would be a cost effective alternative to carbamazepine in the UK.

■ SANAD arm B

Arm B of SANAD recruited 716 patients, 62% of whom were classified as having an idiopathic generalized epilepsy, 27% as having an unclassified epilepsy, 7% as having a cryptogenic or symptomatic partial epilepsy and 5% as having other syndromes. This reflect the current use of valproate for patients with a generalized epilepsy and for patients with epilepsy that is difficult to classify.

Results for time to treatment failure show that valproate is superior to either lamotrigine or topiramate *(Figure 5)*. Lamotrigine has a higher failure rate due to reduced efficacy whilst topiramate has a higher failure rate for both lack of efficacy and tolerability.

Results for time to 12 month remission are summarised in *table IV*. The intention to treat results show that valproate is superior to lamotrigine but that topiramate and valproate may be similar. The per protocol results however show a larger difference between topiramate, with valproate superior. The reason for this apparent disparity is that in the intention to treat analysis patients failing on topiramate and then switching to valproate and achieving a remission have the remission attributed to topiramate, the initial randomized policy. In the per protocol analysis for time to 12 month remission patients are censored at the time of failure of the randomized drug, and hence assesses patients achieving remission on the randomized drug.

As with arm A the quality of life analysis failed to find a difference between treatment policies, and the health economic analysis did not suggest that either lamotrigine or topiramate would be cost effective alternatives to valproate.

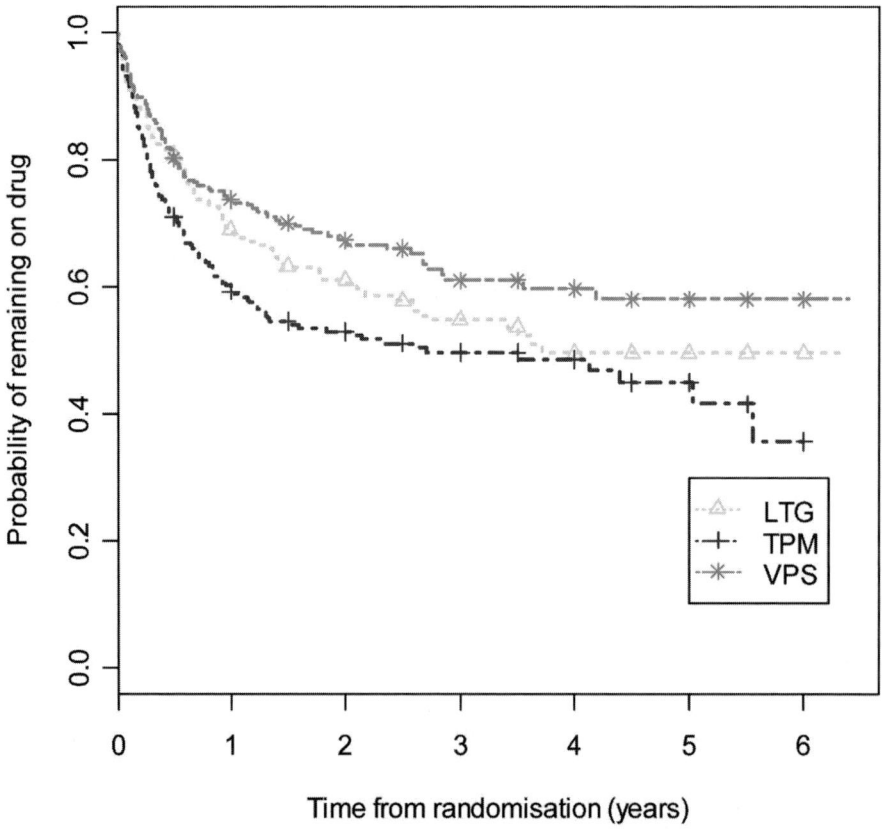

Figure 5. Time to treatment failure SANAD arm B.

Table IV. Time to 12 month remission for SANAD arm B

		Year				
		1	2	3	4	5
Intention to treat						
Valproate	% with a 12 month remission (95% CI)	43 (37,50)	69 (63,76)	81 (75,87)	87 (81,92)	92 (87,98)
Lamotrigine	Difference (95% CI)	−11 (−20,−2)	−7 (−16,2)	−7 (−15,1)	−8 (−16,0)	−9 (−17,0)
Topiramate	Difference (95% CI)	−4 (−13,5)	0 (−9,9)	−1 (−9,7)	0 (−8,7)	0 (−8,9)
Per protocol						
Valproate	% with a 12 month remission (95% CI)	36 (29, 42)	55 (48, 62)	63 (57, 70)	64 (57, 71)	66 (59, 74)
Lamotrigine	Difference (95% CI)	−10 (−19, −1)	−9 (−19, 0)	−12 (−22, −2)	−11 (−21, −1)	−13 (−24, −3)
Topiramate	Difference (95% CI)	−4 (−13, 5)	−7 (−17, 2)	−14 (−23, −4)	−13 (−23, −3)	−15 (−25, −5)

■ Discussion of SANAD results

In the past 20-30 years there have been an increasing number of comparative AED monotherapy studies. The majority of these studies are designed to inform regulatory decisions, and the designs used have a number of limitations for informing clinical practice as outlined in the text above. Few trials have examined QOL and none prior to SANAD examined health economic outcomes. The lack of reliable evidence to inform clinical practice more than 10 year after licensing of drugs such as lamotrigine could be regarded as a failure of strategies to adequately assess the role of newer AEDs.

SANAD has demonstrated that large scale longer term RCTs that are simple and pragmatic design are feasible in epilepsy. The clinical results for SANAD arm A indicate that for patients with partial onset seizures lamotrigine is similar to and probably non-inferior to carbamazepine for the primary efficacy outcome – time to 12 month remission. Lamotrigine was significantly superior to carbamazepine for time to treatment failure due to better tolerability. Thus based in the clinical results, lamotrigine should be considered the first line antiepileptic drug for patients with partial onset seizures. The health economic analysis suggests that lamotrigine would be a cost effective alternative to carbamazepine for a health economy prepared to pay in the region of £30,000 per QALY.

In SANAD arm B, the clinical results show that for patients with an idiopathic generalized epilepsy, or seizures that are difficult to classify, valproate is superior to topiramate and lamotrigine for time to treatment failure and time to 12 month remission. Given the clinical results it is not surprising that the health economic analysis suggest that neither lamotrigine nor topiramate are likely to be cost effective alternatives to valproate. Thus valproate should remain the first line treatment for such patients. Given this result as well as increasing knowledge about the teratogenic effects of valproate and its effect on cognitive development for children exposed in utero (Adab et al., 2004), women of child bearing age remain a difficult group to counsel, although SANAD does now provide robust evidence regarding the efficacy and effectiveness of the main treatment options. In simplistic terms, women can choose between a drug with higher efficacy and higher teratogenic potential (valproate) or a drug with lower efficacy and lower teratogenic potential (lamotrigine). The current lack of knowledge regarding the teratogenic potential of topiramate makes counselling women about the use of this drug in pregnancy difficult. The importance of teratogenicity in treatment choices made by women, and the fact that information about teratogenicity will come from observational studies rather than RCTs highlights the need for robust studies assessing teratogenic effects as well as the development of methodologies to incorporate information from RCTs as well as observational studies to better inform clinical decision making.

■ Individualising treatment choices

The RCTs discussed in this chapter provide data that can be applied to broad groups of patients, primarily those with partial onset seizures, those with generalized onset seizures and those with seizures that are difficult to classify. At present there is an increasing literature on "individualised patient treatment" (Constable et al., 2006; Lunshof et al., 2006). In order to individualise patient treatment, we need to be able to reliably predict the outcome or outcomes for the individual patient with differing treatment alternatives. This will ultimately require multivariate analysis of data using factors that are of prognostic importance in order to produce predictive models. Given the strength of RCTs in minimising bias when making treatment comparisons, the most reliable data will come from multivariate analyses of RCTs. Some multivariate analyses and prognostic models have been reported, including predictive models from the MRC Antiepileptic Drug Withdrawal Study (The Medical Research Council antiepileptic drug withdrawal study group 1993) and the Multi Centre Study of Early Epilepsy and Single Seizures (Kim et al., 2006). The multivariate analyses in both of these studies used clinical factors collected at baseline. Whilst these models can be used to improve outcome prediction for individual patients, a significant amount of heterogeneity of outcome remains unexplained by clinical factors. More recently there has been increasing interest in genetic factors that are associated with treatment outcomes. Most of the positive findings are for polymorphisms that predict serious adverse events (Pirmohamed, 2006), but there has been less success in finding genetic polymorphisms associated with treatment success such as seizure control. For example there has been much interest in the role of drug transporters (e.g. ABCB1) following an initial positive result form a retrospective study (Siddiqui et al., 2003), but a more recent study using prospectively collected data found no association between ABCB1 polymorphisms and seizure control outcomes (Leschziner et al., 2006). Despite this negative finding, it remains likely that genetic polymorphisms are responsible for some of the heterogeneity in outcome that is seen in epilepsy. To do so effectively will require large scale prospective studies, primarily RCTs, with analyses that take into account both clinical and genetic patient factors.

Future challenges

We still have much work to do to assess the place of standard and newer treatments for epilepsy as monotherapy, particularly if we wish to provide robust data that will inform individual patient outcomes utilising both clinical and genetic data. Policy makers will require information about cost effectiveness of treatments as well as any genetic tests that are developed. The studies required will need to recruit many thousands of patients and this can only be achieved by the establishment of effective research networks and by breaking down institutional and geographical barriers. The results of such studies, as with existing studies, are likely to highlight risks of harms and benefits associated with a number of treatment options. The patient and clinician will still need to decide which the preferred outcomes are for the individual patient, and further work assessing decision making in epilepsy is also required.

References

The epilepsies: the diagnosis and management of the epilepsies in adults and children in primary and secondary care. London: National Institute for Clinical Excellence. *Clinical Guideline* 2004: 20.

Adab N, Kini U, Vinten J et al. The longer term outcome of children born to mothers with epilepsy. *J Neurol Neurosurg Psychiatry* 2004; 75: 1575-83.

Anhut H, Greiner MJ, Murray GH, the International GBP Monotherapy Study Group 945-77/78. Double-blind, fixed-dose comparison study of gabapentin (GBP; Neurontin®) and carbamazepine (CBZ) monotherapy in patients with newly diagnosed partial epilepsy. *Epilepsia* 1995; 36 (suppl 4): 67.

Baker GA, Jacoby A, Smith D, Dewey M, Johnson A, Chadwick D. Quality of life in epilepsy: the Liverpool initiative. In: Trimble MR DW, ed. *Epilepsy and Quality of Life*. New York: Raven Press, 1994: 135-50.

Bill PA, Vigonius U, Pohlmann H et al. A double-blind controlled clinical trial of oxcarbazepine *versus* phenytoin in adults with previously untreated epilepsy. *Epilepsy Res* 1997; 27: 195-204.

Brodie MJ, Overstall PW, Giorgi L. Multicentre, double-blind, randomised comparison between lamotrigine and carbamazepine in elderly patients with newly diagnosed epilepsy. The UK Lamotrigine Elderly Study Group. *Epilepsy Res* 1999; 37: 81-7.

Brodie MJ, Bomhof MAM, Kalviainen R, et al. Double-blind comparison of tiagabine and carbamazepine monotherapy in newly diagnosed epilepsy. *Epilepsia* 1997; 38 (suppl 3): 66-7.

Brodie MJ, Richens A, Yuen AWC. Double-blind comparison of lamotrigine and carbamazepine in newly diagnosed epilepsy. UK Lamotrigine/Carbamazepine Monotherapy Trial Group. *Lancet* 1995; 345: 476-9.

Brodie MJ, Wroe SJ, Dean ADP, Holdich TAH, Whitehead J, Stevens JW. Efficacy and safety of remacemide *versus* carbamazepine in newly diagnosed epilepsy: comparison by sequential analysis. *Epilepsy Behav* 2002; 3: 140-6.

Brodie MJ, Perucca E, Ryvlin P, Ben-Menachem E, Meencke HJ; Levetiracetam Monotherapy Study Group. Comparison of levetiracetam and controlled-release carbamazepine in newly diagnosed epilepsy. Neurology. 2007;68:402-8.

Brooks R. EuroQol: the current state of play. *Health Policy* 1996; 37: 53-72.

Chadwick D. Safety and efficacy of vigabatrin and carbamazepine in newly diagnosed epilepsy: a multicentre randomised double-blind study. Vigabatrin European Monotherapy Study Group. *Lancet* 1999; 354: 13-9.

Chadwick DW, Anhut H, Greiner MJ et al. A double-blind trial of gabapentin monotherapy for newly diagnosed partial seizures. International Gabapentin Monotherapy Study Group 945-77. *Neurology* 1998; 51: 1282-8.

Christe W, Kramer G, Vigonius U, et al. A double-blind controlled clinical trial: oxcarbazepine *versus* sodium valproate in adults with newly diagnosed epilepsy. *Epilepsy Res* 1997; 26: 451-60.

Commission on antiepileptic drugs. Considerations on designing clinical trials to evaluate the place of new antiepileptic drugs in the treatment of newly diagnosed and chronic patients with epilepsy. *Epilepsia* 1998; 39: 799-803.

Commission on antiepileptic drugs of the International League Against Epilepsy. Guidelines for the clinical evaluation of antiepileptic drugs. *Epilepsia* 1989; 30: 400-8.

Constable S, Johnson MR, Pirmohamed M. Pharmacogenetics in clinical practice: considerations for testing. *Expert Rev Mol Diagn* 2006: 6; 193-205.

Cramer JA, Westbrook LE, Devinsky O, Perrine K, Glassman MB, Camfield C. Development of the Quality of Life in Epilepsy Inventory for Adolescents: the QOLIE-AD-48. *Epilepsia* 1999; 40: 1114-21.

Dam M, Ekberg R, Loyning Y, Waltimo O, Jakobsen K. A double blind study comparing oxcarbazepine and carbamazepine in patients with newly diagnosed, previously untreated epilepsy. *Epilepsy Res* 1989; 3: 70-6.

de Silva M, MacArdle B, McGowan M et al. Randomised comparative monotherapy trial of phenobarbitone, phenytoin, carbamazepine, or sodium valproate for newly diagnosed childhood epilepsy. *Lancet* 1996; 347: 709-13.

Gamble CL, Williamson PR, Marson AG. Lamotrigine *versus* carbamazepine monotherapy for epilepsy. *Cochrane Database Syst Rev* 2006; CD001031.

Guerreiro MM, Vigonius U, Pohlmann H, et al. A double-blind controlled clinical trial of oxcarbazepine *versus* phenytoin in children and adolescents with epilepsy. *Epilepsy Res* 1997; 27: 205-13.

Heller AJ, Chesterman P, Elwes RD, et al. Phenobarbitone, phenytoin, carbamazepine, or sodium valproate for newly diagnosed adult epilepsy: a randomised comparative monotherapy trial. *J Neurol Neurosurg Psychiatry* 1995; 58: 44-50.

Jones B, Jarvis P, Lewis JA, Ebutt AF. Trials to assess equivalence; the importance of rigerous methods. *BMJ* 1996; 313: 36-9.

Kalviainen R, Aikia M, Saukkonen AM, Mervaala E, Riekkinen PJ Sr. Vigabatrin vs carbamazepine monotherapy in patients with newly diagnosed epilepsy. A randomized, controlled study. *Arch Neurol* 1995; 52: 989-96.

Kim L, Johnson T, Marson A, Chadwick D. Prediction of risk of seizure recurrence after a single seizure and early epilepsy: further results from the MESS trial. *Lancet Neurol* 2006; 5: 317-22.

Leschziner G, Zabaneh D, Pirmohamed M et al. Exon sequencing and high resolution haplotype analysis of ABC transporter genes implicated in drug resistance. *Pharmacogenet Genomics* 2006; 16: 439-50.

Lunshof JE, Pirmohamed M, Gurwitz D. Personalized medicine: decades away? *Pharmacogenomics* 2006; 7: 237-41.

Marson AG, Kadir ZA, Chadwick DW. New antiepileptic drugs: a systematic review of their efficacy and tolerability. *BMJ* 1996; 313: 1169-74.

Marson AG, Williamson PR, Hutton JL, Clough HE, Chadwick DW. Carbamazepine *versus* valproate monotherapy for epilepsy. *Cochrane Database Syst Rev* 2000; CD001030.

Marson AG, Al-Kharusi AM, Alwaidh M, et al. The SANAD study of effectiveness of valproate, lamotrigine, or topiramate for generalised and unclassifiable epilepsy: an unblinded randomised controlled trial. *Lancet* 2007a; 369: 1016-26.

Marson AG, Al-Kharusi AM, Alwaidh M, et al. The SANAD study of effectiveness of carbamazepine, gabapentin, lamotrigine, oxcarbazepine, or topiramate for treatment of partial epilepsy: an unblended randomised controlled trial. *Lancet* 2007b; 369: 1000-15.

Mattson R, Cramer J, Collins J. A comparison of valproate with carbamazepine for the treatment of complex partial seizures and secondarily generalized tonic clonic seizures in adults. The Department of Veterans Affairs Epilepsy Cooperative Study No. 264 Group. *New Engl J Med* 1992; 327: 765-71.

Pirmohamed M. Genetic factors in the predisposition to drug-induced hypersensitivity reactions. *AAPS J* 2006; 8: E20-6.

Privitera MD, Brodie MJ, Mattson RH, *et al.* Topiramate, carbamazepine and valproate monotherapy: double-blind comparison in newly diagnosed epilepsy. *Acta Neurol Scand* 2003; 107: 165-75.

Reunanen M, Dam M, Yuen AW. A randomised open multicentre comparative trial of lamotrigine and carbamazepine as monotherapy in patients with newly diagnosed or recurrent epilepsy. *Epilepsy Res* 1996; 23: 149-55.

Richens A, Davidson DL, Cartlidge NE, Easter DJ. A multicentre comparative trial of sodium valproate and carbamazepine in adult onset epilepsy. Adult EPITEG Collaborative Group. *J Neurol Neurosurg Psychiatry* 1994; 57: 682-7.

Sachdeo RC, Reife RA, Lim P, Pledger G. Topiramate monotherapy for partial onset seizures. *Epilepsia* 1997; 38: 294-300.

Siddiqui A, Kerb R, Weale ME *et al*. Association of multidrug resistance in epilepsy with a polymorphism in the drug-transporter gene ABCB1. *New Engl J Med* 2003; 348; 1442-8.

Steiner TJ, Dellaportas CI, Findley LJ *et al*. Lamotrigine monotherapy in newly diagnosed untreated epilepsy: a double-blind comparison with phenytoin. *Epilepsia* 1999; 40: 601-7.

Taylor S, Tudur Smith C, Williamson PR, Marson AG. Phenobarbitone *versus* phenytoin monotherapy for partial onset seizures and generalized onset tonic-clonic seizures. *Cochrane Database Syst Rev* 2001; CD002217.

The Medical Research Council antiepileptic drug withdrawal study group. Prognostic index for recurrence of seizures after remission of epilepsy. *BMJ* 1993; 22: 1374-8.

Tudur Smith C, Marson AG, Clough HE, Williamson PR. Carbamazepine *versus* phenytoin monotherapy for epilepsy. *Cochrane Database Syst Rev* 2002; CD001911.

Tudur Smith C, Marson AG, Williamson PR. Phenytoin *versus* valproate monotherapy for partial onset seizures and generalized onset tonic-clonic seizures. *Cochrane Database Syst Rev* 2001; CD001769.

Tudur Smith C, Marson AG, Williamson PR. Carbamazepine *versus* phenobarbitone monotherapy for epilepsy. *Cochrane Database Syst Rev* 2003; CD001904.

Verity CM, Hosking G, and Easter DJ. A multicentre comparative trial of sodium valproate and carbamazepine in paediatric epilepsy. The Paediatric EPITEG Collaborative Group. *Dev Med Child Neurol* 1995; 37: 97-108.

Bridging the gap between clinical guidelines and individualized patient treatment

John M. Pellock

Division of Child Neurology, Department of Neurology, Virginia Commonwealth University/Medical College of Virginia Hospitals, Richmond, Virginia, USA

Childhood epilepsy differs from that seen in adults because of age related seizures, their etiology with both benign and malignant epilepsy syndromes being present, and the frequent presence of neurologic abnormality, mental retardation and behavioral difficulties as co-mobidities (Pellock, 1997). They also may respond differently to antiepileptic drugs (AEDs) or have a specific pattern of evolution of seizure types which are not controlled or are even exacerbated by specific medications. Randomized clinical trials of AEDs applicable for the treatment of children with epilepsy are performed initially for adult onset refractory partial seizures. Following these studies, pediatric partial seizure trials are initiated and recommendations follow. Only recently have trials for Lennox Gastaut and childhood absence epilepsy been performed, leading to specific indications for newer AEDs.

Many other epilepsy types are never formally studied regarding the most efficacious therapy. Few, if any, trials have been performed for the treatment of neonatal seizures and the encephalopathic epilepsies including West syndrome (infantile spasms), Dravet syndrome (severe myoclonic epilepsy of infancy) and specific myoclonic syndromes, especially the progressive myoclonic epilepsies. In adolescents recent trials in juvenile myoclonic epilepsy and adolescent/adult onset primary generalized epilepsies have been performed. The procedural difficulties in conducting these studies, particularly in infants and young children are significant. Not only are these trials limited by the number of patients that might be enrolled in a well controlled study but they are also limited by the evolution of seizure types and the perceived urgency for the treatment of epilepsy. Furthermore, many are complicated by clustering of seizures or status epilepticus which typically requires exit from randomized trials.

As guidelines for the treatment of epilepsy using new and classic AEDs have been proposed elsewhere in this symposium and have been well documented, this discussion will concentrate on expert consensus reports and the selection criteria for AED treatment used by many clinicians. It is stressed that arriving at the treatment of choice for an individual patient is dependent upon many factors, some of which are discussed herein.

■ Utility of randomized clinical trials

Adults

Clinicians must decide what AED therapy or combination thereof is best for a given individual when faced with a person with epilepsy. Controlled clinical trials have provided specific information regarding the efficacy and adverse effects of each of these medications as they are introduced and accepted by regulatory authorities with specific indications. Over the past decade multiple studies regarding adjunctive therapy for specific AEDs, monotherapy trials, and some comparative trials have produced highly regulated and encyclopedic reports regarding each drug. The clinician and patient ultimately must use these data comparing newer and classic AEDs, chose the appropriate treatment for the individual and then proceed to administer the drug in a most appropriate manner.

The American Academy of Neurology Practice Guidelines reviewed evidence for the treatment of new onset and refractory epilepsy in 2004 (French 2004, 2004a) concluding that for newly diagnosed partial seizures in adults, gabapentin is an effective treatment. For partial and generalized tonic clonic seizures lamotrigine, topiramate and oxcarbazepine are effective. The newer agents gabapentin, lamotrigine, levetiracetam, oxcarbazepine, tiagabine, topiramate and zonisamide were established as effective as adjunctive therapy for refractory partial seizures in adults. Lamotrigine and topiramate are effective as monotherapy. For adults with generalized epilepsy, topiramate is effective.

In 2000, an expert opinion survey was performed to determine which treatment options were preferred in a number of clinical situations, mostly regarding adults with epilepsy (Karceski, 2000). The survey of United States epileptologists was again performed in 2004 and results were compared (Karceski, 2005). Forty-three of forty eight experts responded to the second survey of which 67% also participated in the original questionnaire. Valproate was rated as the treatment of choice for initial monotherapy for idiopathic generalized epilepsy (generalized tonic-clonic, absence, and myoclonic seizures). For primary generalized idiopathic generalized tonic clonic seizures lamotrigine and topiramate were also identified as usually appropriate for initial monotherapy. For absence, ethosuximide was also the treatment of choice and lamotrigine was felt to be usually appropriate.

Carbamazepine and oxcarbazepine were treatments of choice for symptomatic localized resistant epilepsy, while lamotrigine and levetiracetam were also thought to be appropriate. In complex partial seizures, carbamazepine, lamotrigine and oxcarbazepine were treatments of choice while levetiracetam was felt to be usually appropriate. For women with partial epilepsy, lamotrigine was felt to be the treatment of choice.

Bridging the gap between clinical guidelines and individualized patient treatment

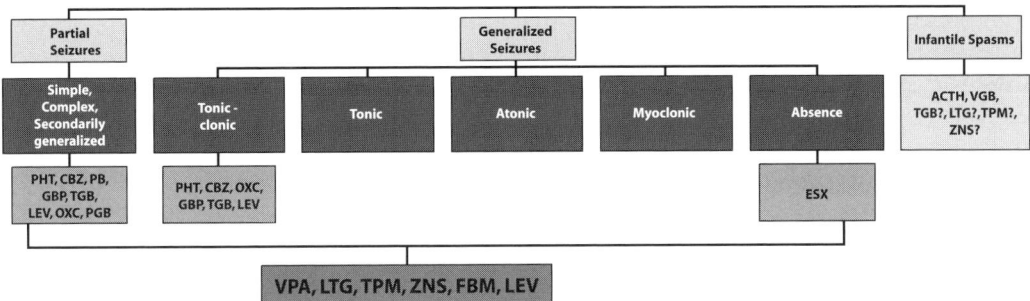

Figure 1. Clinical utility of established and newer AEDs. Treatment options.
CBZ: carbamazepine; ESX: ethosuximide; FBM: felbamate; GBP: gabapentin; LTG: lamotrigine; LEV: levetiracetam; OXC: oxcarbazepine; PB: phenobarbital; PGB: pregabalin; PHT: phenytoin; TGB: tiagabine; TPM: topiramate; VGB: vigabatrin; VPA: valproic acid; ZNS: zonisamide.

In the elderly, lamotrigine was felt to be the treatment of choice, while levetiracetam was felt to also be usually appropriate, along with gabapentin, especially when persons had co-morbid medical illness. Lamotrigine and levetiracetam were thought to be usually appropriate in persons with HIV and epilepsy. For those persons with co-morbid depression, lamotrigine was felt to be the treatment of choice. Renal disease influenced the choice for the treatment of partial seizures such that lamotrigine was felt to be appropriate, while valproate was also appropriate for idiopathic generalized epilepsy with this co-morbidity. For those with hepatic disease, levetiracetam and lamotrigine were felt to be usually appropriate for idiopathic generalized epilepsy whereas levetiracetam was the treatment of choice with gabapentin also usually appropriate for those with localization related epilepsy. The authors felt that the survey results could be helpful to clinicians but should not, of course, replace clinical judgment. Rather they suggested that the experts identified first line therapies which would form a (menu(of appropriate therapies and then separated them from a group of equivocal treatment options. The treating physician could use this information to help them consider appropriate options for treatment.

Childhood

Fewer randomized clinical trials have been carried out in childhood epilepsy, as they are a heterogenous group of conditions that differ significantly from those seen in adults. Still, seizures are primarily classified as partial or generalized. As noted above, the evolution of childhood epilepsy syndromes and their age relationship makes them more difficult to study. Classic studies demonstrated the near equipoise of treatment with phenobarbital, carbamazepine, phenytoin and valproate, however the intolerability of barbiturates was quickly identified as other agents became available (Pellock 1997). Thus, phenobarbital became recommended as a second line drug because of its lack of tolerability rather than its efficacy. Of the newer drugs, FDA approval exists for childhood use of lamotrigine, oxcarbazepine, and topiramate for partial onset seizures and lamotrigine has been added to the prior approvals of ethosuximide and valproate for absence. AAN Guidelines noted above are consistent with these findings. Recently topiramate and levetiracetam have been given approval for the treatment of primary generalized epilepsy (juvenile myoclonic epilepsy). Felbamate, topiramate and lamotrigine have also undergone randomized clinical trials and proven efficacious for seizure types associated with Lennox Gastaut syndrome. In the case of infantile spasms, the American Academy of Neurology has published a guideline establishing ACTH as probably effective and vigabatrin as possibly effective for the treatment of this disorder; significant side effects of both agents were stressed in that report (McKay, 2006).

Because of the heterogeneity of the epilepsies in childhood and the fact that many are age related and thus relatively rare when considering numbers needed to perform a well designed randomized clinical trial, many syndromes go without well designed trials to aid clinicians in treating these children.

Neonatal seizures, the encephalopathic epilepsies of infancy with and without myoclonus, severe myoclonic epilepsy of infancy, and Landau Kleffner syndrome are some of the examples. Certainly additional studies are needed in these syndromes. When reviewing isolated reports the patient numbers are limited and inclusion criteria are frequently disparate.

Recommendation s from the National Institute of Clinical Excellence (NICE, 2004) state that the newer AEDs gabapentin, lamotrigine, oxcarbazepine, tiagabine, topiramate, and vigabitrin (as adjunctive for partial seizures), within their licensed indications are recommended for the management of epilepsy in children who have not benefitted from treatment with older agents (carbamazepine or valproate) or for whom the older AEDs were unsuitable. Vigabitrin is recommended as first line for infantile spasms. In addition, NICE guidelines provide recommendations for the syndrome of childhood and juvenile absence, JME, generalized tonic-clonic seizures only, cryptogenic and symptomatic focal epilepsies, infantile spasms, benign epilepsy with centro-temporal spikes, benign epilepsy with occipital paroxysms, severe myoclonic epilepsy, continuous spike wave of slow sleep, Lennox Gastaut, Landau-Klenner syndrome and myoclonic astatic epilepsy *(Table I)* (NICE, 2004).

Wheless et al. (2005) published the results of an expert opinion survey performed using similar methodology as that done in adults. Of 41 physicians specializing in pediatric epilepsy invited to participate, 39 responded. Valproate was the treatment of choice for symptomatic myoclonic and generalized tonic clonic seizures except in the very young, with lamotrigine and topiramate being also rated as first line. Zonisamide was first line only in children with myoclonic seizures. For initial monotherapy of complex partial seizures, oxcarbazepine and carbamazepine were treatments of choice with lamotrigine and levetiracetam also felt to be first line. As initial therapy for infantile spasms associated with tuberous sclerosis, vigabatrin was the treatment of choice with ACTH also first line. When infantile spasms were symptomatic in etiology (other than tuberous sclerosis) ACTH was the treatment of choice with topiramate also considered a first line agent. Valproate was the treatment of choice for Lennox Gastaut syndrome with topiramate and lamotrigine also first line. For the acute treatment of prolonged febrile seizures and clusters of seizures was felt best treated by rectal diazepam as first choice. For benign childhood epilepsy with centro temporal spikes (BECTS) oxcarbazepine and carbamazepine were treatment of choice with gabapentin, lamotrigine and levetiracetam also first line. Ethosuximide was rated as the treatment of choice for childhood absence epilepsy with valproate and

Table I. Comparaison of recommendations for the treatment of pediatric epilepsy

Seizure Type or Epilepsy Syndrome	Pediatric Expert Consensus Survey[a]	ILAE[b]	SIGN[c]	NICE[d]	French Study[e]	FDA approved[f]
Partial-onset	OXC, CBZ	A: OXC B: none C: CBZ, PB, PHT, TPM, VPA	PHT, VPA, CBZ, LTG, TPM, OXC, VGB, CLB	CBZ, VPA, LTG, OXC, TPM	OXC, CBZ, LTG (adult males)	PB, PHT, CBZ, OXC, TPM
Benign epilepsy of childhood with centro-temporal spikes	OXC, CBZ	A, B: none C: CBZ, VPA	Not specifically mentioned	CBZ, OXC, LTG, VPA	Not surveyed	None
Childhood Absence Epilepsy	ESM	A, B: none C: ESM, CBZ, VPA	VPA, ESM, LTG	VPA, ESM, LTG	VPA, LTG	ESM, VPA, LTG*
Juvenile Myclonic Epilepsy	VPA, LTG	A, B, C: none	VPA, LTG, TPM	VPA, LTG	VPA, LTG	TPM, LEV*
Lennox-Gastaut Syndrome	VPA, TPM, LTG	Not reviewed	Not Specifically mentionned	LTG, VPA, TPM	Not surveyed	FLB, TPM, LTG

* Recently approved after publication cited. Modified from: Whelss JW et al. J Child Neuro 2005; 20: S1-S56.
See references for b-e.

lamotrigine also first line. For juvenile absence epilepsy, valproate and lamotrigine were treatments of choice. For juvenile myoclonic epilepsy in adolescent males, valproate and lamotrigine were treatments of choice with topiramate also first line, whereas in adolescent females lamotrigine was the treatment of choice with topiramate and valproate other first line options. For the treatment of neonatal status epilepticus intravenous phenobarbital was the treatment of choice with lorazepam and fosphenytoin also first line.

For the initial therapy of all other types of pediatric status epilepticus, lorazepam was the treatment of choice with intravenous diazepam also a first line agent. For generalized tonic clonic status epilepticus, rectal diazepam and fosphenytoin were also first line whereas, fosphenytoin was also felt first line for complex partial status epilepticus while intravenous valproate was first line for absence status epilepticus. Thus, expert opinion for pediatric epilepsy inquired about additional epilepsy syndromes and seizure types seen more commonly by pediatric neurologists. *Table I* from Wheless (2005) shows how this pediatric expert consensus survey compares with recommendations from the International League Against Epilepsy (Glauser, 2006), Scottish Intercollegiate Guideline Network, National Institute for Clinical Excellence, the French study by Semah, *et al.* and current FDA approvals. Survey of European colleagues regarding pediatric epilepsy treatment suggests that valproate is more commonly the drug of choice than in the United States. Michelucci *et al.* (2006) have recently published guidelines of the Italian League Against Epilepsy for the treatment of status epilepticus in adults, which also stresses the importance as using benzodiazepine as a first line therapy.

▪ Beyond guidelines

The physician treating epilepsy must frequently go beyond guidelines and expert opinion publication in the treatment of individual patients. It is here where clinical experience, expertise, depth of knowledge and truly discussing considering all aspects of an individual patient become most important. Co-morbidities of epilepsy are present at every age, either as etiologic factors for the epilepsy itself or as a part of the total medical history, age, gender and life situation of the individual patient. The co-morbidities of epilepsy frequently encountered are listed in *table II*. Additionally, the neuropsychiatric co-morbid symptomatology associated with epilepsy is only beginning to be recognized and certainly some of the main behavioral difficulties seen may be significantly influenced by anti-epileptic drug treatment. Perhaps the most obvious example is the association of symptoms of depression with phenobarbital use. While the epilepsy itself may be of the same etiology as that of co-morbid neuropsychiatric disturbance, medications may influence these symptoms in a positively or negatively way (Rogawski, Loscher 2004; Weintraub, 2007).

Women, infants, elderly and all those with associated medical and psychiatric illness require that special considerations be given when treating their epilepsy. Women have different needs than men. Obviously, teratogenic and hormonal factors play a large part in choice of an anticonvulsant medication. Women's issues are many but frequently center around hormonal effects of epilepsy and AEDs and the potential for childbearing. Birth control hormonal preparations are frequently affected by enzyme inducing AEDs and only recently has the interaction between hormonal therapy and lamotrigine clearance been appreciated (Christensen *et al.*, 2007). Teratogenesis has been more commonly reported with older AEDs, but the balance of seizure control *versus* the potential for fetal malformation is multifactorial and needs to be balanced. More recently the potential for in-utero exposure to certain AEDs, particularly valproate, has been linked to cognitive effect in children of women with epilepsy (Meador, 2006). In later years, bone metabolism is a major concern in women, but it is during childhood that primary bone is established and treatment with enzyme inducing AEDs should be avoided whenever possible (Morrell, 2006).

In children, neonates and infants rapidly developing CNS present both theoretical and real challenges. The effects of AEDs on brain development are just beginning to be understood. Recent evidence suggesting that classic medications used for the treatment of neonatal seizures may actually promote apoptosis is bothersome (Bittigau *et al.*, 2002), and requires careful consideration for both acute and chronic treatment of these infants, but information regarding alternatives is lacking. In young infants seizure identification and evolution through various syndromes makes the potential worsening or seeming precipitation of certain seizures types a real consideration for using more broad spectrum AEDs. Frequent re-evaluation may become necessary.

Table II. National Collaborating Centre for Primary Care. Clinical Guideline 20. The epilepsies: the diagnosis and management of the epilepsies in adults and children in primary and secondary care. London, UK: National Institute for Clinical Excellence; 2004

Epilepsy syndrome	First-line drugs	Second-line drugs	Other drugs	Drugs to be avoided (may worsen seizures)
Childhood absence epilepsy	Ethosuximide Lamotrigine[b] Sodium valproate	Levetiracetam Topiramate[a]		Carbamazepine[a] Oxcarbazepine[a] Phenytoin Tiagabine Vigabatrin
Juvenile absence epilepsy	Lamotrigine[b] Sodium valproate	Levetiracetam Topiramate[a]		Carbamazepine[a] Oxcarbazepine[a] Phenytoin[a] Tiagabine Vigabatrin
Juvenile myoclonic epilepsy	Lamotrigine[b] Sodium valproate	Clobazam Clonazepam Levetiracetam Topiramate[a]	Acetazolamide	Carbamazepine[a] Oxcarbazepine[a] Phenytoin[a] Tiagabine Vigabatrin
Generalised tonic-clonic seizures only	Carbamazepine[a] Lamotrigine[b] Sodium valproate Topiramate[a,b]	Levetiracetam	Acetazolamide	Tiagabine Vigabatrin
Focal epilepsies: cryptogenic, symtomatic	Carbamazepine[a] Lamotrigine[b] Oxcarbazepine[a] Sodium valproate Topiramate[a,b]	Clobazam Gabapentin Levetiracetam Phenytoin[a] Tiagabine	Acetazolamide Clonazepam Phenobarbital[a] Primidone[a,c]	
Infantile spasms	Steroids[c] Vigabatrin[b]	Clobazam Clonazepam Sodium valproate Topiramate[a]	Nitrazepam	Carbamazepine[a] Oxcarbazepine[a]
Benign epilepsy with centrotemporal spikes	Carbamazepine[a] Lamotrigine[b] Oxcarbazepine[a] Sodium valproate	Levetiracetam Topiramate[a]	Sulthiame[e]	

Table II. National Collaborating Centre for Primary Care. Clinical Guideline 20. The epilepsies: the diagnosis and management of the epilepsies in adults and children in primary and secondary care. London, UK: National Institute for Clinical Excellence; 2004

Syndrome				
Benign epilepsy with occipital paroxysms	Carbamazepine[a], Lamotrigine[b], Oxcarbazepine[a,b], Sodium valproate	Levetiracetam, Topiramate[a]		
Severe myoclonic epilepsy of infancy	Clobazam, Clonazepam, Sodium valproate, Topiramate[a,b]	Levetiracetam, Stiripentol[e]	Phenobarbital[a]	Carbamazepine[a], Lamotrigine, Oxcarbazepine[a], Vigabatrin
Continuous spike wave of slow sleep	Clobazam, Clonazepam, Ethosuximide, Lamotrigine[b], Sodium valproate, Steroids[d]	Levetiracetam, Topiramate[a]		Carbamazepine[a], Oxcarbazepine[a], Vigabatrin
Lennox-Gastaut syndrome	Lamotrigine[b], Sodium valproate, Topiramate[a,b]	Clobazam, Clonazepam, Ethosuximide, Levetiracetam	Felbamate[e]	Carbamazepine[a], Oxcarbazepine[a]
Landau-Kleffner syndrome	Lamotrigine[b], Sodium valproate, Steroids[d]	Levetiracetam, Topiramate[a]	Sulthiame[e]	Carbamazepine[a], Oxcarbazepine[a]
Myoclonic astatic epilepsy	Clobazam, Clonazepam, Sodium valproate, Topiramate[a,b]	Lamotrigine, Levetiracetam		Carbamazepine[a], Oxcarbazepine[a]

[a] Hepatic enzyme-inducing AED.
[b] Should be used as a first choice under circumstances as outlined in the NICE technology appraisal of newer AEDs – see page 47.
[c] Should rarely be initiated – if a barbiturate is required, phenobarbital is preferred.
[d] Steroids: prednisolone or ACTH (adrenocorticotrophic hormone).
[e] Not licensed in the UK, but available by importation.

Seizures/syndrome	CBZ	PHT	LTG	GBP	VGB	TGB	BDZ
Absence seizures	X	X		X	X	X	
Myoclonic seizures	X	X	X	X	X		
JME	X	X	X				
LGS / MAE	X	X	X	X	X		X
BECTS	X		X				
SMEI	X		X		X		
LKS / ESES	X	X					
Unverricht-Lundborg disease	X						

Figure 2. Aggravation of seizures or epilepsy syndromes.

Also, drug utilization patterns will change with age from neonate to infant, school-age and then puberty and adolescence (Pellock, 1997). In those with the comorbidities of cerebral palsy and mental retardation multiple medications may be administered for conditions such as spasticity or aberrant behaviors with their attendant drug interactions, both pharmacokinetic and pharmacodynamic. As discussed herein, seizure type and epilepsy syndrome need to be constantly re-visited in those with refractory epilepsy. A plan for seizure emergencies and rapid treatment of prolonged seizures is mandatory (Pellock, Shinnar, 2007). However, as demonstrated in the chapter by Hersdorfer, even those children who appear normal and are diagnosed with benign epilepsy, cognitive and behavioral effects of the epilepsy itself and its treatment must be carefully monitored.

Whereas cognitive factors have been stressed for children attending school, adults must be protected from cognitive dulling, memory deficits and depression in order for them to be successful in their life's work. Memory difficulties are among the most frequent complaints. The elderly, who are likely to have multiple co-morbid medical disorders and concomitant medications prescribed (Ramsey, et al., 2004) especially need to have special considerations regarding drug interactions and tolerability at the forefront when physicians chose a medication for their epilepsy treatment. Those with cancer and stroke must not be prescribed AEDs that severely decrease the efficacy of primary disease treatment.

■ An approach to treatment

Upon the presentation of someone with presumptive first seizure or established epilepsy, the clinician must decide first whether treatment should be initiated at all and, secondly, which is the best mode of treatment. Other sections of this symposium have addressed considerations for the treatment of the first seizure and the relative risks of not treating that seizure. It is noted however, that frequently a person who presents with what is thought to be a first seizure in fact, in fact, has had numerous other episodes which were not recognized to be seizures. This is of course, especially true in those with non-convulsive seizures or with myoclonic jerks which were not perceived to be seizures as in juvenile myoclonic epilepsy. Once a diagnosis of epilepsy is ascertained, the physician must guide the patient and arrive at the most well tolerated efficacious medication for the treatment of epilepsy. This requires the identification of the epilepsy syndrome over and above the seizure type. In children this is extremely important because of the eventual development of other seizure types which may or may not be controlled or seemingly made worse by the initial medication (Pellock, 1997). In adults, co-morbidities *(Table III)* along with careful identification of possible surgical candidates with considerations for precise semiology description is the main challenge. All of those with partial epilepsy or presumptive symptomatic epilepsy should be evaluated early for the possibility of surgical therapy.

As noted above, besides establishing AEDs which would be appropriate based on seizure type, one must be sure to use medications that will not exacerbate associated or yet to appear seizure types, or ones that have not yet been well identified even though they are present. Reviews by Perucca (2001) and Sazgar and Bourgeois (2005) have discussed the likelihood for seizure exacerbation by particular AEDs. In general, those medications with broader spectrum of activity rarely lead to seizure exacerbation, unless patients are made toxic with too high a dose. Those AEDs typically used for the treatment of partial seizures have mostly been identified as those leading to the exacerbation with the appearance of generalized seizures, particularly myoclonic and absence spells.

Figure 2 summarizes this data. Only after a period of use will it be known whether newer AEDs, such as pregabalin, will join similar agents regarding possible exacerbation of certain seizure types.

At initiation the likelihood of efficacy against an identified seizure type is the predominant reason for picking a specific AED. *Figure 1* demonstrates the general efficacy of AEDs for partial or generalized seizures (Pellock, 2006). Early identification of the entire epilepsy syndrome enhances AED choice and directs expectations regarding seizure control, development of other seizure types, length of treatment and perhaps even an estimate of amount of medication needed for continued seizure control. Specific side effect profiles or the potential for these side effects appearing in a specific patient usually lead to choice of the first medication selected for treatment. It is extremely important to involve the patient and/or family in the discussion so that they understand risks and benefits of the proposed medications. At present with the number of new and classic compounds available there is rarely only one drug of choice for an individual. Rather, discussion centers around two or more

Table III. Co-morbidities of epilepsy

• Renal	• Stroke
• Hepatic	• Anoxic ischemic encephalopathy
• Connective tissue	• Endocrine/reproductive
• Cardiac/cerebrovascular	• Infection/immunizations
• Immunodeficiency (HIV)	• Degenerative/dementia
• ETOH and drugs	• Trauma
• Pulmonary	• Migraine
• Metabolic abdnormalities	• Behavioral/Psychiatric
– Glucose, Na Ca	– Mental retardation
• Bone	– Depression
• Cerebral palsy	– ADHD

possibilities and a choice is selected because of co-morbidity, or potential cause for seizure control balanced with tolerability, or the perception of adverse side effects by both physician and patient (family).

Specific examples of the use of balancing efficacy *versus* potential adverse effect are numerous. In women of child bearing age potential for teratogenesis must be discussed and frequently leads to the selection of first choice drug. If however, that agent does not lead to seizure freedom or it is not well tolerated, an alternative drug should be chosen. In children, phenobarbital has been used less and less when other medications are available because of the high likelihood of mood and behavioral disturbances. In both children and adults, bone metabolism and formation will be highly affected by AEDs inducing cytochrome P450 activity. Immobility of a patient may further complicate bone formation. In the elderly the highest etiology of new onset epilepsy is that associated with cerebral vascular disease. They must have careful consideration of medications already prescribed that might be significantly influenced by AED interactions. As shown in the Veteran's Administration Cooperative Study (Rowan, Ramsay 2004), persons who are older may require lower dosing of both new and classic AEDs because of seemingly decreased tolerability.

Those with refractory epilepsy should have a careful review of all medications and procedures previously performed as part of their re-evaluation. One important question for the patient and family is whether there seemed to be a better response or worsening to any specific medication used in the past. One needs to establish how much, how high and how fast mediations were introduced, titrated and eventually dosed or done as adjunctive therapy. Frequently one finds that a potentially good treatment was not given an adequate trial or was titrated upward or downward too rapidly, causing false information regarding its efficacy. Re-evaluation with imaging is extremely important in refractory patients as it may lead to an alternative approach. Even in the refractory patient monotherapy or at most two medications should be the goal for treatment. AED polytherapy is of limited advantage over monotherapy but many of these patients receive multiple medications the combination of which leads to greater adverse effects. Rescue medication, typically a benzodiazepine, can be used for clusters or seizure exacerbations. During transitions from one to another medication removal of the ineffective drug should occur. This will only improve tolerability and perhaps remove an agent which has been causing exacerbation of seizures, either directly because of the drug itself or because of combined AED toxicity.

In conclusion, the choice of the best AED for each patient really requires the art of medicine to be practiced. One takes all of the information available regarding efficacy and tolerability and then during a discussion with the family decides upon the best approach. The clinician should outline a plan, discuss reasons for AED therapy and the consequences of not treating or being non-compliant. The patient should be given or referred to information to help guide the decisions and further care. The physician should propose an understanding or contract with the patient and family. This final step may be the single most important factor in the successful management of patients with epilepsy. Following proper diagnosis, randomized clinical trials and expert opinions aid the clinician in choosing the proper first choice therapy; individualization and clinical discussion best insure success.

References

Bittigau P, Sifringer M. Genz K et al. Antiepileptic drugs and apoptotic neurodegeneration in the developing brain. *Proc Natl Acad Sci USA* 2002 12; 99 (23): 15089-94.

Christensen J, Petrenaite V, Atherman J et al. Oral contraceptives induce lamotrigine metabolism: Evidence from a double-blind, placebo-controlled trial. *Epilepsia* 2007; 48: 484-9.

French JA, Kanner AM, Bautista J et al. Efficacy and tolerability of the new antiepileptic drugs I: Treatment of new onset epilepsy: Report of the Therapeutics and Technology Assessment Subcommittee and Quality Standards Subcommittee of the American Academy of Neurology and the American Epilepsy Society. *Neurology* 2004; 62: 1252-60.

French JA, Kanner AM, Bautista J et al.. Efficacy and tolerability of the new antiepileptic drugs II: Treatment of refractory epilepsy: Report of the Therapeutics and Technology Assessment Subcommittee and Quality Standards Subcommittee of the American Academy of Neurology and the American Epilepsy Society. *Neurology* 2004; 62: 1261-73.

Glauser TA. Purpose and development of the guidelines. Presented as part of a session titled Impact of ILAE Guidelines: Initial monotherapy treatment of epileptic seizures and syndromes with antiepileptic drugs, at the 26th International Epilepsy Congress, Paris, France, September 1, 2005. Abstract in *Epilepsia* 2005; 46 (suppl 6): 47-8.

Glauser T, Ben-Menachem E, Bourgeois B, Cnaan A, Chadwick D, Guerreiro C et al. ILAE treatment guidelines: evidence-based analysis of antiepileptic drug efficacy and effectiveness as initial monotherapy for epileptic seizures and syndromes. *Epilepsia* 2006; 47 (7): 1094-120.

Karceski S, Morrell M, Carpenter D. The expert consensus guideline series: treatment of epilepsy. *Epilepsy Behav* 2001; 2 (suppl): A1-A50.

Karceski S, Morrell MJ, Carpenter D. Treatment of epilepsy in adults: expert opinion, 2005. *Epilepsy Behav* 2005; 7 (suppl 1): S1-64.

Mackay MT, Weiss SK, Adams-Webber T, Ashwal S, Stephens D, Ballaban-Gill K, Baram TZ, Duchowny M, Hirtz D, Pellock JM, Shields WD, Shinnar S, Wyllie E, Snead III, OC. Practice.

Parameter: Medical Treatment of Infantile Spasms. Report of the American Academy of Neurology and Child Neurology Society. *Neurology* 2004; 62 (10): 1668-81.

Meador KJ. Cognitive effects of epilepsy and antiepileptic medications. In: Wyllie E (ed), *The Treatment of Epilepsy*, 4th Edition, Philadelphia: Lippincott 2006: 1185-96.

Minicucci, F, Muscas G, Perucca E et al. Treatment of status epilepticus in adults: guidelines of the Italian League Against Epilepsy. In: *Italian League against Epilepsy (LICE) Official Reports 2005-2006 and Proceedings of the 28th National Congress*, Bari, Italy, May 18-21, 2005. *Epilepsia* 2006; 47 (suppl 5): 9-15.

Morrell MJ. Hormones, Catamenial epilepsy and reproductive and bone health in epilepsy. In: Wyllie E ed, *The Treatment of Epilepsy*, 4th Edition, Philadelphia: Lippincott 2006: 695-704.

NICE Guidelines. Clinical Guideline 20. The epilepsies: the diagnosis and management of the epilepsies in adults and children in primary and secondary care. NICE website (www.nice.org.uk/CG020NICEguideline). Issue date: October 2004.

Pellock, JM, Shinnar S. Foreward: A Framework for the Treatment of Prolonged or Repetitive Seizures. JCN, in press 2007.

Pellock JM. Epilepsy in Patients with Multiple Handicaps. In: Wyllie E ed. *The Treatment of Epilepsy: Principles and Practice*, 4th Edition. Baltimore:Lippincott Williams and Wilkins, 2006.

Pellock JM, Drug Treatment in Children. In Engel J, Pedley T ed. *Epilepsy: A comprehensive Textbook*, Lippincott-Raven, Philadelphia. 1997: 1205-10.

Perucca E. The management of refractory idiopathic epilepsies. *Epilepsia* 2001; 42 (suppl 3): 31-5.

Rogawski MA, Loscher W. The neurobiology of antiepileptic drugs fro the treatment of nonepileptic conditions. *Nat Med* 2004; 10: 685-92.

Rowan AJ, Ramsay RE, Pryor FM. Special considerations in treating the elderly patient with epilepsy. *Neurology* 2004; 9; 62 (5 suppl 2): S24-9. Review.

Sazgar M, Bourgeois BF. Aggravation of epilepsy by antiepileptic drugs. *Pediatr Neurol* 2005; 33 (4): 227-34.

Scottish Intercollegiate Guideline Network: Diagnosis and management of epilepsies in children and young people: A national clinical guideline. Edinburgh, Scottish Intercollegiate guidelines network, March 2005 (Copies available at http://www.sign.ac.uk/pdf/sign81.pdf).

Semah D, Picot MC, Derambure P, et al: The choice of antiepileptic drugs in newly diagnosed epilepsy: A national French survey. *Epileptic Disord* 2004; 6: 255-65.

Weintraub D., Buchsbaum R, Resor SR, Jr., Hirsch LJ. Psychiatric and behavioral side effects of the newer antiepileptic drugs in adults with epilepsy. *Epilepsy & Behavior* 2007; 10, Issue 1, 2007: 105-10.

Wheless JW, Clarke DF, Carpenter D. Treatment of pediatric epilepsy: expert opinion, 2005. *J Child Neurol*. 2005; 20: S1-S56.

Section VI:
Future Challenges

What types of trials and studies do we need for early treatment of epilepsy?

Elinor Ben Menachem, Frederik Azstely

Institute for Clinical Neuroscience and Physiology, Göteborg University, Sahögrenska University Hospital, Göteborg, Sweden

---

Monotherapy trials for new onset epilepsy have been performed for the last 60 years with progressive and more sophisticated methodology. An analysis of the monotherapy studies up until 2006 are presented in the ILAE Treatment Guidelines: Evidence based analysis of antiepileptic drug efficacy and effectiveness as initial monotherapy for epileptic seizures and syndromes (Glauser et al., 2006). The trials that have been done have either been superiority trials with forced exit criteria, comparative trials, or titration down to monotherpay in patients with refractory epilepsy participating in trials when the investigational drug or placebo was added on initially. These trials have either been open label or double-blind but most have been randomized. In spite of the plethoria of studies, and even in the few that were identified as Evidence Class I, the results seem always to be the same. After one year of treatment, irrespective of the drugs having different mechanisms of action, about 50% of patients will become seizure free and the rest will continue to have seizures and be refractory for the first drug. (Glauser *et al.*, 2006; Brodie *et al.*, 2007).

In analyzing the existing trials most appear to be designed to qualify for registration from the FDA or EMEA and do not necessarily answer questions that help the clinician treat patients. For example, most of the comparative studies with carbamazepine are done with the non-slow release formulation. These studies will then show that the comparative drug is better tolerated even if not more effective. This is, however, often not the case when the retard formulation is used which is what actually occurs in the clinic, of course.

In a recently published monotherapy study comparing levetiracetam (LEV) and carbamazepin (CBZ) slow release, the results demonstrated that efficacy was the same for the two groups for the one year period regardless of mechanism of action and tolerability. This study was the first of its kind which was a more useful pragmatic study, especially for the clinician. (Brodie *et al.*, 2007) In a double blind design patients were started on either a low dose of CBZ (400 mg) or LEV (1,000 mg). If not seizure free during 6 months, they received a medium dose of the drug and then if not seizure free during another 6 months they were given a high dose of LEV or CBZ, thus reflecting what a doctor would do in clinical practice. Patients were followed for one year. In the study design new information was obtained. Besides showing with a power of 90% that CBZ and LEV were equivalent, it became obvious that most patients became seizure free on the lowest dose of either drug and that increases had only a marginal effect. This is in accordance with the retrospective study of Brodie et al. (2000) and the results of the VA cooperative study (Mattson et al., 1985) even when using other drugs. The other interesting observation was that after 6 months 72-73% of both populations were seizure free but at one year only 56-58% were seizure free. This indicates that declaring someone seizure free after 6 months is not acceptable and may even have implications on the decision to drive after such a short time of seizure freedom. As a result of the LEV monotherapy study, most new monotherapy studies, at least in Europe, are comparative and use the same study design as it seems this is so far the most successful and provides Level 1 evidence of equivalency according to the ILAE Guidelines. In the ILAE guidelines only phenytoin (PHT) and CBZ were judged to have Class 1 evidence but probably after further analysis LEV will also be included in this category.

▪ The problems

So now we have an adequate design for new onset epilepsy to test new AEDs to see if they are as good as the Class 1 drugs or not, and we know how to conduct these studies so that there will be adequate power to be able to determine non-inferiority. Still, there are many unanswered problems.

1. Tolerability and side effect profiles are always analysed in trials but it is difficult to compare side effects in an evidence based fashion when patients usually only report the adverse events spontaneously.

2. Still superiority trials are the only acceptable in the USA by the FDA,

3. There is still no drug that prevent or slow down the process of epileptogenesis, although some of the existing drugs might actually do it but have not been tested appropriately.

4. Most of the studies, such as those published by the group of Martin Brodie (2000, 2006) and the recent MESS study (Marson et al., 2005; Kim et al., 2006), have used old generation drugs except for lamotrigine (LTG). Results from those studies do not necessarily reflect what might happen with the newer AEDs, especially when patients are treated for longer periods of time than 1 year.

5. Still no study follows hormonal levels in patients or bone measurements – which would not be a hard task, although more expensive. Blood samples could easily be obtained in order to determine biochemical parameters (calcium, phosphorus, alkaline phosphates, parathormone, and 25-hydroxyvitamin D). Bone mineral density could easily be measured for example with the dual-energy x-ray absorptiometry method as have been done in other studies (Babayigit et al., 2006).

6. In all clinical trials, not to mention monotherapy studies, therapeutic drug monitoring is done but not revealed and analyses not forthcoming. It could be that blood concentrations of the drug make a difference in effect and tolerability and not just the dose. It should be a requirement in all published clinical trials that these data are presented since they are available in the drug company's database.

7. Quality of Life and depression scales are now a common and necessary component of clinical trials. Most patients will have a better quality of life if they are seizure free and side effect free so how does it reflect on the drug's other characteristics like a potential antidepressant effect? Are the tests sensitive enough to pick up those subtle differences? Neuropsychological testing is probably more important to pick up cognitive deficits that can be concealed. These are much more time consuming and costly but could help in revealing cognitive side effects that are not obvious.

Seizure severity assessment is not an issue in monotherapy studies for new onset epilepsy as the goal of the treatment is seizure freedom and so this aspect will not be discussed here.

▪ Designing new trials for the future

1. In designing new trials cost is always a major factor and inhibits the design of the ideal study. So are inclusion and exclusion criteria. An AED trial is more valid if it addresses only one seizure type and aetiology. However, to design the ideal study with a homogeneous group of patients, the inclusion criteria could be so strict that only a few patients would ever be able to participate. In order to recruit ample patients to be able to have adequate power and to be able to determine non-inferiority (as in the LEV study) in a comparative trial, inclusion needs to be wide enough to find enough patients. Therefore restricting patients to only post-traumatic seizures or only stroke or mesial temporal sclerosis is not feasible. It would be interesting indeed to include only a certain group of patients and then more information would be forthcoming about on how they react and if there is any particular AED that would be especially effective. To get such an answer, however, there would have to be a worldwide effort to include only specific groups of patients. Even then there would be discussions on just how homogeneous these groups really are. Thus, pragmatically I am for a broad inclusion as is currently done for most of the clinical trials.

2. Being that there are so many new drugs all with the same efficacy in partial onset seizures, it is necessary to look at the other characteristics of a drug to see if there is room for improvement in either efficacy or tolerability. Gene analyses might be a way to begin.

3. One of the most important goals in treating epilepsy is to try to prevent or decrease the process of epileptogenesis. So far no drug has shown this ability in humans, but it is not clear if some of the existing drugs such as LEV or topiramate (TPM) might have such properties. In order to evaluate antiepileptogenic effects, the following protocol could be implemented.

Patients could participate in the usual comparative trails for monotherapy and new onset seizures. At the end of one year of treatment on one of the two drugs being compared, patients would be offered blinded continuation for another year. If at the end of 2 years if the patient is still seizure free while taking the drug (and had less than 3 seizures totally before treatment), he/she would be offered the opportunity to be randomised to either down-titration of the study drug or continuation with treatment. Now there would be four parallel groups to follow for one to two years as open label/(or blinded which is preferable but not really realistic). At the end of 1 or 2 years, the groups (two still being treated and 2 now without drug) could be compared to see if the patients without drug were no worse in regards to recurrence of seizures than the treated groups. If one seizure had occurred after down titration or even with continuation of the drug, then the patient would leave the study and receive another treatment. If there are more patients without drug, but who were previously treated with the new drug, still seizure free in comparison to CBZ- previously treated group, and this is statistically significant, then the conclusion could be that the new drug has in some way prevented or delayed the progress of epileptogenesis. This would be an important finding and one that would justify using the drug as first line therapy. Another variation would be to use historical data for CBZ (Chadwick et al., 1999) and have only two arms: continued treatment with the new drug and no drug at all after being downtitrated from the drug after 2 years of treatment and seizure freedom.

This protocol has an advantage of not having to enter too many patients and follow them for many years as in the post traumatic epilepsy trials which have always failed to show a difference between treatment and not.

The disadvantages with this trial are that the patient population still needs to be considerable and the trials are costly because of the length of follow-up. However, if patients without the test drug remain seizure free in spite of no treatment but the other group with the comparative drug does not, then there would be form of superiority outcome between the test and comparator drug.

3. Hormonal dysfunctions and bone density are subjects that are constantly being addressed, often after a drug is already marketed. With only marginal costs bone density studies and hormonal levels in both men and women could be followed throughout the study with baseline levels providing valuable information.

■ Can placebo trials be done ethically?

Another problem discussed for many years without finding an appropriate solution, especially in communication with the FDA, is the type of comparative studies needed for obtaining a monotherapy license. The FDA still believes that only superiority studies are appropriate. My solution to this problem would be the following protocol: This would be based on the results from the MESS study showing that delaying treatment with one seizures does not significantly reduce the prospects for long term seizure freedom if the patient does not have EEG and MRI changes and if they have not had more than 2 seizures (Kim et al., 2006). If we add to the inclusion criteria that only patients with complex partial seizures (CPS) and never generalized tonic-clonic seizures (GTC) may enter, then patient safety would not be jeopardised either and all ethical concerns would then addressed. Recruitment would be harder than a usual monotherapy trial but such a design would satisfy the FDA requirements.

My suggestions are now open for discussion:
- Is it possible for placebo-controlled trials for monotherapy indication for epilepsy to be conducted?
- Do we have existing study protocols to determine epileptogenesis properties of AEDs? Is my proposal possible?
- Can questions about bone health and hormonal changes be addressed in existing protocols? Are they necessary and should we insist on their implementation?
- What about therapeutic drug monitoring?
- Should we include formal side effect questionnaires in clinical trials or continue to rely on spontaneous reports of side effects?

All of my questions are very concrete and pragmatic unanswered problems and should be addressed now and not in some distant future.

References

Babayigit A, Dirik E, Bober E, Cakmakci H. Adverse effects of antiepileptic drugs on bone mineral density *Pediatr Neurol* 2006; 35 (3): 177-81.

Chadwick D, Taylor J, Johnson T. Outcomes after seizure recurrence in people with well-controlled epilepsy and the factors that influence it. The MRC Antiepileptic Drug Withdrawal Group. *Epilepsia* 1996; 37 (11): 1043-50.

Chadwick D. Does withdrawal of different antiepileptic drugs have different effects on seizure recurrence? Further results from the MRC Antiepileptic Drug Withdrawal Study. *Brain* 1999; 122: 441-8.

Glauser T, Ben-Menachem E. Bourgeois B. Cnana A, Chadwick D, Guerreiro C, Kalviainen R, Mattson R, Perucca E, Tomson T. ILAE treatment guidelines: evidence-based analysis of antiepileptic drug efficacy and effectiveness as initial monotherapy for epileptic seizures and syndromes. *Epilepsia* 2006; 47 (7): 1094-120.

Kim LG, Johnson TL, Marson AG, Chadwick DW, MRC MESS study Group. Prediction of risk of seizure recurrence after a single seizure and early epilepsy: further results from the MESS trial. *Lancet Neurology* 2006; 5: 317-22.

Marson A, Jacoby A, Johnson A, Kim Lm, Gamble C, Chadwick D, Medical Research Council MESS study Group. Immediate *versus* deferred antiepileptic drug treatment for early epilepsy and single seizures: a randomised controlled trial. *Lancet.* 2005; 365: 2007-13.

Mattson RH et al., Comparison of carbamazepine, phenobarbital, phenytoin, and primidone in partial and secondarily generalized tonic-clonic seizures. *N Engl J Med* 1985; 313 (3): 145-51.

Mattson RH, Cramer JA, Collins JF. A comparison of valproate with carbamazepine for the treatment of complex partial seizures and secondarily generalized tonic-clonic seizures in adults. The Department of Veterans Affairs Epilepsy Cooperative Study No. 264 Group *N Engl J Med* 1992; 327 (11): 765-71.

From prediction of medical intractability to early surgical treatment

Jerome Engel Jr[1], Anne T. Berg[2]

[1] Departments of Neurology, Neurobiology and Psychiatry and Biobehavioral Sciences and the Brain Research Institute, David Geffen School of Medecine at UCLA, Los Angeles, USA

[2] Department of Biological Sciences, Northern Illinois University, DeKalb, USA

The modern history of surgical treatment for epilepsy began in the latter half of the nineteenth century with the elucidation of functional localization in the brain (Engel, 1993). John Hughlings Jackson (Taylor, 1958) is credited with mapping primary cortical areas by corrrelating ictal behaviors with post mortem examinations of the brain, and Ferrier (1874) confirmed these clinical observations by stimulating the brains of monkeys. Based on this work, neurosurgeons were able to find "invisible" epileptogenic lesions that could be seen intraoperatively, and surgically removed, as a treatment for focal seizures (Horsley, 1886; Macewen, 1881). Surgical therapy thus became available for a limited number of patients whose seizures were due to localized structural abnormalities that could be visualized intraoperatively, if their location was predictable preoperatively by seizure semiology, and later pneumoencephalography (Dandy, 1919), and cerebral arteriography (Moniz, 1934). Many more patients became eligible for surgical treatment in the mid twentieth century with the demonstration of the localizing value of epileptiform EEG abnormalities (Bailey and Gibbs, 1951; Jasper *et al.*, 1951), greatly expanding the availability of surgical treatment, particularly for temporal lobe epilepsy (TLE). As the number of antiepileptic drugs (AEDs) was limited, it was an easy matter to demonstrate that seizures were refractory to pharmacotherapy; therefore, medical intractability, as a criterion for early surgery, was not an issue.

In the 1980s and '90s, two major advances in clinical epileptology markedly altered consideration of surgery as an alternative treatment for epilepsy. On the one hand, first positron emission tomography (PET) (Engel *et al.*, 1982a;b;c) and then magnetic resonance imaging (MRI) (Cascino *et al.*, 1991; Jackson *et al.*, 1990) made it possible to localize hippocampal sclerosis, malformations of cortical development, and other localized surgically resectable epileptogenic lesions that were not previously identifiable extraoperatively. Consequently, a large number of patients with so-called "cryptogenic" epilepsy who previously were either not considered candidates for surgery, or would have required expensive, potentially risky intracranial EEG telemetry became eligible for surgery based on noninvasive presurgical evaluation. While this greatly increased the number of potential surgical candidates, there was a simultaneous increase in the number of new AEDs. As a result, it became impossible to determine medical intractability definitively, given that it would literally take a lifetime to prove that every AED, alone and in all conceivable combinations, was ineffective in a given patient. In response to this quandary, an alternative approach based on the concept of surgically remediable epilepsy syndromes was advocated (Engel and Shewmon, 1993; Engel, 1996). A surgically remediable epilepsy syndrome is a condition for which there is a known pathophysiology and a predictable natural history, including unresponsiveness to AEDs and an excellent surgical outcome. Most of these syndromes have progressive features, such as developmental delay in infants and small children, interictal behavioral disorders in older children and adults, or structural alterations, as occurs with hippocampal sclerosis, implying that early surgical intervention is necessary to reverse or avoid enduring disabling consequences.

Surgical therapy for surgically remediable epilepsy is cost-effective because presurgical evaluation can usually be performed noninvasively and, by definition, there is a 60-80% chance of complete elimination of disabling seizures in appropriately selected patients. Mesial temporal lobe epilepsy is the prototype of a surgically remediable epilepsy syndrome, but other examples include focal epilepsies due to discrete resectable structural lesions, and catastrophic secondary epilepsies due to diffuse hemispheric disturbances such as hemimegencephaly, Rasmussen's encephalitis, Sturge-Weber syndrome, and large porencephalic cysts.

Although the application of surgical treatment for epilepsy continued to increase towards the end of the twentieth century, in large part due to an emphasis on identifying surgically remediable epilepsy syndromes, there was an average delay of over 20 years between onset of epilepsy and surgery (Berg et al., 2003). The important question of when to consider early surgical intervention in these patients persists. While early surgery would presumably provide the best opportunity for complete psychological and social rehabilitation, there remains no reliable diagnostic means to establish the existence of pharmacoresistance – that is, a situation where subsequent medication trials would never result in satisfactory seizure control.

■ Natural history of medical intractability

In addition to the fact that the large number of available AEDs has made it impractical, if not impossible, to establish true medical intractability in individual patients, there is no accepted definition for the concept of medical intractability or pharmacoresistance (French, 2006; Berg and Kelly, 2006). Whereas these terms might imply that epileptic seizures do not respond at all to pharmacotherapy, this is rarely the case. Most patients who are considered to have medically refractory epilepsy experience some benefit from pharmacotherapy, perhaps fewer seizures, or less severe seizures, although treatment is unsatisfactory because disabling seizures remain. On the other hand, patients are usually *not* considered medically intractable if pharmacotherapy eliminates disabling seizures even when auras (experiental or sensory simple partial seizures) continue to occur. In this case, the remaining ictal events are still pharmacoresistant.

For purposes of surgical treatment, an operational, rather than absolute, definition of medical intractability is necessary, and this is usually based on the expectation that an unacceptable number of disabling seizures will remain despite treatment with appropriate AEDs at adequate dosages. Even this definition, however, is subject to considerable variability, based on the needs and expectations of individual patients. For instance, a single complex partial or secondarily generalized seizure a year could be unacceptable for someone wishing a normal, independent lifestyle, as it would prevent obtaining a driver's license, and perhaps other important occupational or social activities, while much more frequent recurrence of such seizures may not adversely affect the lifestyle of an individual with cognitive impairment in an assisted living situation.

Furthermore, seizure control and intractability are not steady state phenomena. Patients may be in remission for long periods of time and then experience seizure relapse, while those with difficult-to-control seizures may eventually achieve full remission. A certain percentage of patients can cycle between remission and relapse with unpredictable patterns (Berg, 2004; Arts, 2004). This variability in drug responsiveness poses a particular problem relevant to selecting surgical candidates. How long do you continue trials of AEDs before deciding that a patient is unlikely to enter remission and therefore should be considered for surgical therapy? Although a number of different operational definitions have been used to determine medical intractability for surgical therapy (Berg and Kelly, 2006), a more important factor in the consideration of when to recommend surgery is the degree to which persistent seizures interfere with the patient's ability to achieve or maintain a desired lifestyle.

Infants and young children with surgically remediable syndromes often have very frequent seizures that are associated with developmental delay and can be life-threatening. It is not difficult, in this situation, to opt for early surgery that could prevent these serious consequences. In older children, recurrent seizures can interfere with the acquisition of vocational and social skills necessary for them to lead an independent life, while in adults such seizures can threaten the maintenance of their livelihood and lifestyle. Consequently, once seizures begin to interfere with schoolwork, or interpersonal relationships, successful surgical intervention could avert a lifetime of disability. Unfortunately, such patients with surgically remediable syndromes often experience a stuttering course of easily treated seizures, which then return, but with long periods of remission and relapse (Berg *et al.*, 2003), making it difficult to identify a time when the risk of continuing seizures is greater than the risk of surgical intervention.

Retrospective data from a surgical cohort of adults provide descriptive information relevant to the natural history of surgically remediable epilepsy syndromes (Berg *et al.*, 2003). In this study, the average adult surgical patient first began having seizures during childhood or early adolescence (average age at onset was 14.6 years and the average age of surgery was 36.7 years). This delay of over 20 years before surgical referral is typical of published surgical cohorts (Berg, 2004). More important for this discussion, however, on average, it took nine years for patients to fail two AED trials, but there was considerable variation in this pattern. A quarter of the patients experienced remissions of one year or longer, and some longer than ten years. The younger the age of seizure onset, the more likely remissions would occur, and the longer it took to fail two AED trials. Although most patients in this study had TLE, the relationship between this diagnosis and the occurrence of remissions was not analyzed. The impression that continued seizures, particularly during critical periods of adolescence and early adulthood, increased the risk of irreversible disability also has been derived from retrospective studies from surgical centers (Sperling, 2004). Such studies, however, concern a subpopulation of patients with medically refractory epilepsy who are sufficiently disabled by their disorder to seek surgical intervention, and cannot be extrapolated to the entire population of newly intractable TLE patients. Many of those who never seek surgical intervention may ultimately enter long-term remission, or continue to have seizures that do not sufficiently interfere with daily activities to consider surgery an option.

Available population-based studies of epilepsy in adults or in groups of all ages (but not limited to children) all demonstrate that the majority of patients experience substantial periods of remission (1 to 5 years). For example, a study from Rochester, MN (Annegers et al., 1979), found that almost 80% of patients had experienced a minimum 5 year remission by 20 years after diagnosis, and 70% were at least five years seizure free at that time. The difference is due to patients who relapsed. In Sweden, Lindsten et al. (2001) reported that by 10 years after initial diagnosis, 58% of patients were at least five years seizure-free. Comparable findings have been reported from studies in Italy (Collaborative Group, 1982), and the UK (Hart et al., 1990). Other community- or population-based studies of new-onset epilepsy (e.g., Jallon et al., 2001) do not involve prospective follow-up. None of these studies, however, specifically focused on factors that influence a surgical decision, such as accuracy of diagnosis, localizability of the epileptogenic region, social and psychological consequences of continuing seizures, and evidence of progressive deterioration of cerebral structure and function. These observational studies, in fact, were designed to show that most patients with epilepsy have a benign course and are not surgical candidates.

These studies demonstrated that, in the majority of individuals with epilepsy, long-term remission is the most common outcome. They fall short of explaining intractable epilepsy, however, because there is no information about reasons for not being in remission. For example, one cannot distinguish lack of remission due to absence of treatment, noncompliance, and deliberate discontinuation of AEDs *versus* failure of reasonable trials of AEDs. Related to that, there are no attempts to measure appropriateness of AED treatment and whether, by current standards, patients not in remission would be considered to have failed a certain number of trials of appropriate AEDs.

Another shortcoming with these studies from the perspective of understanding pharmacoresistant epilepsy is that patients are not sufficiently characterized with respect to type of epilepsy or epilepsy syndrome. At most, patients are divided into those with partial onset *versus* generalized onset seizures. Such designations are made based upon medical records, sometimes only those available from a general practitioner. As a final point, these studies were done largely prior to the era of MRI, many prior to CT scans, or such evaluations were not employed routinely enough to provide consistent information for the cohort.

It may be true that the most reliable predictor of pharmacoresistance is failure of seizures to respond to the first AED (Kwan and Brodie, 2000; 2004); however, while many assume that intractability is evident from the outset, and that seizures follow a relentlessly intractable course, this in fact is not the case. Although the typical surgical patient has had epilepsy for over 20 years, the average duration of intractable epilepsy is only about half that time (Berg, 2003). Many experienced prolonged periods of remission during that time. A similar observation was made by French (1993). In a prospective cohort of children followed from initial diagnosis of epilepsy, 24% (72/300) with focal epilepsy continued to have seizures after two trials of AEDs during a median follow-up period of 9.7 (8.6-11.1) years (Berg et al., 2006). In 40% (29/72) of cases, the criteria for intractability were not met for more than three years after initial diagnosis of epilepsy, and three-quarters of these had been in remission for at least one year. Of those who eventually failed a second AED trial, almost half experienced a subsequent period of remission lasting one year, and approximately one-third remained in remission at the time of last contact.

While the pattern of well-controlled seizures followed later by intractable seizures has now been documented prospectively in children, many patients with newly intractable epilepsy will subsequently experience periods of relative or complete seizure control (Berg and Kelly, 2006; Arts, 2004). For observations of these patients to be useful in devising standardized guidelines for early surgical intervention, it is not only necessary to characterize them in detail, but to identify clinical factors that predict remission and seizure persistence, as well as risk factors for disabling consequences of continuing seizures. Past and current population studies have demonstrated the phenomenon but were not designed to study in detail these more complex issues. A well designed prospective observational study is needed to clearly describe the natural history of surgically remediable epilepsies and to identify reliable predictors of pharmacoresistance that could be used to select candidates for early surgical treatment.

■ Surgical decisions

There are many factors that go into a decision to treat an epileptic condition surgically, but the one that concerns this discussion is the determination of medical intractability. What are the advantages and disadvantages of using a liberal operational definition of medical intractability to select patients for early surgical intervention? On the one hand, an unknown number of patients so selected would have eventually gone into remission without surgery, and it could be argued that they were unnecessarily exposed to the risks of surgical treatment. On the other hand, in many of these patients, early surgical intervention might avoid the development of irreversible deleterious psychological and social consequences of recurrent disabling seizures, that would prevent full rehabilitation after successful surgical treatment at some later date. It might be that early surgical intervention is preferable even in patients who would ultimately have gone into remission many months or years later without surgery, because continued disabling seizures *during* this time could still have serious adverse effects on later life. The primary argument for surgical intervention is that surgical treatment for appropriately selected patients is indeed effective; while the primary arguments for *early* intervention are that seizures not only lead to irreversible psychological and social decline, but also that surgically remediable epilepsies are progressive disorders.

Epilepsy surgery is effective

Patients with pharmacoresistant TLE are most easily and effectively treated surgically; 60-80% can expect to become free of the disabling seizures postoperatively (Wiebe et al., 2001; Engel et al., 1993; 2003). A landmark randomized controlled trial carried out at the University of Western Ontario was published in 2001 and unequivocally proved the superiority of surgical treatment over continued pharmacotherapy in patients with longstanding TLE (Wiebe et al., 2001). At the end of one year, 64% of patients treated surgically were free of disabling seizures compared to only 8% who continued with pharmacotherapy. Furthermore, health-related quality of life (HRQOL) was significantly better for patients treated surgically, and there was a trend towards improved school and work performance in this group as well. The figure of two-thirds seizure free after surgical treatment is remarkably similar to a retrospective multicenter survey of surgery performed between 1985 and 1990 (Engel et al., 1993), and a critical review of the surgical literature between 1990 and 2000 (Engel et al., 2003). Successful surgical outcome is also associated with positive gains in employment (Chin et al., 2005; Sperling, 2004), HRQOL (Mikati et al., 2006; Spencer et al., 2003; Vickrey et al., 1995; Wiebe et al., 2001), and psychiatric outcomes (Devinsky et al., 2005).

Based on the Western Ontario trial, and a literature review, the American Academy of Neurology (AAN), in association with the American Epilepsy Society (AES) and the American Association of Neurological Surgeons (AANS), published a Practice Parameter recommending surgery as the treatment of choice for TLE when pharmacotherapy fails (Engel et al., 2003). Neither this Practice Parameter nor the Western Ontario RCT, however, found sufficient data to determine when pharmacotherapy has failed and surgical treatment should be considered. Although the AAN Practice Parameter also reviewed published reports of neocortical resections, and found similar beneficial results, no formal recommendation could be made because of the absence of a randomized controlled trial. Nevertheless, there is consistent evidence in the literature for the efficacy of surgical treatment for conditions other than temporal lobe epilepsy, including hemispherectomy and multilobar resections for secondary generalized epilepsies of infancy and early childhood due to diffuse unilateral disturbances (Engel and Shewmon, 1993).

Surgically remediable epilepsies are progressive

The typical natural history of TLE, beginning with seizures that are easily controlled by medication which then become pharmacoresistant over time, suggests, but does not prove, that TLE is a progressive condition. Although there is ample evidence from animal research to indicate that focal seizures are progressive (Corcoran and

Moshé, 2005; Morrell, 1959/60; Heinemann et al., 1996), stronger evidence of progression in patients, particularly if risk factors for progression could be identified, would greatly help to determine when surgical intervention should be considered in pharmacoresistant patients. There are limited data suggesting that: 1) hippocampal atrophy can progress as a result of recurrent seizures in patients with TLE (Cendes, 2005; Mathern et al., 1995a;b); 2) some types of seizures can injure the human brain (Sutula and Pitkänen, 2002); 3) recurrent seizures make subsequent seizures more frequent (Hauser and Lee, 2002); and 4) surgical treatment is more likely to eliminate all seizures when performed early (Engel and Cahan, 1986).

When temporal lobe seizures become refractory to medication, particularly when they are frequent and disabling, interictal behavioral disturbances can occur, most commonly depression (Kanner and Balabanov, 2002; Mendez et al., 1986; Victoroff et al., 1994). Although behavioral disorders may merely reflect the social and psychological consequences of disabling seizures (Sperling, 2004), there is evidence from both animal and human studies (Adamec et al., 2004; Engel et al., 1991; Engel and Taylor, 1998) to suggest that recurrent epileptic seizures in limbic structures could also contribute to enduring, if not irreversible, disturbances in brain function and structure, causing behavioral disorders such as depression and psychosis. Furthermore, material-specific memory and learning disturbances are common in patients with MTLE, and these can improve following successful surgical treatment (Hermann et al., 1995; Langfitt and Rausch, 1996), indicating that they are, to some degree, related to the occurrence of epileptic seizures.

It is true that none of these largely indirect or cross-sectional clinical studies provide definitive evidence of progressive disturbances as a result of pharmacoresistant seizures which could be used to justify early surgical intervention. A longitudinal observational study of such patients is needed not only to determine the risk factors for irreversible psychological and social consequences of recurrent disabling seizures, but to determine the risk factors for progressive deleterious disruption of brain function and structure.

■ Future goals

Biomarkers of epileptogenicity and epileptogenesis are a "holy grail" of clinical epileptology. A biomarker of epileptogenicity that accurately identifies tissue capable of generating spontaneous seizures could be used to determine the extent of surgical resections without the need for video-EEG recordings of ictal events using scalp, and sometimes intracranial, electrodes. A biomarker of epileptogenicity that measures the severity of the epileptic condition, specifically the risk of occurrence of a subsequent seizure, could be used to determine the effectiveness of a therapeutic intervention such as a specific AED, or vagus nerve stimulation, without the need to wait for another seizure to occur. A biomarker of epileptogenesis could be used to determine which patients are likely to develop epilepsy following a potential epileptogenic cerebral insult, such as head trauma or intracranial infection, in order to introduce antiepileptogenic treatments. A biomarker of epileptogenicity could also be used to determine which patients have seizures that will not respond to *any* medications or other alternative treatments, while a biomarker of epileptogenesis could be used to predict which patients *with* epilepsy have progressive disorders that will require early surgical intervention.

The recent benchmarks for epilepsy research published by the American Epilepsy Society and the National Institutes of Neurological Disorders and Stroke identified biomarkers as a primary goal (Jacobs et al., 2001); however, only a few putative biomarkers have so far been identified. Alpha-methyl-tryptophan (AMT) has been used as a PET ligand to identify the epileptogenic region in a variety of conditions (Duchowny et al., 2003; Fedi et al., 2001; Juhasz et al., 2003; 2004; Kagawa et al., 2005; Natsume et al., 2003), but its role as a biomarker remains controversial. High frequency (200-600 Hz) oscillations, termed "Fast Ripples" (FR) appear to delineate epileptogenic hippocampal tissue in patients with temporal lobe epilepsy (Bragin et al., 1999; 2002a; b; Staba et al., 2002), and animal models of this condition (Bragin et al., 2004), and predict which animals will develop epilepsy after intrahippocampal kainate treatment (Bragin et al., 2004), but FR can be detected only by electrodes implanted directly into the brain and therefore are not yet useful as a screening tool in most patients.

The development of microarray technology for detection of gene expression profiles which are altered in various disease states has raised the possibility that genomics could provide the biomarkers needed to reliably identify potential surgical candidates as pharmacoresistant. At some point in the future, it may not be entirely inconceivable that changes in brain structure and function underlying the development of medically intractable epilepsy, and the progression of epileptic disorders, will be associated with uniquely altered expression of specific genes that could be measured in peripheral blood. If so, it would then be possible to identify candidates for early surgical intervention with a simple finger stick.

■ Conclusions

Tremendous advances in the safety and efficacy of surgical therapy for epilepsy have occurred, particularly in recent decades, greatly increasing the population of patients who can be considered to have surgically remediable epilepsy syndromes, and greatly expanding the availability of surgical treatment. There remains, however, an average delay of over 20 years between onset of epilepsy and referral for surgical therapy, despite recommendations that *early* surgical intervention provides the best opportunity to avoid or reverse the development of irreversible disabling psychological, social, and neurobiological consequences of recurrent seizures. The major obstacle to appropriate early referral for surgical treatment is the inability to reliably identify, let alone predict, medical intractability. Surgically remediable epilepsies, particularly TLE, can have a fluctuating course with long periods of remission, and no guidelines exist to help physicians decide when the risk of continued pharmacotherapy is greater than the risk of surgical intervention. It is possible that current research on biomarkers of epileptogenicity and epileptogenesis, such as AMT PET and FR, as well as future investigations of gene expression profiles in peripheral blood, could eventually provide diagnostic tools to definitively determine pharmacoresistance early in the course of an epileptic disorder. Until then, however, a carefully designed prospective observational study is needed to define the natural history of specific surgically remediable syndromes, such as TLE, and identify clinical and diagnostic factors that reliably predict medical intractability.

Acknowledgments

Original research reported by the author was supported in part by Grants NS-02808 (JE); NS-15654 (JE); NS-33310 (JE); NS-31146, (ATB); NS-32375 (ATB) from the National Institutes of Health.

References

Adamec R, Shallow T, Blundell J, Burton P. Contribution of pre kindling affective state to hemispheric differences in the effects on anxiety of basolateral amygdala kindling. In: Corcoran ME, Moshé SL, eds. *Kindling 6*. New York: Springer Science, 2005: 263-71.

Annegers JF, Hauser WA, Elveback LR. Remission of seizures and relapse in patients with epilepsy. *Epilepsia* 1979; 20: 729-37.

Arts WFM, Brouwer OF, Peters ACB, Stroink H, Peeters EAJ, Schmitz PIM *et al*. Course and prognosis of childhood epilepsy: 5-year follow-up of the Dutch study of epilepsy in childhood. *Brain* 2004; 127: 1774-84.

Bailey P, Gibbs FA. The surgical treatment of psychomotor epilepsy. *J Am Med Assoc* 1951; 145: 365-70.

Berg AT. Understanding the delay before epilepsy surgery: Who develops intractable focal epilepsy and when? *CNS Spectrums* 2004; 9: 136-44.

Berg AT, Kelly MM. Defining intractability: comparisons among published definitions. *Epilepsia* 2006; 47: 431-6.

Berg AT, Langfitt J, Shinnar S, Vickrey BG, Sperling MR, Walczak T *et al*. How long does it take for partial epilepsy to become intractable? *Neurology* 2003; 60: 186-90.

Berg AT, Vickrey BG, Testa FM, Levy SR, Shinnar S, DiMario F *et al*. How long does it take for epilepsy to become intractable? A Prospective Investigation. *Ann Neurol* 2006; 60: 73-9.

Bragin A, Engel J Jr, Wilson CL, Fried I, Mathern GW. Hippocampal and entorhinal cortex high frequency oscillations (100-500 Hz) in kainic acid-treated rats with chronic seizures and human epileptic brain. *Epilepsia* 1999; 40: 127-37.

Bragin A, Mody I, Wilson CL, Engel J Jr. Local generation of fast ripples in epileptic brain. *J Neurosci* 2002; 22: 2012-21.

Bragin A, Wilson CL, Almajano J, Mody I, Engel J Jr. High frequency oscillations after status epilepticus: epileptogenesis and seizure genesis. *Epilepsia* 2004; 45: 1017-23.

Bragin A, Wilson CL, Staba RJ, Reddick MS, Fried I, Engel J Jr. Interictal high frequency oscillations (80-500 Hz) in the human epileptic brain: entorhinal cortex. *Ann Neurol* 2002; 52: 407-15.

Cascino GD, Jack CR Jr, Parisi JE, Sharbrough FW, Hirschorn KA, Meyer FB *et al*. Magnetic resonance imaging-based volume studies in temporal lobe epilepsy: pathological considerations. *Ann Neurol* 1991; 30: 31-6.

Cendes F. Progressive hippocampal and extrahippocampal atrophy in drug resistant epilepsy. *Curr Opin Neurol* 2005; 18: 173-7.

Chin P, Berg AT, Spencer SS, Sperling M, Shinnar S, Langfitt J *et al*. Employment following resective epilepsy surgery. *Epilepsia* 2005; 46 (suppl 8): 255.

Collaborative Group for the Study of Epilepsy. Prognosis of epilepsy in newly referred patients: a multicenter prospective study of the effects of monotherapy on the long-term course of epilepsy. *Epilepsia* 1992; 33: 45-51.

Corcoran ME, Moshé SL, eds. *Kindling 6*. New York: Springer Science, 2005, 415 p.

Dandy WE. Roentgenography of the brain after injection of air into the spinal canal. *Ann Surg* 1919; 70: 397-403.

Devinsky O, Barr WB, Vickrey BG, Berg AT, Bazil CW, Pacia SV *et al.* Changes in depression and anxiety after resective surgery for epilepsy. *Neurology* 2005; 65: 1744-9.

Duchowny MS. A potential role for alpha-Methyl-l-tryptophan PET in seizure localization in patients with intractable epilepsy. *Epilepsy Curr* 2003; 3: 184-6.

Engel J Jr. Historical perspectives. In: Engel J Jr, ed. *Surgical treatment of the epilepsies, second edition*. New York: Raven Press, 1993: 695-705.

Engel J Jr. Current concepts: surgery for seizures. *N Engl J Med* 1996; 334: 647-52.

Engel J Jr. The emergence of neurosurgical approaches to the treatment of epilepsy. In: Waxman S, ed. *From neuroscience to neurology: neuroscience, molecular medicine, and the therapeutic transformation of neurology*. Amsterdam: Elsevier, 2005: 81-105.

Engel J Jr, Bandler R, Griffith NC, Caldecott-Hazard S. Neurobiological evidence for epilepsy-induced interictal disturbances. *Advances in Neurology, Vol 55*. New York: Raven Press, 1991: 97-111.

Engel J Jr, Brown WJ, Kuhl DE, Phelps ME, Mazziotta JC, Crandall PH. Pathological findings underlying focal temporal lobe hypometabolism in partial epilepsy. *Ann Neurol* 1982; 12: 518-28.

Engel J Jr, Cahan L. Potential relevance of kindling to human partial epilepsy. In: Wada J, ed. *Kindling 3*. New York: Raven Press, 1986: 37-51.

Engel J Jr, Kuhl DE, Phelps ME, Crandall PH. Comparative localization of epileptic foci in partial epilepsy by PCT and EEG. *Ann Neurol* 1982; 12: 529-37.

Engel J Jr, Kuhl DE, Phelps ME, Mazziotta JC. Interictal cerebral glucose metabolism in partial epilepsy and its relation to EEG changes. *Ann Neurol* 1982; 12: 510-7.

Engel J Jr, Shewmon DA. Overview: Who should be considered a surgical candidate? In: Engel J Jr, ed. *Surgical Treatment of the Epilepsies, 2nd Edition*. New York: Raven Press, 1993: 23-34.

Engel J Jr, Taylor DC. Neurobiology of behavioral disorders. In: Engel J Jr, Pedley TA, eds. *Epilepsy: A Comprehsive Textbook*. Philadelphia: Lippincott-Raven, 1998: 2045-52.

Engel J Jr, Wilson C, Bragin A. Advances in understanding the process of epileptogenesis based on patient material: what can the patient tell us? *Epilepsia* 2003; 44 (suppl 12): 60-71.

Fedi M, Reutens D, Okazawa H, Andermann F, Boling W, Dubeau F *et al.* Localizing value of alpha-methyl-L-tryptophan PET in intractable epilepsy of neocortical origin. *Neurology* 2001; 57: 1629-36.

Ferrier D. On the localisation of the functions of the brain. *Br Med J* 1874; 2: 766-7.

French JA. Refractory epilepsy: one size does not fit all. *Epilepsy Currents* 2006; 6: 177-80.

French JA, Williamson PD, Thadani VM, Darcey TM, Mattson RH, Spencer SS *et al.* Characteristics of medial temporal lobe epilepsy: I. results of history and physical examination. *Ann Neurol* 1993; 34(6): 774-80.

Hart YM, Sander JWAS, Johnson AL, Shorvon SD. National general practice study of epilepsy: recurrence after a first seizure. *Lancet* 1990; 336: 1271-4.

Hauser WA, Lee JR. Do seizures beget seizures? *Prog Brain Res* 2002; 135: 215-9.

Heinemann U, Engel J Jr, Meldrum BS, Wasterlain C, Avanzini G, Mouritzen-Dam A, eds. *The Progressive Nature of Epilepsy, Epilepsy Research (Supplement 12)*. Amsterdam: Elsevier, 1996, 385 p.

Hermann BP, Seidenberg M, Dohan FC, Wyler AR, Haltiner A, Bobholz J *et al.* Reports by patients and their families of memory change after left anterior temporal lobectomy: Relationship to degree of hippocampal sclerosis. *Neurosurgery* 1995; 36: 39-45.

Horsley V. Brain surgery. *Br Med J* 1886; 2: 670-5.

Jackson GD, Berkovic SF, Tress BM, Kalnins RM, Fabinyi G, Bladin PF. Hippocampal sclerosis can be reliably detected by magnetic resonance imaging. *Neurology* 1990; 40: 1869-75.

Jacobs MP, Fischbach GD, Davis MR, Dichter MA, Dingledine R, Lowenstein DH. Future directions for epilepsy research. *Neurology* 2001; 57: 1536-42.

Jallon P, Loiseau P, Loiseau J. Newly diagnosed unprovoked epileptic seizures: presentation at diagnosis in CAROLE study. *Epilepsia* 2001; 42: 464-75.

Jasper H, Pertuisset B, Flanigin H. EEG and cortical electrograms in patients with temporal lobe seizures. *Arch Neurol Psychiatr* 1951; 65: 272-90.

Juhasz C, Chugani DC, Mizik O, Shah A, Asano E, Mangner TJ et al. Alpha-methyl-L-tryptophan PET detects epileptogenic cortex in children with intractable epilepsy. *Neurology* 2003; 60: 960-8.

Juhasz C, Chugani DC, Padhye UN, Muzik O, Shah A, Asano E et al. Evaluation with alpha-[11C]methyl-L-tryptophan positron emission tomography for reoperation after failed epilepsy surgery. *Epilepsia* 2004; 45: 124-30.

Kagawa K, Chugani DC, Asano E, Juhasz C, Muzik O, Shah A et al. Epilepsy surgery outcome in children with tuberous sclerosis complex evaluated with alpha-[11C]methyl-L-tryptophan positron emission tomography (PET). *J Child Neurol* 2005; 20: 399.

Kanner AM, Balabanov A. Depression in epilepsy: how closely related are they? *Neurology* 2002; 58 (suppl 5): S27-39.

Kwan P, Brodie MJ. Early identification of refractory epilepsy. *New Engl J Med* 2000; 342: 314-9.

Kwan P, Brodie MJ. Drug treatment of epilepsy: When does it fail and how to optimize its use? *CNS Spectrums* 2004; 9: 110-9.

Langfitt JT, Rausch R. Word-finding deficits persist after left anterotemporal lobectomy. *Arch Neurol* 1996; 53: 72-6.

Lindsten H, Stenlund H, Forsgren L. Remission of seizures in a population-based adult cohort with a newly diagnosed unprovoked epileptic seizure. *Epilepsia* 2001; 42: 1025-30.

Macewen W. Intra-cranial lesions – illustrating some points in connexion with the localisation of cerebral affections and the advantages of aseptic trephining. *Lancet* 1881; ii: 544 and 581.

Mathern GW, Babb TL, Vickrey BG, Melendez M, Pretorius JK. The clinical-pathogenic mechanisms of hippocampal neuron loss and surgical outcomes in temporal lobe epilepsy. *Brain* 1995a; 118: 105-18.

Mathern GW, Pretorius JK, Babb TL. Influence of the type of initial precipitating injury and at what age it occurs on course and outcome in patients with temporal lobe seizures. *J Neurosurg* 1995b; 82: 220-7.

Mendez MF, Cummings JL, Benson DF. Depression in epilepsy: significance and phenomenology. *Arch Neurol* 1986; 43: 766-70.

Mikati MA, Comair YG, Rahi A. Normalization of quality of life three years after temporal lobectomy: a controlled study. *Epilepsia* 2006; 47: 928-33.

Moniz E. *L'angiographie cérébrale*. Paris: Masson et Cie, 1934.

Morrell F. Secondary epileptogenic lesions. *Epilepsia* 1959/60 ; 1 : 538-60.

Natsume J, Kumakura Y, Bernasconi N, Soucy JP, Nakai A, Rosa P et al. Alpha-[11C] methyl-L-tryptophan and glucose metabolism in patients with temporal lobe epilepsy. *Neurology* 2003; 60: 756-61.

Spencer SS, Berg AT, Vickrey BG, Sperling MR, Bazil CW, Shinnar S et al. Initial outcomes in the multicenter study of epilepsy surgery. *Neurology* 2003; 61: 1680-5.

Sperling MR. The consequences of uncontrolled epilepsy. *CNS Spectrums* 2004; 9: 98-109.

Staba RJ, Wilson CL, Bragin A, Fried I, Engel J Jr. Quantitative analysis of high frequency oscillations (80-500 Hz) recorded in human epileptic hippocampus and entorhinal cortex. *J Neurophysiol* 2002; 88: 1743-52.

Sutula T, Pitkänen A, eds. Do seizures damage the brain? *Progress in Brain Research, Vol. 135*. Amsterdam: Elsevier, 2002, p. 520.

Taylor J, ed. *Selected writings of John Hughlings Jackson. Vol 1*. New York: Basic Books Inc, 1958, p 499.

Vickrey B, Hays R, Engel J Jr, Spritzer K, Rogers W, Rausch R *et al*. Outcome assessment for epilepsy surgery: the impact of measuring health-related quality of life. *Ann Neurol* 1995; 37: 158-66.

Victoroff JI, Benson DF, Grafton ST, Engel J Jr, Mazziotta, JC. Depression in complex partial seizures: electroencephalography and cerebral metabolic correlates. *Arch Neurol* 1994; 51: 155-63.

Wiebe S, Blume WT, Girvin JP, Eliasziw M. A randomized, controlled trial of surgery for temporal lobe epilepsy. *N Engl J Med* 2001; 345: 311-8.

Achevé d'imprimer par Corlet, Imprimeur, S.A.
14110 Condé-sur-Noireau
N° d'Imprimeur : 105060 - Dépôt légal : juin 2007

Imprimé en France